THE ROLE OF NON-SPECIFIC IMMUNITY
IN THE PREVENTION AND TREATMENT OF CANCER

PONTIFICIAE ACADEMIAE SCIENTIARVM SCRIPTA VARIA

---- 43 ----

SEMAINE D'ETUDE

SUR LE THÈME

THE ROLE OF NON-SPECIFIC IMMUNITY IN THE PREVENTION AND TREATMENT OF CANCER

17-21 octobre 1977

ÉDITÉ PAR MICHAEL SELA

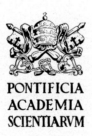

PONTIFICIA
ACADEMIA
SCIENTIARVM

EX AEDIBVS ACADEMICIS IN CIVITATE VATICANA

--

MCMLXXIX

THE ROLE OF NON-SPECIFIC IMMUNITY IN THE PREVENTION AND TREATMENT OF CANCER

PROCEEDINGS OF A STUDY WEEK
AT THE
PONTIFICAL ACADEMY OF SCIENCES

October 17-21, 1977

EDITED BY MICHAEL SELA

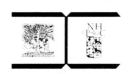

ELSEVIER/NORTH-HOLLAND BIOMEDICAL PRESS
AMSTERDAM - NEW YORK - OXFORD
1979

Elsevier/North-Holland Biomedical Press
Jan van Galenstraat 335
P.O. Box 211, Amsterdam, The Netherlands

Elsevier North Holland, Inc.
52 Vanderbilt Avenue
New York, New York 10017, U.S.A.
ISBN 0-444-80156-1

Printed in Italy

INDEX

SCIENTIFIC PAPERS

CONCLUSION

FOREWORD

The Pontifical Academy of Sciences organized in October 1977 a meeting on: " The Role of Non-Specific Immunity in the Prevention and Treatment of Cancer ".

This meeting was the realization of a wish of His Holiness Pope Paul VI, who expressed the desire to see the Pontifical Academy of Sciences deal with the all-engaging subject of cancer research. After due consideration, reflection and consultation with fellow-Academicians and various specialists, I decided to focus the attention of the Study Week on the role that immunogenic factors may play in the evolution of malignant processes. Therefore the title of the Study Week and the choice of the participants.

The Study Week may be judged a scientific success not only for the quality of the papers presented but also for the lively discussions undertaken. Papers and discussions are all included in the present Volume.

Due to factors beyond our control, the present publication was delayed. It is my belief, however, that it will be of great interest because it concerns a field wherein progress, albeit slow, has been necessary.

The participants in the Study Week were received in a private Audience by His Holiness Pope Paul VI. The rather small but beautiful site where he generously received us, as well as the simple way he conversed with the participants and their families, showed again and very strongly the interest His Holiness has always given to the work of the Academy. We could not imagine that the frail Sovereign who so kindly received us and was able to diffuse a feeling of intimacy which all of us appreciated would no longer be among us for the next meeting of the Academy. It is with great emotion that I remember his last direct contact with our activity and the prestige and strength with which he supported the work the Academy carried on during his reign.

Together with the help given to us by the Vatican authorities, I wish to acknowledge the cooperation from Professors Michael Sela, Sheldon Wolff and William Terry who helped plan the meeting before the responsibility of its realization was given to Prof. Sela. A thankful message must also be recorded to Rev. Father di Rova-senda, Director of the Chancellery of the Academy and to Filippo Colelli — without their assistance the meeting could not have been held.

A special word, however, must go to Michelle Porcelli-Studer, Secretary of the Academy. Her zeal during the Study Week and the great task undertaken in assembling the papers and discussions and all the proof corrections were invaluable.

Finally I also want to thank Gilda Massa for her help in preparing the transcriptions of the discussions, Prof. M. Barcinski for his assistance in the final editing of the proceedings and Prof. Paolo Merucci for his cooperation during the Study Week.

CARLOS CHAGAS
President of the Pontifical
Academy of Sciences

LIST OF THE PARTICIPANTS
IN THE STUDY WEEK

Prof. R. W. Baldwin, The University of Nottingham - Cancer Research Campaign Laboratories, University Park, *Nottingham* NG7 2RD - England.

Dr. M. A. Barcinski, Universidade Federal do Rio de Janeiro, Centro de Ciencias da Saude, Instituto de Biofisica, *Rio de Janeiro*, R. J. - 20.000 - Brazil.

Prof. C. Chagas, Instituto de Biofisica, Centro de Ciencias da Saude, Universidade Federal do Rio de Janeiro, Ilha do Fundão, *Rio de Janeiro* - Brazil.

Dr. L. Chedid, Institut Pasteur, Immunothérapie Expérimentale, Rue du Docteur Roux 28, 75015 *Paris* - France.

Prof. E. Clerici, Cattedra di Immunologia, Università degli Studi, Via Venezia n. 1, 20133 *Milano* - Italy.

Prof. D. A. L. Davies, G. D. Searle & Co. Ltd., Research Division, P. O. Box 53, Lane End Road, *High Wycombe*, Bucks., HP12 4HL - England.

Prof. Ch. De Duve, I. C. P., International Institute of Cellular and Molecular Pathology, Avenue Hippocrate 75, *Bruxelles* - Belgium.

Prof. J. De Marsillac, National Cancer Institute, *Rio de Janeiro* - Brazil.

Prof. J. M. Dewdney, Beecham Pharmaceuticals, Research Division, Chemotherapeutic Research Centre, Brockham Park, *Betchworth*, Surrey RH3 7AJ - England.

Prof. J. U. Gutterman, M. S. Anderson and Tumor Institute, Texas Medical Center, *Houston*, Texas 77030 - U.S.A.

Prof. Ed. KLEIN, Roswell Park Memorial Institute, Department of Health, 666 Elm Street, *Buffalo*, New York 14263 - U.S.A.

Dr. EVA KLEIN, Karolinska Institutet, Department of Tumor Biology, S-104 01 *Stockholm* 60 - Sweden.

Prof. G. KLEIN, Karolinska Institutet, Department of Tumor Biology, S-104 01 *Stockholm* 60 - Sweden.

Prof. R. LEVI-MONTALCINI, Laboratorio di Biologia Cellulare del C.N.R., Via G. Romagnosi 18/A, 00196 *Roma* - Italy.

Prof. G. B. MARINI-BETTÒLO, Istituto di Chimica, Facoltà di Medicina, Università Cattolica del Sacro Cuore, Via Pineta Sacchetti 644 and Istituto di Chimica generale, Università, *Roma* - Italy.

Prof. G. MATHÉ, I.C.I.G., Institut de Cancérologie et d'Immunogénétique, Groupe Hospitalier Paul-Brousse, 14 & 16 Avenue Paul-Vaillant-Couturier, 94800 *Villejuif* - France.

Prof. P. MERUCCI, Istituto Regina Elena, Viale Regina Elena 291/295, *Roma* - Italy.

Prof. R. J. NORTH, Trudeau Institute, Inc., Immunobiological Research Laboratories, P. O. Box 59, *Saranac Lake*, N. Y. 12983 - U.S.A.

Prof. G. NOSSAL, The Walter and Eliza Hall Institute of Medical Research, Post Office, Royal Melbourne Hospital, *Victoria* 3050 - Australia.

Prof. H. F. OETTGEN, Memorial Sloan-Kettering Cancer Center, 1275 York Avenue, *New York*, N. Y. 10021 - U.S.A.

Prof. H. J. RAPP, Department of Health, Education and Welfare, Public Health Service, National Institutes of Health, National Cancer Institute, *Bethesda*, Maryland 20014 - U.S.A.

Prof. A. ROJAS, Chiclana 560, Moreno 1744, Pcia. *Buenos Aires* - Argentina.

Prof. S. A. ROSENBERG, Department of Health, Education and Welfare, Public Health Service, National Institutes of Health, National Cancer Institute, *Bethesda*, Maryland 20014 - U.S.A.

Prof. M. SELA, The Weizman Institute of Science, P. O. Box 26, *Rehovot* - Israel.

Prof. F. SPREAFICO, Istituto di Ricerche Farmacologiche « Mario Negri », Via Eritrea 62, 20157 *Milano* - Italy.

Prof. H. STRANDER, Radiumhemmet, Karolinska Sjukhuset, 104 01 *Stockholm* - Sweden.

Prof. W. D. TERRY, Department of Health, Education and Welfare, Public Health Service, National Institutes of Health, National Cancer Institute, Division of Cancer Biology and Diagnosis, *Bethesda*, Maryland 20014 - U.S.A.

Prof. D. WEISS, The Hebrew University-Hadassah Medical School, The Lautenberg Center for General and Tumor Immunology, P. O. Box 1172, *Jerusalem* - Israel.

Prof. O. WESTPHAL, Max-Planck-Institut für Immunbiologie, Stübeweg 51, Postfach 1169, 78 *Freiburg-Zähringen* - Germany.

Prof. S. M. WOLFF, Tufts University School of Medicine, New England Medical Center Hospital, Department of Medicine, 171 Harrison Avenue, *Boston*, Massachusetts 02111 - U.S.A.

**

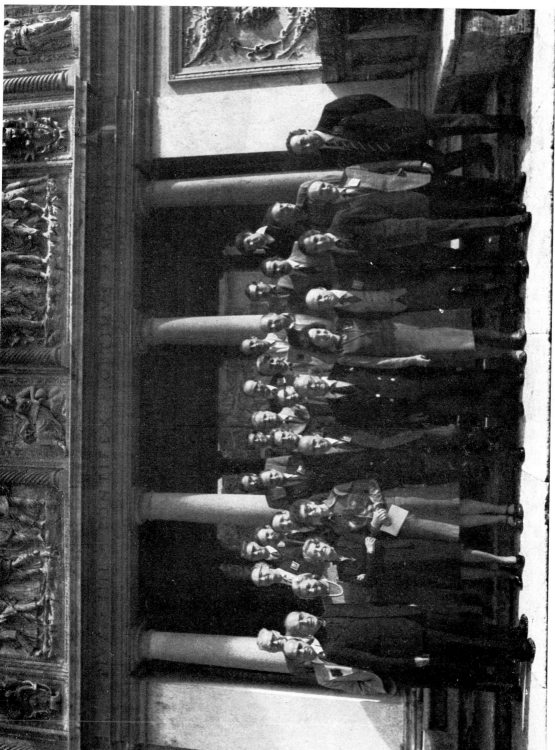

Participants in the Study Week

AUDIENCE OF THE HOLY FATHER

October 22nd, 1977 at 12 noon, at the conclusion of the Study Week, the Holy Father Pope Paul VI received in special Audience in the Vatican Palace all the Participants in the meeting together with their families and the Council of the Academy. The group was guided by the President of the Pontifical Academy of Sciences, His Excellency Prof. CARLOS CHAGAS and the Director of the Chancellery, Rev. Father ENRICO DI ROVASENDA.

The President delivered the following address of homage to the Holy Father:

Your Holiness,

In answer to your wishes, the Pontifical Academy of Sciences has organized a Study Week on the problem of cancer, tackling one of the ways of research which seems to be able to contribute to knowledge of cancerogenic mechanisms and consequently to bring results to the improvement of the ways of combatting this terrible affliction.

Thirty scientists from eleven countries during five days of intense work, have discussed the data they had obtained. They have endeavoured, through an exchange of ideas, theories and results, to promote the progress of scientific knowledge as regards this set of diseases that is called cancer. The ardour with which the participants in the Study Week set about this task, shows their dedication and their eagerness to overcome one of the most frequent causes of man's death.

Allow me, therefore, Holy Father, to assure you that the intensity of the work carried out in all freedom, as well as its multidisciplinary character in convergence on the same target, are the guarantee that the effort made by Your Academy will yield its fruit and contribute to the development of the struggle against cancer.

By deigning to receive the Council of the Academy, the participants in the Study Week, and their wives, and thus enabling us to present to you our heartiest thanks for the support which you give our work, you indicate once more your deep interest in science and its applications, and you comfort the spirit and the heart of those who have dedicated their lives to the laborious and often fruitless work, which is the very lot of scientific research.

The Holy Father Pope Paul VI deigned answer in these terms:

Mr. President,

Ladies and Gentlemen,

We are very happy to receive your visit. And the reason is a double one: the presence of the Council of the Pontifical Academy of Sciences and that of eminent cancerologists.

We are always ready, in fact, to encourage the activity of our Academy, stimulated zealously by its President and its Council. The Holy See is anxious to honour in this way, in the person of the members of this Pontifical Institution, and through them, all those who in a worthy way, shed lustre on science. For, by examining objectively the immense field of physical and biological realities, they contribute to ensuring the real progress of scientific knowledge, according to the Creator's invitation, and to preparing technical progress in harmony with man's vocation and complete good, and therefore under the responsibility of conscience.

But this morning, our interest takes on concrete form and increases since, with the specialists that we are happy to greet, you have just dedicated a week of studies to what is, rightly, the object of deep concern on the part of our contemporaries: the way of preventing and treating cancer.

You have concentrated your attention on non-specific immunity in this field. We ourself attribute great importance to this work, for we share the anxiety of our brothers and Christ's ardent desire to see the sick relieved or cured of their infirmities. And it is a question of a terrible affliction, which strikes, still too often irremediably and in the midst of cruel sufferings, a large number of people, even comparatively young persons, from every country. The disease is all the more redoubtable in that its mechanisms seem closely linked with the normal processes of cellular reproduction, in which they create grave anarchy.

In addition to surgical operations and radiological treatments which have already made great progress, at the risk, however, of acting on normal cells as well as on cells of cancerous tumours, you have wished to study the exploration of a new way, by utilizing immunological and immunochemical means, to activate the defences of the organism or stop the proliferation of neoplastic cells. We thank you heartily for informing us of the result of your work. We hope that it will help to prepare the medical progress to which so many people aspire, physicians, patients and the relatives of patients. We congratulate you on this high service to humanity and we willingly implore on you and on the members of your families the blessings of God, the source of life and Saviour.

SCIENTIFIC PAPERS
AND
DISCUSSIONS

INTRODUCTORY REMARKS

MICHAEL SELA

I would like first of all to join in welcoming this august body of specialists in the areas of cancer, of immunology, as well as of the interaction between immunology and cancer. I would like, not less, to welcome those from adjacent fields of science who were agreeable to give us of their time and wisdom and came to join us here for the next few days.

Is the lack of an adequate immune response one of the causative reasons for cancer? Few would agree with this statement, but — on the other hand — few would disagree with the statement that there is definitely an immunological component in the development of cancer. I hope that at the end of this Study Week we shall have a clearer picture concerning this question.

Both experimental and clinical studies in the last dozen years or so, have suggested that a non-specific increase in general immunity is helpful in combating at least some types of cancer. How far have the laboratory results already been successfully translated to the patients? And what are the main limitations, if any?

The most significant results seem to have been obtained with adjuvants derived from — or including — mycobacteria. How do mycobacteria, or corinobacterium parvum, compare with fractions isolated therefrom, or even with synthetic glycopeptides derived from the bacterial cell wall? What about the manifold soluble factors such as endotoxins, interferon, double-stranded RNA, thymic factors, transfer factors, etc.? And what about the role of such defined small molecules as levamisole? We have a most interesting week before us and, hopefully, shall have a clearer picture at its end, both concerning what can, and what cannot be done.

We must remember well one thing: we are dealing here with matters of paramount importance, and under no circumstances should our devotion and our enthusiasm run ahead of our carefully checked and statistically evaluated data. Immunology has — I deeply believe — a lot to contribute to the cure and prevention of cancer. Let us not diminish its importance through hasty claims. Rather, let us take a more cautious — but beneficial road which may be slower but will ultimately lead us to a significant progress and lasting achievements.

ANIMALS, TEST-TUBES AND CANCER: IN VIVO VERITAS, IN VITRO MENDACIUM

HERBERT J. RAPP and JAMES T. HUNTER

Tumor immunology consists at one extreme of purely "mechanistic" immunologic studies and at the other of clinical trials of the "immunotherapy" of human cancer. Evidence is presented in this report that there is need for less extreme approaches to the question of whether natural host resistance can be manipulated to control cancer.

The demonstration that cells of neoplasms from inbred animals contained antigens capable of inducing tumor specific transplantation resistance in syngeneic recipients [1] has been cited as a basis for the hope that immunotherapy will be useful in the control of human cancer [2]. Subsequent studies, however, revealed a gap between the knowledge that animal tumors induced in the laboratory contained tumor specific rejection antigens (TSRA) and the application of that knowledge to the treatment of established naturally occurring cancers in humans. The ability to immunize normal, healthy, tumor-free animals against subsequent tumor challenge has had no direct or obvious application to the elimination of growing neoplasms in cancer patients. Moreover, there has been no unequivocal demonstration of the existence of TSRA in human agnogenic cancers.

Perhaps also premature has been the attempt to study in vitro "mechanisms" of tumor immunity as they may relate to the diagnosis and treatment of cancer in humans and animals. Optimism derived from these studies in the 1960s has given way to pessimism in the 1970s as the disappointing results of clinical trials of cancer immunotherapy have continued to accumulate [3] and as it has become evident that the immunodiagnosis of cancer is still little more than a hope. In vitro mechanistic studies of so-called tumor immunity, therefore, may provide false leads and generate false hopes. Interest in immunologic studies on the in vitro killing of cancer cells from human patients [4] has turned into skepticism about what significance those investigations have to in vivo events [5]. Indeed, there is some justification for the view that at present the only measure of tumor immunity that has validity in studies of cancer immunotherapy is prolongation of the life of individuals with cancer [6].

The fact that reputedly immunotherapeutic procedures have cured animals with experimental cancer [7] or caused the regression of some malignant growths in outbred species [8, 9] does not justify the conclusion that TSRA were at the basis of these observations. The demonstration that experimental cancer was cured by the systemic transfer of cells from appropriately immunized donors [10] provided neither proof that TSRA were needed in active cancer immunotherapy nor a practical method for the treatment of cancer. Immune cells from syngeneic but not from allogeneic donors were effective. If this observation is generally valid it would mean that appropriate donors for the treatment of cancer in outbred species such as humans would be virtually impossible to find.

The notion that current in vitro studies of so-called correlates of tumor immunity will eventually provide a means to control human cancer now seems questionable. Fundamental knowledge of immunobiology and immunochemistry has not yet had direct application to cancer immunotherapy, and there is no assurance that it ever will. Rational cancer immunotherapy may require fundamental knowledge unique to tumor immunology. If so, there would be little to support the view that studies aimed at the advancement of immunology in general without focusing on the immunology of cancer will eventually solve the cancer problem.

It has been suggested that additional empirical information from experimental and naturally occurring animal cancers may be required as a basis for mechanistic studies of tumor immunology and the immunotherapy of human solid tumors [6]. This view was derived from studies with an animal model consisting of intradermal implants of a syngeneic guinea pig hepatoma that metastasizes to lymph nodes [11]. In many experiments all guinea pigs with a growing intradermal tumor and metastasis confined to the capsule of the regional lymph node were cured by a single injection into the dermal implant of a sufficiently high dose of living *Mycobacterium bovis* (strain BCG) or a specially prepared vaccine containing the cell walls of BCG. When metastasis was permitted to spread to the interior of the draining lymph node before treatment with BCG, the cure rate decreased; treatment given at a time when metastasis was grossly evident (detectable by palpation of the regional lymph nodes) was usually ineffective.

Attempts to find in vitro or in vivo correlates of cure by BCG in the guinea pig hepatoma model have failed [12]. In one study it was suggested that one or more of the mediators of tumor specific delayed cutaneous hypersensitivity were distinct from those responsible for immunotherapy or the development of specific resistance to the growth of tumor transplants [13]. Indeed, it is not known whether immunotherapy and specific resistance to tumor growth are due to the same mediators. The search for correlates of cancer immunotherapy is at an early stage and progress may require new information. Under present circumstances it seems advisable to base this search on successful animal analogs of cancer immunotherapy in which established tumors as well as metastases were eliminated. In vitro studies of tumor immunology in the absence of such analogs have little chance of providing guides to the design of clinical protocols of cancer immunotherapy.

More than 90 percent of the cancer mortality in the United States has been due to metastasizing solid tumors. Many of these cancers have metastasized to lymph nodes and through hematogenous spread to other organs. The results of a study of malignant melanoma of the limbs indicated that in cases with clinically uninvolved regional lymph nodes, the survival rate following surgery was the same whether primary treatment consisted of local excision and lymph node dissection or local excision alone followed by dissection only after appearance of palpable metastases at the regional nodes [14]. Of those patients initially classified as Stage 1 and later found to have had occult microscopic regional lymph node metastases, only about 30 percent survived for five years. By contrast more than 95 percent of guinea pigs with growing intradermal transplants of a syngeneic hepatoma and microscopic regional lymph node metastases were cured by local excision of the tumor and dissection of the regional lymph nodes [15]. While there are many differences between human malignant melanoma and the guinea pig hepatoma model, perhaps the absence of hematogenous spread in the animal model was mainly responsible for the difference in the survival rates following surgery at times when microscopic but not palpable regional lymph node metastases were present. Results of studies with the guinea pig hepatoma model, therefore, may not be applicable to human cancer in which death is a consequence of hematogenous spread. Some information from this animal model may be relevant to Stage 1 human cancer under special circumstances in which currently accepted therapies may be inappropriate. On that basis, studies have been performed to delineate the limits of intralesional BCG therapy of the guinea pig hepatoma, and to establish whether immunotherapy might influence the results of surgery. In those studies clinical staging was substituted for time as the independent variable; 4 to 6 months survival was the dependent variable. Animals at different stages of disease were treated either by intralesional BCG alone, by surgery alone, or by a combination of surgery and immunotherapy. A summary of the results of this study in several different experiments is given in table 1.

The experimental results outlined in tables 1 and 2 show that immunotherapy may not be useful as a means of preventing recurrence of malignant disease following surgery. The guinea pig model studies suggest that intralesionally administered BCG cell walls might be useful for patients with Stage 1 cancers in which other treatments are either ineffective or inappropriate. Among cancers that may be in this category are lung cancer occurring at the carina, Clark's level 4 malignant melanoma, cancers in which mutilation due to surgery might be unacceptable and cancers of the esophagus, liver and stomach. Whether carcinomas beyond Stage 1 will respond to immunotherapy is still a question that needs to be answered by studying appropriate animal analogs of human malignant disease. In one study 70 percent of cows with naturally occurring Stage 1 primary, agno-

TABLE 1 - *Comparison of Cure Rates[a] by Immunotherapy and by Surgery of Line 10 Guinea Pig Hepatoma[b] at Different Stages of Malignant Disease.*

Regional Lymph Node Metastasis	Percent Survival (120 days)	
	Immunotherapy [c]	Radical Surgery [d]
None	>95	>95
Microscopic	>95	>95
Early Palpable (3-4 mm)	55	90
Palpable (6-7 mm)	<10	50
Palpable (>10 mm [e])	0	<10

[a] These data are averages from at least three independent experiments and are consistent with our general experience with this model.

[b] 10^6 line 10 tumor cells were injected intradermally into syngeneic guinea pigs; clinical stage was determined by palpation of regional lymph nodes.

[c] Treatment consisted of a single intralesional injection of BCG cell walls incorporated into mineral oil droplets. In each case a dose was used that produced more than 95 percent cure when microscopic but not palpable regional lymph node metastasis was present.

[d] Surgery consisted of excision of the dermal tumor, and where appropriate, dissection of the regional (superficial distal axillary) and the proximal axillary (PA) lymph nodes.

[e] When the regional lymph node was 10 mm or greater there was microscopic metastasis in the PA node.

genic, ocular, squamous cell carcinoma have had either regression of disease or prolonged survival after a single intralesional injection of BCG cell wall vaccine [9]. Studies are in progress to determine whether this treatment will be effective when the disease has reached Stage 2 and whether hematogenous metastases can be affected. Among additional analogs of human cancer that seem appropriate for study are naturally occurring equine melanoma, canine mammary carcinoma and bovine lymphosarcoma. Empirical knowledge gained from these studies may provide the means to study fundamental mechanisms of tumor immunity and provide guides for the design of clinical protocols of cancer immunotherapy that have a greater chance of success than those being followed, currently.

TABLE 2 - *Survival of Guinea Pigs with Stage 2 Malignant Disease (6-7 mm Regional Lymph Nodes). Treated by Surgery or Immunotherapy Alone and in Combination.*

Treatment	Percent Survival (120 days)
Radical Surgery [a]	60 – 70
Modified Radical Surgery [b]	<10
Intralesional BCG-CW [c]	<10
Intralesional BCG-CW Followed by Radical Surgery	30 – 70
Intralesional BCG-CW Followed by Modified Radical Surgery	<10
Modified Radical Surgery Plus Active Immunization [d]	<10
Modified Radical Surgery Plus Adoptive Immunization [e]	<10

[a] Radical surgery consisted of excision of the dermal tumor, and dissection of the regional (superficial distal axillary) and the proximal axillary lymph nodes.

[b] Modified radical surgery consisted of excision of the primary tumor and the superficial distal axillary nodes. Microscopic metastasis was present in the proximal axillary lymph nodes.

[c] A single intralesional injection of BCG cell walls incorporated into mineral oil droplets was given one week before surgery at a dose that in previous studies produced more than 95 percent cures when microscopic but not palpable regional lymph node metastasis was present.

[d] Active immunization consisted of intradermal injection of a vaccine containing 3×10^6 living or x-irradiated line 10 tumor cells mixed with 212 µg of emulsified BCG cell walls contralaterally or ipsilaterally near the involved lymph nodes.

[e] Adoptive immunization was given on the day of surgery and consisted of intracardiac injection of 200×10^6 peritoneal exudate cells from immunized syngeneic donors. Donors were immunized by intradermal injection of line 10 tumor mixed with BCG cell wall vaccine followed by 5 weekly intradermal injections of 1×10^6 line 10 tumor cells alone.

REFERENCES

[1] PREHN R.T. and MAIN J.M., *Immunity to methylcholanthrene induced sarcomas.* « J. Natl. Cancer Inst. », *18*, 769 (1957).

[2] RAPP H.J., *Immunology and Cancer.* In « Sixth National Cancer Conference Proceedings ». Philadelphia and Toronto, J.B. Lippincott Co., 1970, pp. 39-43.

[3] TERRY W.D. and WINDHORST D. (Eds.), *Immunotherapy of Cancer: Present Status of Trials in Man.* Volume 6 in « Progress in Cancer Research and Therapy Series » New York, Raven Press, (1978).

[4] HELLSTROM I., HELLSTROM K.E. and SHEPARD T.H., *Cell-mediated immunity against antigens common to human colonic carcinomas and fetal gut epithelium.* « Int. J. Cancer », *6*, 346-351 (1970).

[5] TAKASUGI M., MICKEY M.R. and TERASAKI P.I., *Reactivity of lymphocytes from normal persons on cultured tumor cells.* « Cancer Res. », *33*, 2898 (1973).

[6] RAPP H.J., *Immunotherapy of cancer: Theory and practice.* « Proc. Inst. Med. Chic. », *30*, 251-255, 274-275 (1975).

[7] BAST R.C. Jr., BAST B.S. and RAPP H.J., *Critical review of previously reported animal studies of tumor immunotherapy with non-specific immunostimulants.* « Ann. N. Y. Acad. Sci. », *277*, 60-93 (1976).

[8] RAPP H.J., KLEINSCHUSTER S.J., LEUKER D.C. and KAINER R.A., *Immunotherapy of experimental cancer as a guide to the treatment of human cancer.* « Ann. N. Y. Acad. Sci. », *276*, 550-556 (1976).

[9] KLEINSCHUSTER S.J., RAPP H.J., LEUKER D.C. and KAINER R.A., *Regression of bovine ocular carcinoma by treatment with a Mycobacterial vaccine.* « J. Natl. Cancer Inst. », *58*, 1807-1814 (1977).

[10] SMITH H.G., HARMEL R.P., HANNA M.G. Jr., ZWILLING B.S., ZBAR B. and RAPP H.J., *Regression of established intradermal tumors and lymph node metastases in guinea pigs after systemic transfer of immune lymphoid cells.* « J. Natl. Cancer Inst. », *58*, 1315-1322 (1977).

[11] ZBAR B., RIBI E., MEYER T., AZUMA I. and RAPP H.J., *Immunotherapy of cancer: Regression of established intradermal tumors after intralesional injection of mycobacterial cell walls attached to oil droplets.* « J. Natl. Cancer Inst. », *52*, 1571-1577 (1974).

[12] LITTMAN B.H., MELTZER M.S., CLEVELAND R.P., ZBAR B. and RAPP H.J., *Tumor specific cell-mediated immunity in guinea pigs with tumors.* « J. Natl. Cancer Inst. », *51*, 1627-1635 (1973).

[13] SMITH H.G., BAST R.C. Jr., ZBAR B. and RAPP H.J., *Eradication of microscopic lymph node metastases after injection of living BCG adjacent to the primary tumor.* « J. Natl. Cancer Inst. », 55, 1345-1352 (1975).

[14] VERONESI U., ADAMUS J., BANDIERA D.C., BRENNHOVD I.O., CACERES E., CASCINELLI N., CLAUDIO F., IKONOPISOV R.L., JAVORSKJ V.V., KIROV S., KULAKOWSKI A., LACOUR J., LEJEUNE F., MECHL Z., MORABITO A., RODE I., SERGEEV S., VAN SLOOTEN E., SZCZYGIEL K., TRAPEZNIKOV N.N. and WAGNER R.I., *Inefficacy of immediate node dissection in stage 1 melanoma of the limbs.* « N. Engl. J. Med. », 297, 627-630 (1977).

[15] HUNTER J.T., OKUDA T. and RAPP H.J., *Immunotherapy of metastatic cancer in guinea pigs: Failure of intralesional BCG to influence the results of radical surgery.* « J. Natl. Cancer Inst. », 59, 1435-1439 (1977).

DISCUSSION

CLERICI

I am somewhat skeptical about the BCG treatment. I would like to point out that some of the data that you have presented are controversial with some others. For instance, you stated that the treatment with BCG is not effective when the tumour has a dimension over 6 to 7 mm while in the case of ocular carcinoma of cattle you said that the injection of BCG intralesionally reduces and cures the tumor. I would like to recall that BCG was used about 50 years ago for the treatment of tumors and it was demonstrated that you can get some results when the BCG is administered before the graft of a transplantable tumor, but not after the tumor is already growing. I would say that the use of BCG in the treatment of human tumors is a question of faith more than a question of scientific utility.

RAPP

I am sorry; obviously I did not make myself clear because your two points are not relevant to what I said. First, we did not treat 6 to 7 mm primary tumors; we treated animals in which lymph nodes measured more or less 6 to 7 mm. The primary transplants were larger. Your second point is that BCG works only before challenge. However, I presented two examples in which intralesionally administered BCG eliminated growing tumors and produced permanent cures.

CLERICI

Yes, probably I misunderstood what you said; but I would like to ask you an odd question: among people who have been vaccinated with BCG, is the incidence of tumors significantly modified as compared to the control population?

RAPP

Claims have been made that children vaccinated with BCG within three days of birth have less death from leukemia than unvaccinated children. But these data have been seriously challenged. There has been one study indicating that lymphomas may be more prevalent in BCG-vaccinated individuals than in unvaccinated individuals. In my opinion this difference is of questionable significance.

ROSENBERG

You began your talk by mentioning that there was not good correlation between *in vitro* assays and *in vivo* effects, but you did not show us any *in vitro* data. Could you enlarge this point? What *in vitro* tests do not correlate? More specifically, have you looked at a variety of assays that measure cytotoxic lymphocytes specific cytotoxic for the line 10 hepatoma, and the correlation between the presence of those cytotoxic lymphocytes and survival of animals following therapy?

RAPP

We had difficulty in finding cytotoxic lymphocytes against the line 10 hepatoma, so we have been unable to make the correlation. We can produce cytotoxic lymphocytes in line 10 *in vitro*, but they are not specific.

ROSENBERG

What assay was used?

RAPP

Direct cytotoxicity by terminal labeling with a radioisotope. We can also find blastogenesis, the production or migration inhibition factor and tumor specific antibodies. There is no correlation between these findings and the fate of treated animals. Our inability to detect cytotoxic lymphocytes against line 10 in treated animals has made this comparison impossible.

[2] *Rapp, Hunter* - p. 10

MATHÉ

I would like to make three comments. First, in previously irradiated areas it rarely works. Is there a local immunotherapy inhibitor process related to irradiation? My second remark is: we are starting to combine local injection of bleomycin in oil and BCG alternatively, and it seems encouraging, maybe because both work on different stages of the cell cycle. And my third comment is: surgeons do not like to inject things in the primary tumors. So we wondered if something between local and systemic immunotherapy would not be accepted by them. We studied the effect of surgery for the primary tumor and local injection of BCG between the tumor and the lymph node in the case of EAKR lymphosarcoma and of BIG melanoma. This regional immunotherapy in complement of surgery in the first case, and in complement of surgery and systemic immunotherapy in the second case is promising.

RAPP

Dr. Zbar has tried paralesional injection of BCG and the only way we can make it work is to inject the BCG between the tumor and the lymph node before surgery. If surgery is done before BCG treatment, it does not work. I should have mentioned that among the investigators responsible for much of the work I have presented, are Drs. Hunter, Smith, Borsos, Hanna and others. Dr. Zbar has done some experiments in which he injects line 10 hepatoma in the skin over the midline of the back, so that the metastasis is going in two directions at the same time. If BCG is injected between the tumor and the lymph node on both sides and the primary transplant removed later, a significant number of cures are obtained. The cure rate, however, is not as good as when BCG is injected directly into the primary transplant. However, if BCG is injected on only one side between the tumor and the lymph node, the animals are not cured.

MATHÉ

When the site was irradiated — submitted to radiotherapy before — have you noticed that it works experimentally?

[2] *Rapp, Hunter* - p. 11

RAPP

No, because if we selectively irradiate the primary tumor with a shield and the lymph node, that alone can be curative.

MATHÉ

Have you alternated local chemotherapy and local immunotherapy?

RAPP

Our preliminary attempts to do this have not yielded encouraging results.

GUTTERMAN

Dr. Mathé has brought up one of the two points I wanted to ask you. Your group has published data with local chemotherapy, and it seems as if certain agents but not all are useful. But you have not tried any accommodation experiments?

RAPP

We have but there is not much to talk about.

GUTTERMAN

The second question is: the guinea pigs are not sensitive to BCG, at the time they receive the BCG. Would the results with surgery, in the guinea pigs with metastatic tumors, be improved by using an agent to which the guinea pig has already been sensitized as, for example, some endotoxin material rather than BCG?

RAPP

I do not know the answer but it is certainly worth looking into.

NOSSAL

I have one comment with one question regarding the work with cattle. I can report on behalf of colleagues in Queensland, that extremely analogous results have been observed in what appears to be an identical tumor — really quite remarkable and encouraging cures of these quite dreadful malignancies. My question relates to a criticism I heard that was made of your work two or three years ago — well not so much of your work but as to its general significance in the hepatoma story. When it appeared, it was claimed that there was an antigenic cross reactivity between the hepatoma line and constituents of the BCG. What is the current status of that criticism?

RAPP

I never considered that as a criticism. We were hopeful that this cross reaction, which is real, would have something to do with why immunotherapy is successful. But apparently it does not; it is just another one of those non-correlates that goes along with our other disappointments. It does not mean that this general idea may not be useful elsewhere, but it just does not seem to have anything to do with why BCG works.

OETTGEN

I have two questions. First, if you compare living BCG and BCG cell walls would you say the latter are at least as effective as BCG if not more effective? What about just-killed BCG organisms?

RAPP

They do not work at all, unless you put them in oil.

OETTGEN

If you put them in oil?

RAPP

Yes, just as good as cell wall. The only reason we use cell wall is that Edgar Ribi made large amounts of it and we get it from him.

OETTGEN

So the simpler preparation is effective against tumors?

RAPP

Yes.

OETTGEN

The second question: I am a bit puzzled — you said you have lymphocyte cytotoxicity in the treated guinea pigs but that it is not related to survival. But you also said that when you transfer lymphocytes from sensitized guinea pigs, you think there may be prolongation of survival.

RAPP

We know there is.

OETTGEN

But about lymphocyte cytotoxicity in these transferred preparations, does it correlate with their efficacy? And if so, how do you explain the discrepancy?

RAPP

We have not done that yet because I have assumed that lymphocytes from hyperimmunized normal animals will kill line 10 hepatoma cells *in vitro*. But we are looking for lymphocytes in cured animals that are cytotoxic and these are almost never found. We have produced cytotoxic lymphocytes *in vitro*, but they are not specific. They kill normal cells, and hepatomas other than line 10.

EVA KLEIN

I gather from the discussion that you have been looking for some cytotoxic lymphocytes mainly from the spleen, I guess.

[2] *Rapp, Hunter* - p. 14

RAPP

No, from peritoneal exudates induced by mineral oil.

CHEDID

I wish to congratulate you not only for having developed a fascinating guinea pig model a few years ago but also for offering today a "clinical" veterinarian therapeutic system in cattle. Could you please clarify a technical point concerning one of your first slides: You showed us that guinea pigs treated by both BCG and surgery developed delayed hypersensitivity in all cases, whereas they had enhanced immunity only if the BCG had been inoculated into the tumor lesion. Since cross reacting antigens have been described between the hepatoma cells and BCG, could you tell us what happens in controls who have received BCG only, that is without tumor implantation? Do they develop protection or even just delayed hypersensitivity?

RAPP

No, there is no protection.

Actually that experiment is a little bit of a set-up because I think the delayed hypersensitivity would have developed without BCG.

As a matter of fact if you just leave the tumors in place for about sixteen days — about the time you just begin to get palpable lymph nodes — and then you do radical surgery, these animals invariably develop the ability to reject a tumor challenge on the other side. And this may explain why surgery alone is effective, because when you leave the tumor in there long enough, presumably to get a large enough antigenic mass, and you remove it at the right time, you do get a specific immune response. The only problem is: we do not know whether that specific rejection contributes to the therapy. We have no direct evidence that it does.

CHEDID

I suppose Dr. North will have some comments also on this type of question: the relevance or non-relevance between delayed hypersensi-

[2] *Rapp, Hunter* - p. 15

2

tivity and immunity in different systems. More particularly, in your bovine system it is interesting to remember that BCG is pathogenic for bovines. Since your cell wall vaccine can be made artificially with cell walls of other mycobacteria, I was wondering if you did really need BCG for your cell wall vaccine or if you could use cell walls of other mycobacterial strains?

RAPP

We have not tried anything but BCG so far.

CHEDID

Do you know if there is some sort of antigenic privileged situation of BCG in your bovine cancer? And also — this is such a wonderful model — I was wondering if you should not try additional chemotherapy.

RAPP

I think of it more as an analogue.

CHEDID

Yes, as an analogue, since "model" is derogatory in your opinion. Did you try and see the incidence of chemotherapy on that analogue?

RAPP

We started to do that because of the other work in our laboratory with interlesional chemotherapy and we tried a couple of animals, but we are in a stage right now where we are trying to find our way to establish the biology of the system so that we can compare surgery with BCG.

SELA

We are going to discuss in the next few days quite a lot the role of BCG and various materials derived from it, and it would be nice — at least for myself — to have a clearer picture as to how many different

[2] *Rapp, Hunter* - p. 16

types of cancer have been claimed or have been reported to involve an immunological cross-reactivity between mycobacteria and those particular tumor lines. I am aware that there is at least one line of rats in which the normal cells are cross-reactive with mycobacteria. I think it would be good for all of us to have this picture as we listen to the various presentations in the next few days. Is it really a bona fide immunochemical cross-reaction? Is anything known about the chemical nature of the determinant, and in how many cases has it already been reported?

RAPP

I would like Dr. Gutterman to answer that question.

GUTTERMAN

Mike Hanna originally reported on the human element, as Dr. Rapp said, but by immunolectromicroscopy. Percy Linden reported the binding assay with human melanoma — that has been reported in the literature — and also has a fair amount of data with acute myeloid leukemia of the adult. I think there are about eight or nine preparations from our own clinic in which there is cross-reactivity with AML and BCG. There is also some reactivity, I believe, between AML and pseudomonas vaccine, a material that Dr. Oettgen has used and we ourselves are using as well. Linden also looked by the binding technique with adult lymphocytic leukemic cells, AL and L cells, and there was no cross-reactivity in two or three preparations. So, as far as Linden's data and Hanna's data go, that would be summarized as human melanoma, acute myeloblastic leukemia, but not adult lymphocytic leukemic blasts.

BALDWIN

I would like to make one or two points about the discussion of squamous cell carcinoma in cattle. I had the opportunity to see the cattle at the University of Queensland. If I remember correctly, tumors recurred some six to nine months after the initial regression, so the question I put to you in that respect is: how effective is the regression? I take it from what you said that you are getting essentially complete regression in the cow.

[2] *Rapp, Hunter* - p. 17

RAPP

Yes. Some animals have complete regressions with no recurrence for more than two years. The disease has been arrested in other animals also for more than two years. In Australia, the cows were treated by intramuscular injection of tumor extract?

BALDWIN

The tumor extracts are injected intramuscularly.

RAPP

It is hard to see how that works, but if it works, I am ready to accept it.

BALDWIN

I think you have to consider how the immunological mechanisms are involved in those responses. They are particularly concerned now with looking at an anti-virus immunity in cattle.

RAPP

My first impression is: if they do recur in six months, I would not be very interested in it. So I would not concern myself with the mechanism, but it could be a hint, and one could improve on it, but I prefer to work on something that looks like a permanent cure.

BALDWIN

We are looking at the cytotoxicity of lymphocytes taken from tumors. With tumor immune donors something like 50-100 effector cells tumorall is needed to get cytotoxicity. These tumor lymphocytes are cytotoxic at about 25 effector cells per tumor cell, and at that level you get both specific and non-specific cytotoxicity.

WEISS

To add to what Dr. Gutterman said a moment ago, when Dr. Lin-

[2] *Rapp, Hunter* - p. 18

den worked for a year in our laboratories in Jerusalem he also demonstrated cross-reactivity between BCG fractions and Rous sarcomas as well as several other mouse neoplasms. To this might be added the fact that in his recent work, Linden also has found such cross-reactivities involving several other families of microorganisms. The key question is: what is the biological significance, if any, of these very widely prevalent cross-reactivities between tumor cells and different microorganisms? I do not think there is any information at this time suggesting whether they do or do not have any significance in terms of resistance to tumors induced by immune modulators of microbial origin.

RAPP

In our own work we have used the C-1 fixation and transfer test to demonstrate this so-called cross-reactivity, and Dr. Linden is using radioimmunoassay. Both of these are methods that are at the limits of detection of immune reactions in immunochemistry. You are detecting a really minute quantity of reactivity. I think it is possible that what we are looking at might be called chance complementarity, that somewhere deep in the structure of almost all macromolecules there must be similarities that are very subtle, and I think this is what we are picking up. I doubt that we are ever going to find that these minor reactivities have anything at all to do with something as gross as getting rid of a large tumor. I could be wrong but that is my impression.

OETTGEN

Regarding the question of cross-reactivity between BCG and human cancer cell antigens, I think when we begin to discuss this topic we have to state quite clearly by which reagents cross reactivity is defined. In an extensive serological analysis of human melanoma cell surface antigens based on autoimmune antibodies we have not yet found an example of cross-reactivity between BCG and melanoma. It does not seem to be a common occurrence.

RAPP

I am not ready to take any view and I do not think that we should discard specificity because I think the separations are artificial, much like the separation between basic and applied research.

[2] *Rapp, Hunter* - p. 19

ACTIVE IMMUNOTHERAPY:
EXPERIMENTAL AND RATIONAL BASIS.
EXAMPLES OF CLINICAL RESULTS

G. MATHE

Institut de Cancérologie et d'Immunogénétique, Hôpital Paul-Brousse (*)
and Département d'Hématologie de l'Institut Gustave-Roussy (**)
94800 Villejuif, France

Abstract

Systemic active immunotherapy (SAI) is able to cure mice inoculated with an experimental tumour usually only when the number of grafted cells is small ($\leqslant 10^5$), which suggested that its best situation in the strategy of cancer treatment is the residual minimum imperceptible diseases left by a first treatment.

SAI when applied alone is usually more efficient when consisting of BCG + cells than when consisting of BCG or cells only.

When applied after chemotherapy, BCG alone or C. parvum alone is usually strongly efficient. BCG may also be efficient when given after local radiotherapy or after surgery.

As a growth of a tumour treated by SAI may became a plateau which finally gives way to relapse, as SAI kills only the cells in Gl, one is tempted to intersperse SAI and chemotherapy. This interspersion may be unfavourable when immunosuppressive cytostatics (CTS) are used, but favourable when non immunosuppressive CTS are used.

(*) 14-16, avenue Paul-Vaillant Couturier.
(**) 16bis, avenue Paul-Vaillant Couturier.

Regional AI may be efficient under the form of s.c. injection of BCG near to tumour before its surgical removal.

These notions as well as the dose effect, and that of the differences of effects according to the immunomodulating materials and their combinations are illustrated by results of personal experiments.

The development concerning immunotherapy with the use of neuraminidase treated cells, cells produced by culture, and extracted tumor associated antigen, and that concerning the use of new adjuvants (brucella and pseudomonas) is presented briefly.

Some clinical data, especially concerning our personal results in acute lymphoid leukaemia and bronchus cancer are discussed in correlation with the experimental data.

Introduction

Active immunotherapy of cancer is at the stage where chemotherapy was 20 years ago. The experimental data which prove that active immune manipulation maybe an effective treatment of neoplasias are, to-day, very numerous. The clinical trials, the conclusions of which are in favour of immunotherapy action in man, are still few. There might be more if experimental data were known by physicians who conduct randomized trials.

I - *Active immunotherapy alone applied as a treatment of minimal residual disease left by other cancer treatment(s)*

1 - *Basic experimental data.* The treatment of minimal residual disease was our objective when we embarked, 15 years ago, on the cancer immunotherapy adventure, for two reasons:

a) Many patients relapse after local tumour treatment(s) from the growth of the few cells already emigrated at the time of operation, and/or after chemotherapy, because chemotherapy obeys first order kinetics [1] and therefore often leaves a few cells alive. We had predicted, from our study on the murine L1210 leukaemia mean inductive cell number, that surgery, radiotherapy, or chemotherapy must leave no more than 10 cells, if they are not immunosuppressive, to cure the disease [2]. Moreover, they are often immunodepressive [3]. Hence the need for an effective treatment of minimal residual disease.

b) Attempts at immunoprophylaxis, using a specific vaccine made of irradiated tumour cells and systemic immunity adjuvant such as BCG, increased the mean inductive cell number of leukaemia to 10^5 [2].

2 - Hence our first question was: are similar immuno-interventions efficient in prevention, also efficient in *therapy, after* the tumour is established? We conducted experiments on several tumours (L1210 leukaemia [4, 5], RC 19 and AkR [see 2]) and demonstrated that immunotherapy, that is the immuno-intervention applied after the tumour is established, is able to eradicate such tumours, at least in certain conditions which we will define.

3 - Some of the *conditions of action* concern the modality of active immunotherapy: the combination of irradiated tumour cells as the specific stimulus and of BCG as a non specific immunity adjuvant is often more active than leukaemic cells or BCG alone (in the case of some tumours such as L1210 leukaemia) [4, 5].

Other conditions concern the size of the tumour cell population: active immunotherapy is only able to cure mice that have received 10^5 leukaemic cells or less, and has no effect on those grafted with 10^6 or more [4].

For some tumours, especially some leukaemias (EAkr), if the number of inoculated tumour cells is very small, 10^3 or 10^2, the specific stimulus induced by repeated injections of irradiated tumour cells may be efficient by itself to cure animals, while BCG is not effective [6].

On the contrary, if the tumour cell number has been reduced by a previous treatment, the non specific immune application of a systemic immunity adjuvant may be sufficient to cure animals: BCG is highly effective after chemotherapy with cyclophosphamide of L1210 leukaemia [7]; it is slightly effective after radiotherapy of Lewis tumour [8]; this mycobacterium applied i.v. after tumour and draining lymph-node surgery in the case of melanoma B16 is able to cure animals in conditions where surgery does not cure any animals [9].

In all these experiments, BCG was injected i.v. at the dose
of 1 mg/mouse, which we had showed to be the optimal dose to
stimulate immune reactions in the haemolytic plaque forming assay.
Higher doses such as 3 or 5 mg induce immunodepression [2], the
mechanism of which is the stimulation of suppressor cells as shown
by GEFFARD and ORBACH [10] in our laboratory.

Injected at a dose of 1 mg/mouse i.v., BCG induces a septicemia, the presence of which we have shown to be necessary for
the antitumor effect [11]. Among the other efficient modalities
of administration is the application of BCG by scarifications or via
the Heaf gun [12]. Not only the s.c. route of administration,
which does not induce such a septicemia, does not cause tumour
rejection, but it may in fact produce enhancement of the Lewis
tumour [13].

Not all BCG preparations work: submitting ten preparations
to our experimental screening for immunity systemic adjuvants [13],
we observed that only the fresh Pasteur preparation is efficient in
all tests [14].

4 - In conclusion, immune manipulation may eliminate some
neoplasias, provided the tumour cell number is small, which is
the condition of minimum residual disease left by the first treat-
ment(s), and provided some conditions concerning modalities of
preparations used for specific and non specific stimuli and of methods of application, are respected. However, as illustrated by
the dose-effect correlation of BCG which is immunosuppressive at
high doses [2], and by the enhancement of Lewis tumour growth
after s.c. injection of BCG [13], one must underline the importance
of monitoring during any attempt at immunotherapy, non specific
immune reactions as well as specific reactions. As far as the specific reactions are concerned, we compared the effect of active
immunotherapy with BCG and cells in two groups of EAkR carrying mice, one in which it was effective, one in which it was not,
and we could only correlate the antitumor efficiency with an increase of antibody-dependent cell-mediated cytotoxicity [15].

5 - *First clinical attempts.* This experimental data gives a rational basis for our trials of clinical active immunotherapy of mi-

nimal residual disease left by chemotherapy in acute lymphoid leukaemia, and by surgery in bronchus cancer.

a) In 1962, we conducted the first comparative (randomized) trial on active immunotherapy of acute lymphoid leukaemia previously maintained in remission by chemotherapy [16]. We compared the length of remission and survival of patients submitted to active immunotherapy, consisting of the application after chemotherapy was stopped, of BCG as a non-specific immunity adjuvant applied by scarification and/or irradiated leukaemic cells injected i.d. as the specific stimulus. After the introduction of 30 patients into the trial, we noted a significant difference in favour of immunotherapy, and therefore stopped introducing more patients into the trial, which we were not authorized to prolong and/or repeat for ethical reasons. Then all the immunotherapy patients were submitted to both BCG and irradiated cells. Fourteen years later, seven patients out of 20, and eight out of 20 of the immunotherapy group are still, respectively, in remission and alive, as opposed to zero out of 10 control patients not submitted to immunotherapy after maintenance chemotherapy [17].

Since this trial, we have conducted several successive protocols, adapting the pre-immunotherapy chemo-radio-therapy according to the progress accomplished by the different groups in the world and by ourselves [3], and comparing different immunotherapy modalities applied to patients randomized after the end of post-remission cell reducing complementary chemotherapy.

Among the recent results which we have registered are those of three successive protocols [18] which concern very similar populations of children as far as the prognostic factors are concerned (cytological types and tumour volume), hence are validly comparable, and which differ by the respective lengths of their pre-immunochemotherapy: 9 months in protocol ALL 9, 25 months in protocol ALL 10, and 19 months in protocol ALL 11.

The remission rate was 29 out of 31 (94%) for protocol 9, 14 out of 14 (100%) for protocol 10, and 13 out of 14 (93%) for protocol 11.

The curves of duration of the first remission present a break tending towards a plateau at about the 24th month. This plateau includes about 50% of the children submitted to protocol 9 (only one relapse between the 24th and 54th months), 43% of those submitted to protocol 10, and 54% of those submitted to protocol 11. The differences between these three percentages are not significant. No correlation is therefore found between the results and the length of the pre-immunotherapy chemotherapy, and one can conclude that the long-term first remission rate is of the order of 50% for three protocols.

The cumulative survival curves also form plateaux for 60% (protocol 9), 50% (protocol 10) and 71% (protocol 11) of the patients, respectively.

We cannot exclude that a 9 month chemotherapy does the maximum that maintenance chemothcrapy can do on the remission curves. But this is not the generally accepted concept, at least, that used for exclusive maintenance chemotherapy treatments [19, 20]. Thus the fact that between the 9th and the 25th month the curve of protocol 9 is identical, under immunotherapy, to the curve of protocol 11, under chemotherapy, is in favour of the similarity of actions of immunotherapy and maintenance chemotherapy (MC) during this period. The results, to-day, of an EORTC Haemopathy Working Party [21] randomized trial, which compared, after one year's chemotherapy, active immunotherapy comprising BCG and irradiated cells, with further maintenance chemotherapy, are in favour of this last conclusion.

We know that two controlled studies [22, 23] have failed to confirm the efficiency of active immunotherapy in children. Their conclusions should be restricted to the preparations and modalities of application of BCG used in their trials. Hence these interesting trials do not contraindicate active immunotherapy applied under other modalities such as those employed in our trials: application of a preparation of the living Pasteur BCG which is active in our experimental screening [14], inducing a bacteriemia shown experimentally as a necessary condition for its action [11] and only considered as correct in man if it is followed by a slight increase in temperature (about 38°C for at least one day). Negative results have also been registered in immunotherapy trials of other diseases especially acute myeloid leukaemia, melanoma or bronchus cancer on which the results of other trials have shown the efficiency of the therapeutic weapon [see 24].

Moreover, we know to-day that acute lymphoid leukaemia patients can be stratified in two groups according to prognosis [25]: *a*) one comprising the microlymphoblastic type and the V-macrolymphoblastic and prolymphoblastic types, with a good prognosis: 65 to 80% belong to the long term plateau of the remission curve and 90% to the plateau of survival curve, and *b*) the other one with a very poor prognosis (comprising the prolymphoblastic type and the V+ macrolymphoblastic and prolymphocytic types; only 15 to 25% belong to the remission plateau and 30 to 40% to the survival plateau [18]. Hence the absence of stratification before randomization may explain the negative result of trials conducted with powerful chemotherapy transitorily active on the severe prognosis group. In our first trial [16, 17], the chemotherapy of which was not very powerful (comprising one drug only a time and several drugs poorly or not active in acute lymphoid leukaemia), it is highly probable that the poor prognosis patients had all relapsed before the randomization for immunotherapy, which was compared to abstention on the rather homogeneous group of good prognosis patients.

Finally two differences between acute lymphoid leukaemia patients submitted to systemic active immunotherapy and those submitted only to maintenance chemotherapy are: *a*) the absence of any lethal toxicity of immunotherapy compared to the variable but high mortality in remission under chemotherapy [see 26]; *b*) the absence of relapse after the fifth year in the immunotherapy patients compared to their incidence in most maintenance chemotherapy trials [19, 26].

b) Among the favourable results obtained with active immunotherapy on bronchus cancer are those of the first trial which we have conducted on patients operated for stage I or II, among which half were submitted to BCG for two years [27, 28].

The trial began in June 1973 and included 43 patients operated for squamous cell carcinoma of the bronchus. Twenty-two patients were selected at random and submitted to BCG application, whereas 21 patients received no further treatment after surgery. The distribution according to age, sex and stage is identical in the two groups.

The actual comparison of the 18th month is in favour of the group submitted to immunotherapy. Using the modified Wilcoxon test, the difference is significant at 7%. In the immunotherapy group, the chance of surviving for two years is over 60%, while it is only 38% in the non-treated group.

c) Short term tolerance of immunotherapy is good though we consider a slight increase in temperature for at least one day, as a test of the correct application of BCG. We have found liver granuloma at systematic biopsy, but we have not seen any clinical or biological liver manifestations which would have obliged us to stop. Immunotherapy has not been responsible for one death among more than 400 treated patients. No long term effects have been observed in patients submitted to 5 years immunotherapy [see 2].

d) Our attempt at monitoring the immune functions of the patients has been limited to non specific responses. It has shown an increase: a) of the skin DHS responses to secondary antigens [29]; b) of circulating immunoblasts [29]; c) of circulating leukocyte inhibitor factor (LIF) (observed in the case of bronchus epidermoid carcinoma [30]) and, d) of circulating null cells [31], a population including K-cells which have not been shown to increase significantly (not published).

We have summarized the state of clinical research by our group on systemic active immunotherapy applied alone in the attempts to eradicate the minimal residual disease left by other cancer treatment.

Other medical researchers have obtained a significant improvement in the prognostic of the minimal residual disease left by local treatment, using the same modality of immunotherapy with the same or another adjuvant: BCG in melanoma [32, 33], levamisole in breast cancer [34] and in bronchus carcinomas [35].

II - *Interspersion of intermittent chemotherapy and immunotherapy*

Another approach which we have also studied experimentally, was introduced by the Anderson Hospital Group [36]: the interspersion of chemotherapy and immunotherapy.

1 - There were several *reasons* for the combination and inter-spersion of chemotherapy and immunotherapy.

a) In most of the experiments mentioned above, some mice were cured, but rarely 100%, even with the best conditions of AI application.

Following the tumour volume after AI in the case of s.c. grafted L1210 leukaemia, we observed three kinds of results: a decrease of the tumour volume and cure; an absence of effect on the tumour volume, which increases until death; a plateau in the tumour volume curve which is followed by an increase until death, suggesting an initial effect followed by immunoresistance [2].

b) The results of an experiment of the effect of active immuno-therapy on cells at the different phases of the cell-cycle explain this phenomenon more basically: active immunotherapy only works on cells in G_0 and/or G_1 [37].

These two experiments suggest the possible interest of in-terspersing immunotherapy and chemotherapy: *a*) to try to reduce the number of cells when the tumour volume curve has attained the plateau to the number accessible to immunotherapy, i.e. 10^5 or 10^3;   *b*) in order to increase the number of target cells, immuno-therapy being effective only on cells in the G_0-G_1 phase [37] and chemotherapy mainly on cells in the other phases of the cycle [38].

c) Moreover, we have observed that a given chemotherapy which does not cure leukaemic mice immunodepressed by anti-thymocyte serum may cure leukaemic animals [39] which are not immunodepressed.

d) Another reason in favour of interspersing active immuno-therapy and chemotherapy is the acceleration by immunity adjuvants such as BCG, of blood cell restoration after chemotherapy [40]. This suggests that such adjuvants act on stem cells, and we observed, using the techniques of colony-forming units in the spleen (CFUs), of colony-forming units in agar culture (CFUa) and the tritiated thymidine suicide method, that BCG increases the number of both types of stem cells in the S-phase [41, 42].

e) Finally, there is another reason in favour of the interspersion of very carefully selected chemotherapy and active immunotherapy: immunity systemic adjuvants may, in certain conditions, i.e. at high doses, induce immunosuppression [see 2] through the stimulation of suppressor cells [10]. These cells may be sensitive to cyto-static drugs different from those active on cytotoxic T-cells, helper T-cells, B-cells, K-cells and macrophages.

2 - We were therefore encouraged to conduct immunotherapy-chemotherapy interspersion. In our first *experiments*, we inter-spersed cyclophosphamide (CPM) and BCG in the treatment of L1210 leukaemia on which we had previously seen that the sequence CPM → BCG is much more efficient than CPM alone [7]. We were unpleasantly surprised, however, to observe that two or three interspersion sequences of these two agents were no more efficient than CPM alone and much less efficient than the single sequence of one CPM and one BCG injection [43]. The same result was observed for the solid Lewis tumour [43].

As the single sequence CPM → BCG is more effective than CPM alone [7], we wondered if the reverse sequence BCG → CPM was less effective. As a matter of fact, this is the case: the sequence BCG → CPM is significantly less efficient than CPM alone [7]. As we had shown that the CPM effect is much poorer in immuno-depressed animals [39], we wondered if BCG followed by CPM did not induce immunodepression as BCG pushes the lymphocytes in the cycle, rendering them more sensitive to the lymphostatic action of CPM, a cycle-dependent agent. An experiment on allo-geneic skin grafting [44] demonstrated the validity of this hypo-thesis: the sequence BCG → CPM greatly prolongs allograft sur-vival compared with CPM alone.

The problem was then to investigate whether this phenomenon was true for all chemotherapy agents, or only for those that are known to be immunosuppressive [3]. Hence, we performed a similar experiment using RFCNU [(chloro-2-ethyl-1-ribofuranosyl-isopropylidene-2'-3' paranitrobenzoate-5')-3 nitrosourea], a deri-vative of nitrosoureas which, among those available in practice and a dozen sugar derivatives synthetized in Montpellier and shown to be strongly oncostatic by our experimental screening, is not immunosuppressive at the minimal oncostatic dose [45]. The sequence BCG → RFCNU is more efficient than BCG or RFCNU alone [46].

[3] *Mathé* - p. 10

Thus we may conclude that the interspersion of immunotherapy and chemotherapy may be unfavourable or favourable depending on at least one factor: the effect on immunity of the chemotherapy used. Non-immunosuppressive cytostatics must be chosen according to the available data. This effect on immunity does not eliminate the possible role of other factors, such as the time factor, the dose factor, the phase dependency of the cytostatics, or the adjuvant used for immunotherapy [2].

3 - Some *clinical* immunotherapy-chemotherapy interspersion protocols have been the object of comparative trials for the treatment of minimal residual disease. Their results were compared to those of the same chemotherapy alone: in six trials on acute myeloid leukaemia [36, 47, 48, 49, 50, 51], in one trial on ovarian cancer [52], and in one on bronchus carcinoma [53], the combination was superior to chemotherapy alone.

In the case of advanced tumours, phase II clinical trials of the interspersion of chemo-immunotherapy have given us regression and even apparently complete remission in patients resistant to chemotherapy. Many comparative trials were also conducted: *a)* on melanoma [54, 55]; *b)* on bronchus cancer [56] and *c)* on breast cancer [57, 58] in which the combination of immunotherapy and chemotherapy was superior to chemotherapy.

III - *Immunotherapy applied before other cancer treatment(s)*

1 - Thus, if BCG applied before certain chemotherapies may enhance their immunodepressive effect, hence enhance tumour growth [7] the contrary may be obtained by applying immunotherapy before certain other types of cancer treatment.

a) *Chemotherapy.* We showed that this is true for non immunosuppressive chemotherapies such as RFCNU [46]. Moreover, immunity systemic adjuvants may not only exert an immunostimulating action on normal immune reactions; they may exert an immunorestoration effect [59]. As we showed in mice that a given chemotherapy is much less efficient in immunodepressed animals than in animals with normal immune reactions [39], we attempted immunorestoring with BCG, immunodepressed patients with advanced bronchus cancer. We observed that the survival of the immunorestored subjects was as long as that of patients having initially normal immune reactions and far superior to that of the non immunorestored patients [60].

b) *Surgery*. The above data on the possible enhancing effect of BCG applied before certain therapies led us to study the effect of immunotherapy applied before surgery. BCG administered s.c. before tumour extirpation and between the tumour and the draining lymph-nodes in lymphosarcoma bearing mice may significantly improve the effect of surgery [61].

IV - *Regional immunotherapy*

1 - This observation [61] drew our attention to a new form of immunotherapy, which we called regional immunotherapy. As a matter of fact, the results of this experiment should be compared with those of others in which BCG was applied after surgery for the same lymphosarcoma as above: after surgery, BCG only works if injected i.v. and does not work if injected s.c. (as in all our experiments on systemic immunotherapy [2]); BCG applied before surgery does not work if injected i.v., and only works if injected s.c. near to the tumour [61].

This experimental observation finds a remarkable clinical application in the treatment of bronchus cancer. Mc KNEALLY *et al.* [62], injected lyophilized BCG in the pleura and have obtained a significant prolongation of disease free survival in treated patients compared to his randomized controls.

The operational conditions of regional immunotherapy are not identical in all tumours. Applying BCG s.c. between a local inoculation of B16 melanoma and the draining lymph-nodes invaded at time of treatment, we observed no effect whether the lymph-nodes were extirpated or not at the same time as the tumour. But when combining this presurgical regional immunotherapy with systemic post surgical BCG immunotherapy, we increased the proportion of cure obtained (50% vs 10%), both systemic and sys-

[3] *Mathé* - p. 12

temic plus regional working only if adenectomy was performed at the same time as tumour exeresis (it should be mentioned that draining lymph nodes were invaded at time of surgery) [9].

This observation should encourage the use of the same treatment for human melanoma and bronchus cancer with invaded lymph-nodes.

V - *Local immunotherapy*

Regional presurgical immunotherapy differs from local immunotherapy [63, 64, 65], which consists of intratumoral injection of the agents. It may find many more clinical applications than local immunotherapy, which has yet only found clinical use in very exceptional conditions: for instance, the topical application [63] or local injection [64] of adjuvants or haptens on or in skin tumours which are not eradicable by conventional surgical or radiological treatments, and which are not carried by immuno-depressed patients for whom local immunotherapy is ineffective [64].

VI - *Development*

These are some of the experimental and clinical data which must be borne in mind before setting up any clinical trial.

There are many more questions which the experimentalists have submitted to study and the answers to them may be useful for clinical trials.

1 - Can we improve the efficiency of a *specific immunotherapy* using irradiated tumour cells by treating them with *neuraminidase* [66] or *other enzymes* such as papain? We have not observed such a result either on grafted [67], or spontaneous AkR leukaemia [69]. Thus this manipulation of the cells does not work in all conditions and may facilitate tumour growth.

Can tumour cells produced by *cultures* in permanent lines replace cryopreserved cells and possibly be more efficient? We have several lines of cells produced from leukaemic cell populations which carry several markers of the original leukaemic cells [70]. We are comparing in a randomized trial the use of such cultured and cryopreserved acute lymphoid leukaemia cells in the active immunotherapy of this neoplasia.

The use of soluble *tumour associated antigens*, which may be very effective under some experimental conditions, especially if administered very early [71], may be inefficient in others, for example, if injected later than in the preceding experimental condition.

These antigens may induce tumour rejection or tumour growth enhancement according to the modality of preparation [72].

2 - Can we improve the efficiency and the facility of use of the non-specific manipulation made with *adjuvants*?

Can we replace living BCG by *mycobacterial extracts*? We have observed that if most extracts, including hydrosoluble ones, are efficient in an antibody production test on macrophage activation, only the methanol extracted residue fraction of tubercle bacilli (MER) is active on tumour growth inhibition [73]. But its local tolerance is much poorer than that of living BCG.

What about other dead organisms? I shall not comment on Corynebacteria which have been studied extensively by many other workers [74]. In a randomized clinical trial on acute lymphoid leukaemia, the combination of C. granulosum, BCG and leukaemic cells, was not shown to be more efficient than the binary combination of BCG and leukaemic cells [75].

Conversely, we are enthusiastic about the action of *Brucella* [76] which again illustrates the importance of a phenomenon we noted for BCG, namely that the adjuvant action depends on the strain of microorganism used: only the strain B19R is efficient, and only at certain doses, while the strain B19S is immunosuppressive and enhances tumour growth [77].

Finally, we have recently obtained very promising results with Pseudomonas aeruginosa with our screening in mice [78] and in a clinical study on immunorestoration of immunodepressed patients [79].

The possibility of tumour growth enhancement by certain modalities of immuno-intervention underlines the fact that immunotherapy is not homeopathy and must be based on experimental data. A B-dependent adjuvant, i.e. lipopolysaccharide (LPS) increases antibody production and enhances tumour growth [77].

In conclusion, there is a strong experimental background for clinical immunotherapy which should be considered carefully before establishing any protocol for clinical trials.

REFERENCES

[1] SKIPPER H. E., SCHABEL F. M. and WILCOX W. S., *Experimental evaluation of potential anticancer agents. XIII. On the criteria and kinetics associated with "curability" of experimental leukemia.* « Cancer Chemoth. Rep. », *35*, 1-111 (1964).

[2] MATHÉ G., *Active immunotherapy of cancer: its immunoprophylaxis immuno-restoration. An introduction.* Heidelberg-New York, Springer Verlag, 1976.

[3] CLARYSSE A., KENIS Y. and MATHÉ G., *Cancer chemotherapy. Its role in the treatment strategy of hematologic malignancies and solid tumors.* Heidelberg. New York, Springer Verlag, 1976.

[4] MATHÉ G., *Immunothérapie active de la leucémie L1210 appliquée après la greffe tumorale.* « Rev. Fr. Et. Clin. Biol. », *13*, 881-883 (1968).

[5] MATHÉ G., POUILLART P. and LAPEYRAQUE F., *Active immunotherapy of L1210 leukaemia applied after the graft of tumour cells.* « Brit. J. Cancer », *23*, 814-824 (1969).

[6] OLSSON L., EBBESEN P., KIGER N., FLORENTIN I. and MATHÉ G., *The anti-leukemic effect of systemic non-specific BCG-immunostimulation versus systemic specific immunostimulation with irradiated isogeneic leukemic cells.* Submitted to « Europ. J. Cancer » (1978).

[7] MATHÉ G., HALLE-PANNENKO O. and BOURUT C., *Immune manipulation by BCG administered before or after cyclophosphamide for chemo-immunotherapy of L1210 leukaemia.* « Europ. J. Cancer », *10*, 661-666 (1974).

[8] MARTIN M., BOURUT C., HALLE-PANNENKO O. and MATHÉ G., *BCG immuno-therapy of Lewis tumor residual disease left by local radiotherapy.* « Biome-dicine », *23*, 337-338 (1975).

[9] ECONOMIDES F., BRULEY-ROSSET M., FLORENTIN I. and MATHÉ G., *Treatment of the B16 melanoma with tumorectomy combined or not with adenectomy, systemic or/and regional BCG immunotherapy.* Medical Oncology, *3*, 5-34 (abstract 83), 1977.

[10] GEFFARD M. and ORBACH-ARBOUYS S., *Enhancement of T-suppressor activity in mice by high doses of BCG.* « Cancer Immunol. Immunoth. », *1*, 41-43 (1976).

[11] KHALIL A., RAPPAPORT H., BOURUT C., HALLE-PANNENKO O. and MATHÉ G., *Histologic reactions of the thymus, spleen, liver, lymph-nodes to i.v. and s.c. BCG injections.* « Biomedicine », *22*, 112-121 (1975).

[12] MARTIN M., BOURUT C., HALLE-PANNENKO O. and MATHÉ G., *Routes other than i.v. injection to mice for BCG administration in active immunotherapy of L1210 leukemia.* « Biomedicine », *23*, 339-340 (1975).

[13] MATHÉ G., KAMEL M., DEZFULIAN M., HALLE-PANNENKO O. and BOURUT C., *An experimental screening for "systemic adjuvants of immunity" applicable in cancer immunotherapy.* « Cancer Res. », *33*, 1987-1997 (1973).

[14] MATHÉ G., HALLE-PANNENKO O. and BOURUT C., *BCG in cancer immunotherapy. II. Results obtained with various BCG preparations in a screening study for systemic adjuvants applicable to cancer immuno-prophylaxis or immunotherapy.* « Nat. Cancer. Inst. Monogr. », *39*, 107-112 (1973).

[15] OLSSON L., FLORENTIN I., KIGER N. and MATHÉ G., *Cellular and humoral immunity to leukemia cells in BCG-induced growth control of a murine leukemia.* « J. Nat. Cancer Inst. », *59*, 1297-1306 (1977).

[16] MATHÉ G., AMIEL J. L., SCHWARZENBERG L., SCHNEIDER M., CATTAN A., SCHLUMBERGER J. R., HAYAT M. and DE VASSAL F., *Active immunotherapy for acute lymphoblastic leukaemia.* « Lancet », *1*, 697-699 (1969).

[17] MATHÉ G., AMIEL J. L., SCHWARZENBERG L., SCHNEIDER M., CATTAN A., SCHLUMBERGER J. R., HAYAT M. and DE VASSAL F., *Follow-up of the first (1962) pilot trial on active immunotherapy of acute lymphoid leukaemia. A critical discussion.* « Biomedicine », *26*, 29-35 (1977).

[18] MATHÉ G., DE VASSAL F., SCHWARZENBERG L., DELGADO M., WEINER R., GIL M.A., PENA ANGULO J., BELPOMME D., POUILLART P., MACHOVER D., MISSET J. L., PICO J. L., JASMIN C., HAYAT M., SCHNEIDER M., CATTAN A., AMIEL J. L., MUSSET M., ROSENFELD C. and RIBAUD P., *Results of three protocols for the treatment of A.L.L. of children.* « Med. Pediatr. Oncol. », *4*, 17-27 (1978).

[19] AUR R. J. A., SIMONE J. V., HUSTU H. O., VERZOSA M. S. and PINKEL D., *Cessation of therapy during complete remission of childhood acute lymphocytic leukaemia.* « New Engl. J. Med. », *291*, 1230-1234 (1974).

[20] BAUM E., LAND V., JOO P., STARLING K., LEIKIN S., MIALE T., KRIVIT W., MILLER D., CHARD R., NESBIT M., SATHER H. and HAMMOND D., *Cessation of chemotherapy (Ch) during complete remission (CR) of childhood acute lymphocytic leukaemia (ALL).* « Proc. Amer. Soc. Oncol. », *18*, 290, Abstr. N°C-96 (1977).

[21] Hemopathies Working Party of E.O.R.T.C., *Immunotherapy versus chemotherapy as maintenance treatment of acute lymphoblastic leukemia.* pp. 471-481. In: « Immunotherapy of cancer: present status of trials in man », (W.D. TERRY and D. WINDHORST, eds.) New York, 1978, Raven Press.

[22] Medical Research Council, *Treatment of acute lymphoblastic leukaemia. Comparison of immunotherapy (BCG), intermittent methotrexate, and no therapy after a five month intensive cytotoxic regimen* (Concord trial). «Brit. Med. J. », *4*, 189-194 (1971).

[23] HEYN R., JOO P., KARON M., NESBIT M., SHORE N., BRESLOW N., WEINER J., REED A., SATHER H. and HAMMOND D., *BCG in the treatment of acute lymphocytic leukemia.* pp. 503-512 *in* « Immunotherapy of cancer: present status of trials in man » (W.D. Terry and D. Windhorst, eds), New York, 1978, Raven Press.

[24] TERRY W.D. and WINDHORST D. (eds), *Immunotherapy of cancer: present status of trials in man.* New York, 1978, Raven Press.

[25] MATHÉ G., *Vers le démembrement de la leucémie dite « lymphoïde aiguë ».* « Nouv. Presse Med. », *6*, 2399-2400 (1977).

[26] Mathé G., De Vassal F., Delgado M., Pouillart P., Belpomme D., Joseph R., Schwarzenberg L., Amiel J.L., Schneider M., Cattan A., Musset M., Misset J.L. and Jasmin Cl., *1975 current results of first 100 cytologically typed acute lymphoid leukemia to BCG active immunotherapy.* « Cancer Immunol. Immunoth. », *1*, 77-86 (1976).

[27] Pouillart P., Mathé G., Palangie T., Schwarzenberg L., Huguenin P., Morin P., Gautier M. and Parrot R., *Trial of BCG immunotherapy in the treatment of resectable squamous cell carcinoma of the bronchus* (stages I and II). « Cancer Immunol. Immunoth. », *1*, 271-273 (1976).

[28] Pouillart P., Palangie T., Huguenin P., Morin P., Gautier H., Lededente A., Baron A. and Mathé G., *Attempt at immunotherapy with BCG of patients with bronchus carcinoma*: preliminary results, pp. 225-235. In: « Adjuvant therapy of cancer » (S.S. Salmon and S.E. Jones eds.), Amsterdam, 1977, North Holland Publ.

[29] Schneider M., Mathé G., Schwarzenberg L., Pouillart P., Weiner R., Amiel J.L., Hayat M., Jasmin C., De Vassal F., *Non specific immune responses in hematosarcomas and acute leukemia*, p. 42-53 in: « Investigation and stimulation of immunity in cancer patients » (G. Mathé and R. Weiner. eds.), Heidelberg, New York, Springer Verlag, 1974.

[30] Pouillart P., Personal Communication.

[31] Belpomme D., Joseph R. and Lelarge N., *Increase of null cells in patients submitted to long term immunotherapy.* « Cancer Immunol. Immunoth. », *1*, 113-114 (1976).

[32] Holmes E.C., Eilber F.R. and Morton D.L., *Immunotherapy of malignancy in humans.* « J. Amer. Med. Assoc. », *232*, 1052-1055 (1975).

[33] Beretta G., *Controlled study for prolonged chemotherapy, immunotherapy and chemotherapy plus immunotherapy as an adjuvant to surgery in stage I-II, malignant melanoma*, pp. 65-72 « Immunotherapy of cancer: present status of trials in man ». (W.D. Terry and D. Windhorst, eds). New York, 1978, Raven Press.

[34] Rojas A.F., Feierstein J.N., Glait H.M. and Olivari A.J., *Levamisole action in breast cancer stage III.* pp. 639-645, in: « Immunotherapy of cancer: present status of trials in man ». (W.D. Terry and D. Windhorst, eds). New York, 1978, Raven Press.

[35] Amery W.K., *A placebo-controlled levamisole study in resectable lung cancer.* pp. 191-201, in: « Immunotherapy of cancer: present status of trials in man ». (W.D. Terry and D. Windhorst, eds). New York, 1978, Raven Press.

[36] Gutterman J.U., Rodriguez V., Mavligit G., Burgess M.A., Gehan E., Hersh E.M., Mccredie K.B., Reed R., Smith T., Bodey G.M. Jr. and Freireich E.J., *Chemo-immunotherapy of adult acute leukemia. Prolongation of remission in myeloblastic leukemia with BCG.* « Lancet », *2*, 1405-1409 (1974).

[37] Olsson L. and Mathé G., *A cytokinetic analysis of BCG-induced growth-control of murine leukemia.* « Cancer Res. », *37*, 1743-1749 (1977).

[38] Bruce M.R., Meeker B.E. and Valeriote F.A., *Comparison of the sensitivity of normal hematopoietic and transplanted lymphoma colon-forming cells to chemotherapeutic agents administered in vivo.* « J. Nat. Cancer Inst. », *37*, 233-245 (1966).

[3] *Mathé* - p. 18

[39] MATHÉ G., HALLE-PANNENKO O. and BOURUT C., *Effectiveness of murine leukemia chemotherapy according to the immune state. Reconsideration of correlations between chemotherapy, tumor cell killing and survival time.* « Cancer Immunol. Immunoth. », 2, 139-141 (1977).

[40] MATHÉ G., *Prevention of chemotherapy complications: time, toxicity, pharmacokinetic, pharmacodynamic and logistic factors,* p. 124-139 in « Complications of cancer chemotherapy. (G. Mathé and R. K. Oldham, eds.). Heidelberg, New York, Springer Verlag, 1974.

[41] POUILLART P., PALANGIE T., SCHWARZENBERG L., BRUGERIE H., LHERITIER J. and MATHÉ G., *Effect of BCG on haematopoietic stem cells.* « Biomedicine », 23, 469-471 (1975).

[42] POUILLART P., PALANGIE T., SCHWARZENBERG L., BRUGERIE H., LHERITIER J. and MATHÉ G., *Effect of BCG on hematopoietic stem cells: experimental and clinical study.* « Cancer Immunol. Immunoth. », 1, 163-169 (1976).

[43] MATHÉ G., HALLE-PANNENKO O. and BOURUT C., *Interspersion of cyclophosphamide and BCG in the treatment of L1210 leukaemia and Lewis tumour.* « Europ. J. Cancer », 13, 1095-1098 (1977).

[44] MATHÉ G., HALLE-PANNENKO O. and BOURUT C., *Potentiation of a cyclophosphamide-induced immunodepression by the administration of BCG.* « Transplant. Proc. », 6, 431-433 (1974).

[45] IMBACH J. L., MONTERO J. L., MORUZZI A., SERROU B., CHENU E., HAYAT M., MATHÉ G., *The oncostatic and immunosuppressive action of new nitrosourea derivatives containing sugar radicals.* « Biomed. », 23, 410-413 (1975).

[46] MATHÉ G., HALLE-PANNENKO O., FLORENTIN I. and BOURUT C., *Active immunotherapy and chemotherapy combination using a non-immunosuppressive oncostatic, RFCNU.* In Prep.

[47] BEKESI J.G. and HOLLAND J.F., *Active immunotherapy in leukemia with neuraminidase modified leukemic cells.* pp. 78-89, in « Tactics and strategy in cancer treatment » (G. Mathé, ed.). Heidelberg, New York, Springer verlag, 1977.

[48] POWLES R.L., CROWTHER D., BATEMAN C.J.T., BEARD M.E.J., MACELVAIN T.J., RUSSEL J., LISTER T.A., WHITEHOUSE J.M.A., WRIGLEY P.F.M., PIKE M., ALEXANDER P. and HAMILTON FAIRLEY G., *Immunotherapy for acute myelogenous leukaemia.* « Brit. J. Cancer », 28, 365-376 (1973).

[49] REIZENSTEIN P., BRENNING G., ENGSTEDT L., FRANZEN S., GAHRTON G., GULLBRING B., HOLM G., HOCKER P., HOGLUND S., HORNSTEN P., JAMESON S., KILLANDER A., KILLANDER D., KLEIN E., LANTZ B., LIDEMALM C., LOCKNER D., LONNQVIST B., MELLSTEDT H., PALMBLAD J., PAULI C., SKARBERG K.O., UDEN A.M., VANKY F. and WADMAN B., *Effect of immunotherapy on survival and remission duration in acute, non-lymphatic leukaemia.* pp. 329-339, in: « Immunotherapy of cancer: present status of trials in man », (W.D. Terry and D. Windhorst, eds). New York 1978. Raven Press.

[50] VOGLER W. R. and CHAN Y. K., *Prolonging remission in myeloblastic leukaemia by Ticestrain bacillus Calmette-Guérin.* « Lancet », 2, 128-131 (1974).

[51] WHITTAKER J.A. and SLATER A.J., *Immunotherapy of acute myelogenous leukaemia using intravenous BCG.* pp. 393-403, in: « Immunotherapy of cancer: present status of trials in man », (W.D. Terry and D. Windhorst, eds), New York 1978. Raven Press.

[52] HUDSON C.N., MAC HARDY J.E., CURLING O.M., ENGLISH P.E., LEVIN L., POULTON T.A., CROWTHER M. and LEIGHTON M., *Active specific immunotherapy for ovarian cancer.* « Lancet », 2, 877-879 (1976).

[53] STEWART T.H.M., HOLLINSHEAD A.C., HARRIS J.E., RAMAN S., BELANGER R., CREPEAU A., CROOK A.F., HARTE W.E., HOOPER D., KLAASSEN D.J., RAPP E.F. and SACHS H.J., *Survival study of immuno-chemotherapy in lung cancer.* pp. 203-216, in: « Immunotherapy of cancer: present status of trials in man », (W.D. Terry and D. Windhorst, eds). New York, 1978. Raven Press.

[54] GUTTERMAN J.U., HERSH E.M., MAVLIGIT G.M., BURGESS M.A., RICHMAN S.P., SCHWARZ M., RODRIQUEZ V. and VALDIVIESO M., *Chemo-immunotherapy of disseminated malignant melanoma with BCG: follow-up report.* pp. 103-111, in: « Immunotherapy of cancer: present status of trials in man » (W.D. Terry and D. Windhorst, eds). New York, 1978. Raven Press.

[55] MASTRANGELO M.J., BELLET R.E., BERD D. and LUSTBADER E., *A randomized prospective trial comparing methyl-CCNU + vincristine to methyl-CCNU + Vincristine + BCG + allogeneic tumor cells in patients with metastatic malignant melanoma.* pp. 95-102, in: « Immunotherapy of cancer: present status of trials in man » (W.D. Terry and D. Windhorst, eds). New York, 1978. Raven Press.

[56] YAMAMURA Y., *Immunotherapy of lung cancer with oil-attached cell wall skeleton of BCG.* pp. 173-179, in: « Immunotherapy of cancer: present status of trials in man » (W.D. Terry and D. Windhorst, eds). New York, 1978. Raven Press.

[57] HORTOBAGYI G.N., GUTTERMAN J.U., BLUMENSCHEIN G.R., BUZDAR A., BURGESS M.A., RICHMAN S.P., TASHIMA C.K., SCHWARZ M. and HERSH E.M., *Chemo-immunotherapy of advanced breast cancer with BCG.* pp. 655-668, in: « Immunotherapy of cancer: present status of trials in man » (W.D. Terry and D. Windhorst, eds). New York, 1978. Raven Press.

[58] PINSKY C.M., DEJAGER R.L., WITTES R.E., WONG P.P., KAUFMAN R.J., MIKE V., HANSEN J.A., OETTGEN H.F. and KRAKOFF I.H., *Corynebacterium parvum as adjuvant to combination chemotherapy in patients with advanced breast cancer: preliminary results of a prospective randomized trial.* pp. 647-654, in: « Immunotherapy of cancer: present status of trials in man » (W.D. Terry and D. Windhorst, eds). New York, 1978. Raven Press.

[59] SIMMLER M.C., SCHWARZENBERG L. and MATHÉ G., *Attempts at non specific cell-mediated immunorestoration of immunodepressed cancer patients with BCG.* « Cancer Immunol. Immunoth. », 1, 157-162 (1976).

[60] POUILLART P., MATHÉ G., PALANGIE T., HUGUENIN P., MORIN P., GAUTIER H., BARON A. and LEDEDENTE A., *Pre-chemotherapy (CT) adjuvant immunotherapy of stage III and IV bronchus carcinoma (BCG).* Second National Cancer Institute Conference on Lung Cancer Treatment, Airlie House, Virginia, May 22-24, 1977 (Abstract No. 54).

[61] ECONOMIDES F., BRULEY-ROSSET M. and MATHÉ G., *Effect of pre- and post-surgical active BCG immunotherapies on murine EAkR lymphosarcoma.* « Biomedicine », 25, 372-375 (1976).

[62] MC KNEALLY M.F., MAVER C.M. and KAUSEL H.W., *Intrapleural BCG immunostimulation in lung cancer.* « Lancet », 1, 1003 (one page), 1977.

[63] KLEIN E. and HOLTERMANN O. A., *Immunotherapeutic approaches to the management of neoplasms.* « Nat. Cancer Inst. Monogr. », *35*, 379-402 (1972).

[64] MORTON D. L., EILBER F. R., JOSEPH W. L., WOOD W. C., TRAHAN E. and KETCHAM A. S., *Immunological factors in human sarcomas and melanomas: a rational basis for immunotherapy.* « Ann. Surgery », *172*, 740-749 (1970).

[65] ZBAR B., BERNSTEIN I. D. and RAPP H. J., *Suppression of tumor growth at the site of infection with living Bacillus Calmette-Guérin.* « J. Nat. Cancer Inst. », *46*, 831-839 (1971).

[66] SEDLACEK H. H., SEILER F. R. and SCHWAICK H. G., *Neuraminidase and tumor immunotherapy.* « Klin. Wschr. », *55*, 199-214 (1977).

[67] KIGER N., Unpublished data.

[68] MATHÉ G., HALLE-PANNENKO O. and BOURUT C., *Active immunotherapy in spontaneous leukemia of AkR mice.* « Exp. Hematol. », *1*, 110-114 (1973).

[69] DORE J. F., HADJIYANNAKIS M. J., COUDER A., GUIBOUT A., MARHOLEV L. and IMAI K., *Use of enzyme-treated cells in immunotherapy of leukaemia*, p. 387-388 in: « Investigation and stimulation of immunity in cancer patients » (G. Mathé and R. Weiner eds.). Heidelberg, New York, Springer Verlag, 1974.

[70] ROSENFELD C., GOUTNER A., VENUAT A. M., CHOQUET C., PICO J. L., DORE J. F., LIABEUF A., DURANDY A., DESGRANGES C. and DE THE G., *An effective human leukaemic cell line: Reh.* « Europ. J. Cancer », *13*, 377-379 (1977).

[71] MARTYRE M. C., *Attempt at specific immunotherapy of RC19 leukemia with soluble tumour antigen extracts.* « Biomedicine », *25*, 360-362 (1976).

[72] MARTYRE M. C., WEINER R. and HALLE-PANNENKO O., *The in vivo activity of soluble extract obtained from RC19 leukemia: the effect of the method of extraction*, p. 405-407 in: « Investigation and stimulation of immunity in cancer patients », (G. Mathé and R. Weiner eds.). Heidelberg, New York, Springer Verlag, 1974.

[73] MATHÉ G., HIU I. H., HALLE-PANNENKO O. and BOURUT C., *Methanol extraction residue fraction of tubercle bacilli (MER) and other mycobacterial extracts as systemic immunity adjuvants in cancer immunotherapy.* « Israel J. Med. Sci. », *12*, 468-471 (1976).

[74] HALPERN B., FRAY A., CREPIN Y., PLATICA O., LORINET A. M., RABOURDIN A., SPARROS L. and ISAC R., *Corynebacterium parvum, a potent immunostimulant in experimental infections and malignancies*, p. 217-236 in: « Immunopotentiation » (Ciba Foundation Symp. No. 18), 1 vol., Amsterdam, 1973, Elsevier Excerpta Medica.

[75] MATHÉ G., SCHWARZENBERG L., DE VASSAL F., DELGADO M., PENA-ANGULO J., BELPOMME D., POUILLART P., MACHOVER D., MISSET J. L., PICO J. L., JASMIN C., HAYAT M., SCHNEIDER M., CATTAN A., AMIEL J. L., MUSSET M. and ROSENFELD C., *Chemotherapy followed by active immunotherapy in the treatment of acute lymphoid leukemias for patients of all ages; results of ICIG acute lymphoid leukemia protocols 1, 9 and 10; prognosis factors and therapeutic implications*, p. 451-469, in: « Immunotherapy of cancer: present status of trials in man ». (W.D. Terry and D. Windhorst, eds). New York, 1978. Raven Press.

[76] Toujas L., Sabolovic D., Dazord L., Legarrec Y., Toujas J. P., Guelfi J. and Pilet C., *The mechanism of immunostimulation induced by inactivated brucella abortus*. « Europ. J. Clin. Biol. Res. », *17*, 267-273 (1972).

[77] Mathé G., Halle-Pannenko O., Florentin I., Hayat M., Bruley-Rosset M. and Bourut C., *New agents submitted to E.O.R.T.C.-I.C.I.G. experimental screening for systemic immunity adjuvants applicable to cancer immunotherapy.* In preparation.

[78] Mathé G., Florentin I., Bruley-Rosset M., Hayat M. and Bourut C., *Heat-killed Pseudomonas aeruginosa as a systemic adjuvant in cancer immunotherapy.* « Biomedicine », *27*, 368-373 (1977).

[79] Mathé G., De Vassal F., Gouveia J., Simmler M.C. and Misset J.L., *Comparison of the restoration effect of Pseudomonas aeruginosa, BCG and poly I: poly C in cancer patients non responsive to recall antigen delayed hypersensitivity.* « Biomedicine », *27*, 328-330 (1977).

DISCUSSION

RAPP

We have compared fresh-frozen and freeze-dried preparations of BCG derived from one strain. Most of the organisms in the fresh-frozen preparation were viable while most of the organisms in the freeze-dried preparation were not. The two preparations were equally active immunotherapeutically, provided the dose of the freeze-dried preparation was unvaried in order to give the same number of living organisms as that contained in the fresh-frozen preparation. When you looked at your fresh and dried organisms, did you adjust the dose for the number of living organisms?

MATHÉ

No, it was one milligram of each.

RAPP

But that is not a fair comparison. I think the results you showed are meaningless.

MATHÉ

These were the first obtained comparing different BCG before we showed that bacteremia is the most important factor in BCG immunotherapy.

RAPP

Living organisms are immunotherapeutically active, dead organisms alone are not. Different strains of BCG should be compared on the

basis of number of viable organisms and not on total weight of living
and dead organisms.

MATHÉ

I wish that other BCG were active also.

RAPP

But they are if you compare them on the basis of the number of
living organisms.

MATHÉ

We have to verify it with our tests for systemic immunotherapy
which is not determined by the same factors as local immunotherapy.

GUTTERMAN

Your data on Pseudomonas is interesting. Is that a mutant material
or is it a smooth strain?

MATHÉ

Our material is the organism itself, not an extract. It is in fact a
mixture of 10 serotypes.

GUTTERMAN

The data you showed suggesting that, I believe, the rough strains
were superior to the smooth, I think are confirmed by some of Edgar
Reevy's recent work using the mutant endotoxins. I think the endotoxins
in which the polysaccharide has not been synthesized are much more
active, at least in Herb Rapp's hepatoma model, than the smooth strains
in which the polysaccharides are retained. So there is, I think, something
very crucial about the cell wall properties, at least of endotoxins, in
terms of their anti-tumor properties, both in your screening as well as in
Herb Rapp's model used by Edgar Reevy. Two other points I would

[3] *Mathé* - p. 24

like to bring up: you showed a slide in which the hypotonic membrane preparation may have enhanced leukemia. I would point out that at least in one series of studies from Hera Hollingshead she uses a hypotonic lytic material but she puts these on PAGE or on DEAE and has suggested at least that there may be inhibitory materials in the crude hypotonic materials; so I wondered if you had used a more purified material rather than just the crude hypotonic extract.

MATHÉ

We obtained the favorable effect with the crude hypertonic extract.

GUTTERMAN

The slide you showed with the C1$_9$ binding we can confirm precisely in solid tumors, that is in patients with high C1$_9$ bindings suggesting circulating antigen antibody complexes; clearly there would be much less survival than in those who have lower levels. What this means I am not sure, but in your abstract I believe you mentioned plasmapheresis as a method of immunomodulation prior to therapy. We are beginning to do plasmapheresis based on our findings that high C1$_9$ binding activity does seem to predispose to early death.

MATHÉ

As a matter of fact acute lymphoid-leukemia patients who present high content of antigen-antibody complexes have a poor prognosis. At the present time we are doing a study on antigen-antibody complexes in the serum and we randomize the patients who have a high level of complexes between plasmapheresis and no plasmapheresis before induction remission treatment. We have got one remission with plasmapheresis alone.

GUTTERMAN

Poly-IC conceivably could be immunosuppressive, in certain doses, because it produces enough interferon — one could see a reduction in skin DHS reactions.

MATHÉ

We did not see any suppression of DHS in positive DHS patients.

DAVIES

Could you return for a moment to the previous point? There is no anomaly when Herbert Rapp says: adjust the number of organisms, and you say a milligram of each. A milligram of your freeze-dried preparation must contain an awful lot more organisms than your milligram of fresh.

MATHÉ

But not living.

GUTTERMAN

Are you referring to living organisms in the freeze-dried preparations of BCG?

RAPP

Yes. The proportion of living organisms in freeze-dried preparation of BCG is often as low as 1 in 20.

DAVIES

The other point is the following: I recall that the rough organisms among the enterobacteria were excellent stimulators of what we used to call properdin, to increase the extent of tens or hundreds of times the activity of the smooth ones.

BALDWIN

We recently published a retrospective study on serum immune complexes in breast cancer (Brit. Med. 5, 1977), patients with high immune complex levels compared to normal controls. In this trial patients were

[3] *Mathé* - p. 26

divided into good and bad prognosis groups based upon a number of clinical factors such as triple node biopsies. Patients that were selected as the bad prognosis group had higher levels of immune complexes prior to surgery and these levels were high also 12 months after surgery. Patients that had a good prognosis of surgery also had high levels of immune complexes, but within 12 months their levels fell back to the normal range. I think it would be premature to assume that this has anything to do with a tumor immune reaction and one has to identify the nature of the complexes. The second point — and I will talk on this tomorrow — we have been screening a number of the Trudeau BCG preparations, testing their capacity to inhibit growth of tumor cells when injected together. Using this standard in screening preparations of the Trudeau, Pasteur and Montreal strains we find that they show something like 5 to 10 times greater activity than other preparations such as the Glaxo and Tice strains. Using this screening system, we can differentiate between an increased activity of two bacterial preparations compared to two others.

MATHÉ

In Montreal Turcotte has two phenotypes of the original Pasteur BCG: one is much stronger than the other one for the adjuvant effect and less active for tuberculin effect, and vice versa. So there *is* a strain factor. The protocol for lung cancer is the following: we take stage I and II patients as soon as possible after operation; they are randomized to receive BCG on scarifications according to our usual method, or not.

OETTGEN

I would like to comment on the use of the term specific in immunotherapy. I have no quarrel with using leukemia cell vaccines — allogeneic leukemia cells — particularly if they work. But as far as I know, there is no acceptable proof today, including the serological data that you showed, of leukemia specific antigens in man, individual or shared. I think it is better to keep our thinking straight and not refer to the use of allogeneic leukemia cell vaccines as specific immunotherapy until there is proof that these cells carry such antigens.

[3] *Mathé* - p. 27

4

MATHÉ

I quite agree with you to use the terms tumor cell immunotherapy if you prefer. But I like to remind you of the data collected by Dore on acute lymphoid leukemia and lymphosarcoma associated antigens.

WEISS

I would like to go back for a moment to the question of standardization of living BCG and to point out that more than 25 years ago Pierce and Dubos and their colleagues had made the point that a crucial factor in determining the *specific* immunogenic capacity, vis-a-vis tuberculosis of various strains and sublines of BCG, is the ability of a standard number of living organisms to multiply in the tissues and to disseminate as a function of time. Of course this is very difficult to determine in man, but some suggestive information could come from parallel *in vivo* analyses in experimental animals of viability and reproducibility of BCG preparations. Cell number or weight cannot by themselves serve as the critical determinants of likely efficacy. One other very brief point, with regard to the threat of non-specific stimulation of suppressory cell formation or activity. In our own experience it appears that a variety of "adjuvant" substances stimulate suppressor cell activity, as a function more of the length of time of immune stimulation than of the initial amount of the immuno-stimulator used. The time-of-treatment parameter must be borne in mind. There seems to be a critical point, in man as well as in experimental animals, beyond which further stimulation can turn off immunological capacity even rather precipitously. Thus, a variety of parameters of immunostimulation by non-specific means must be considered from the perspective of the possibly negative, as well as of the hoped-for positive consequences.

MATHÉ

I agree with your two remarks. About dissemination, the work we did with Khalil showed that a BCG septicemia was present in the condition of administration which gave a cure. About the possibility of induction of suppressor cells after a certain time of adjuvant intervention we have clinical data showing the appearance of DHS suppression after

[3] *Mathé* - p. 28

long-term application of high doses of BCG on scarification or short-term application of intravenous injection of BCG. So this may be another reason to use chemoimmunotherapy interspersion with special drugs, which not only would not be immunosuppressive, but would be able to kill suppressor cells.

CHEDID

I wish to stress the following point: in the field of immunostimulation the capacity of a microorganism to proliferate or not in a given species is extremely critical. This is especially true in the case of an immunization model which requires a delayed hypersensitive reaction to increase the resistance of the host. In many cases killed organisms are not effective because they represent a smaller dose of antigen than an inoculum of viable organisms which can proliferate. Such a simple explanation is probably responsible for the differences observed between rough and smooth gram-negative strains since it is well established that lipopolysaccharide endotoxin activity is very similar in both "R" and "S" strains.

MATHÉ

It is exact that in our EAkR model there is a critical dose of tumor cells for specific immunotherapy. As far as immunotherapy with neuraminidase treated cells is concerned, the optimal number in the dog is $2x10^7$ cells according to Sedlacek.

RAPP

I am skeptical about tests for evaluating the anti-tumor effects of adjuvants that do not require the regression of an established tumor. A variety of agents injected together with tumor cells will prevent growth of the tumor, but few will cause regression of an established tumor.

MATHÉ

There are two different models. We need your model for local immunotherapy, but I work on systemic immunotherapy of minimal imperceptible residual disease.

RAPP

But you have not used a minimal residual disease model. Giving a healthy animal the challenge and the adjuvant at the same time, or even one day later, has little relationship to minimal residual disease in humans.

BALDWIN

I cannot agree with Dr. Rapp. At this stage one is asking many questions which the tumor-bearing animal will or will not answer. Unfortunately, there are not yet enough models that are at that stage of development. So that, for example, in our own particular case we are initially evaluating the capacity of different bacterial preparations to cause the rejection of tumor cells when administered in admixture to normal animals. In this case we are evaluating whether agents can mobilize macrophages to cause the tumors to regress.

In studies with transplanted rat hepatomas and sarcomas we have identified tumor specific immune complexes in the serum of tumor-bearing animals. These tumor specific immune complexes can be dissociated and fractionated at acid pH on Sephadex G150 to yield isolated tumor specific antigen. These soluble tumor antigen preparations are immunogenic in syngeneic hosts producing tumor specific antibody responses. Nevertheless, this form of immunization does not elicit tumor rejection response. In this respect, it should be noted that several investigators have established that soluble tumor antigens do not produce an effective tumor specific rejection response.

CLERICI

I would like to go back to the meaning of plasmapheresis. If these immune complexes are found in the serum of poor prognosis patients, that means that they are very pathogenic. Probably most of them are composed of IgG and tumor antigens. If you remove the complexes with plasmapheresis, then you decrease the concentration of IgG, which exerts a negative feedback mechanism on the antibody production. Therefore, after a few days there will be again plenty of complexes in the circulation of your patients, so that the effect of pasmapheresis will be nullified.

[3] *Mathé* - p. 30

MATHÉ

We search for immune complexes in all patients and we submit half of them to plasmapheresis. Interestingly enough we have obtained a remission in all patients after one plasmapheresis.

SPREAFICO

We are all talking about BCG and stimulation of suppressor cells; however, do you have any data on the possible reduction of suppressor cell activity or suppressor cell numbers after treatment with immunostimulants, or for that matter with other pharmacological agents?

MATHÉ

We have been able to suppress the activity of suppressor cells in animals only with methotrexate.

SPREAFICO

So you could never get dosages of drugs which are antitumorally effective in animals and see whether there follows a reduction of suppressor cells?

MATHÉ

No. The only relevant situation I can mention is DHS restoration with pseudomonas seraginase in patients who became DHS negative after long term-high dose BCG application.

WESTPHAL

I should like to come back to Allan Davies' remark and question about the use of bacterial cell walls, of purified extracts, finally of LPS from smooth or rough strains — all these very many different materials. If it is endotoxin which is the active principle of gram-negative organisms, as one can show with purified preparations, then the release of endotoxin and the form in which it will be released *in vivo* plays a great role.

For instance, if you take whole bacteria and you treat them with formaldehyde, you can still prove that endotoxin is present, and by sophisticated means you can extract endotoxin from such bacteria still. But if you inject these formaldehyde-treated bacteria nothing will be released and actually nothing happens. So it is the way in which the bacteria or the materials that you inject undergo dynamic processes *in vivo* which plays a dominant role in its pharmacological actions. Therefore I think we need standardization of whatever materials we are using.

WEISS

I would like to comment on Dr. Spreafico's question. Amounts of MER which will stimulate *in vitro* the specific generation of cytotoxic effector cells against tumor targets, and we are talking about microgram levels, which categorically prevent the appearance of suppressor cell activity in normal lymphoid cell cultures. As shown in Dr. Terry's laboratory, and others, mouse lymphoid cells incubated alone for several days develop strong suppressor activity. Addition of MER to the cultures prevents this almost entirely. In certain cases, at least, immunomodulating agents can thus both stimulate specific immune reactivity and abrogate suppressor function. This appears to hold, for MER, *in vivo* as well as *in vitro*.

SPREAFICO

I was not afraid about that impression; indeed we have data to show that *in vivo* you can get suppression of suppressor cells to the drugs.

GUTTERMAN

I want to come back to the point that Dr. Weiss made earlier regarding the appearance of suppressor cells over time, and I was interested in the comment that George Mathé made regarding at least one patient who was immunosuppressed on BCG and then restored by pseudomonas. We now have over 6 patients we have observed, on BCG over three years, getting BCG every other week, in which their skin tests to recall antigens as well as to PPD became completely negative. On stopping the BCG, the patients were retested 4 to 6 weeks later and I think all

[3] *Mathé* - p. 32

the other variables were excluded, including concomitant viral infections etc. These patients, after stopping their BCG, had a recovery of their immune response. Now with a small number of patients other factors perhaps could be incriminated here, but I think there is a possibility that with chronic use of the same immunoadjuvant as with chronic granulomatous diseases, the patients indeed get immunosuppressed, and I think this needs to be evaluated and of course emphasizes one of the problems in model work and that we really do not have chronic models in which we look at immunomodulation over the course of several weeks, months or even years.

WEISS

What Dr. Gutterman mentioned has been seen recently by Drs. Bekesis and Holland at Mount Sinai Hospital in New York. AML patients treated repeatedly with MER after remission induction, and showing good immunological ability (delayed skin hypersensitivity reactions and strong PHA peripheral lymphocyte transformation capacity) sometimes lost their capacity rather suddenly after 18-24 months. Several such patients also presented indications of incipient relapse at the same time. Cessation of MER treatment was followed after several weeks by a bounce back to good immunological activity, and at least several such patients then remained in prolonged remission, some for over four years. Continuous immunological monitoring and either cessation or change of immunological treatment upon fall of host responsiveness, may thus be a general requirement. Even a substance such as MER, which tends strongly to *prevent* immunosuppression due to a variety of causes, may lead to depressed immunological function after very prolonged administration.

[3] *Mathé* - p. 33

IMMUNOTHERAPY FOR RECURRENT MALIGNANT MELANOMA: THE EFFICACY OF BCG IN PROLONGING THE POSTOPERATIVE DISEASE-FREE INTERVAL AND SURVIVAL.

JORDAN U. GUTTERMAN, STEPHEN P. RICHMAN, CHARLES MCBRIDE,* MICHAEL A. BURGESS, SHELLEY L. BARTOLD,** ANNE KENNEDY,** EDMUND A. GEHAN,** GIORA MAVLIGIT and EVAN M. HERSH

*Departments of Developmental Therapeutics, **Biomathematics and *Surgery, The University of Texas System Cancer Center M. D. Anderson Hospital and Tumor Institute*

Houston - Texas

In this report, we summarize updated results with adjuvant immunotherapy with bacillus Calmette-Guérin (BCG) for patients with recurrent malignant melanoma. This program was initiated in 1971. Preliminary reports have been published elsewhere [1, 2].

MATERIALS AND METHODS

Between November 1971 and March 1976, 107 patients with regional lymph node metastases were entered in the study. All patients had recurrent melanoma in regional lymph nodes and were eligible for the study after surgical removal of all clinical evidence of tumor.

Forty-two patients were entered into the first trial which was conducted between November 1971 and October 1974. Twenty patients received high dose Tice strain BCG and 22 patients received low-dose Tice BCG, as described earlier. In the second trial which was conducted between October 1974 and March 1976, 40 patients received fresh frozen Pasteur strain BCG.

Twenty-five patients were included in another trial conducted between October 1974 and March 1976. These patients received chemotherapy with DTIC, 250 mg/M^2 daily for five days, as well as fresh frozen Pasteur strain BCG, 6×10^8 viable units on days 7, 12, and 17. Cycles were repeated every 21 days.

The surgical control group consisted of 260 patients with stage IIIB melanoma who had been treated with surgery alone at M. D. Anderson Hospital between January 1965 and October 1971. Variables of these patients were examined in a comparable fashion to that of the patients in our study. The natural histories of these surgical control patients will be examined in detail in another report.

The statistical methods used included the generalized Wilcoxon test and a one-tailed analysis for testing differences between disease-free or survival curves [3], and the method of KAPLAN and MEIER for calculating and plotting disease-free and survival curves [4].

RESULTS

The postoperative disease-free interval for the surgically treated control and the BCG treated groups of stage IIIB patients with less than five involved nodes is shown in Figure 1. There has been a statistically significant prolongation of the postoperative disease-free interval for patients treated with either high dose Tice or fresh frozen Pasteur strain BCG compared with the control group. No benefit was derived for those patients treated with low dose Tice BCG. The survival for the group of patients with less than five involved nodes is shown in Figure 2. Patients treated with the high doses of BCG (Tice or fresh frozen Pasteur BCG) have had a highly significant prolongation of survival. Only 4 of 10 patients treated with high dose Tice and 7 of 40 treated with fresh frozen Pasteur BCG have died.

In contrast to these encouraging results, little benefit has been derived for patients with five or more involved nodes. There has been no statistical improvement in the postoperative disease-free

[4] *Gutterman* - p. 2

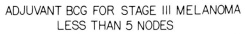

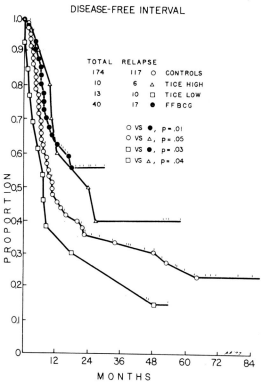

ADJUVANT BCG FOR STAGE III MELANOMA
LESS THAN 5 NODES
DISEASE-FREE INTERVAL

TOTAL	RELAPSE		
174	117	○	CONTROLS
10	6	△	TICE HIGH
13	10	□	TICE LOW
40	17	●	FF BCG

○ VS ●, p = .01
○ VS △, p = .05
□ VS ●, p = .03
□ VS △, p = .04

FIG. 1

interval for patients treated with BCG alone or DTIC plus BCG (Fig. 3). There has been little improvement in the postoperative survival time (Fig. 4).

DISCUSSION

These results suggest that viable BCG given in doses of approximately 6×10^8 colony forming units, is capable of prolonging

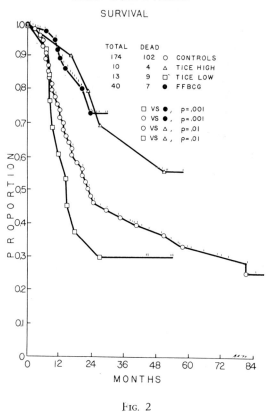

ADJUVANT BCG FOR STAGE III MELANOMA
LESS THAN 5 NODES

SURVIVAL

FIG. 2

the postoperative disease-free interval and survival among patients with small amounts of residual tumor. Patients with five or more nodes, in which the natural history is considerably worse, appeared to have benefitted only slightly or not at all, even with the addition of DTIC chemotherapy to the adjuvant immunotherapy regimen.

Several groups have now reported successful prolongation of postoperative disease-free interval and survival, particularly among patients with small numbers of positive lymph nodes [5-8]. The

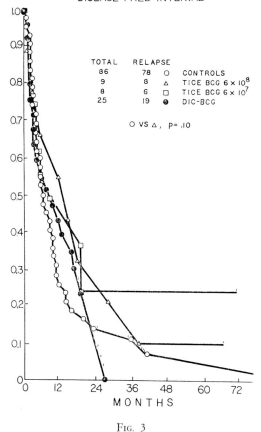

ADJUVANT BCG FOR STAGE III MELANOMA
≥5 NODES
DISEASE-FREE INTERVAL

TOTAL	RELAPSE		
86	78	O	CONTROLS
9	8	△	TICE BCG 6×10^8
8	6	□	TICE BCG 6×10^7
25	19	◉	DIC-BCG

O VS △ , P= .10

MONTHS

FIG. 3

original work of MORTON and EILBER and ourselves, has been confirmed as noted in this conference by several groups.

Despite the promising results, it is clear that BCG immunotherapy for patients with positive nodes is still not ideal treatment since the majority of patients continue to relapse and eventually die of their tumor. Earlier application of BCG therefore seems

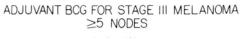

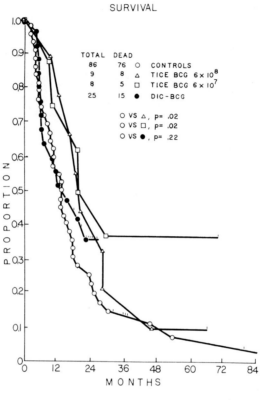

FIG. 4

indicated. Preliminary results of adjuvant BCG in patients with primary melanoma of the trunk in our own experience is promising. This would seem to be the ideal clinical situation in which to investigate adjuvant immunotherapy. Clearly, adjuvant immunotherapy is safe and it appears that benefit has been achieved. Further trials will need to be carried out with other immunotherapeutic modalities to maximize the clinical benefit.

[4] *Gutterman* - p. 6

REFERENCES

[1] GUTTERMAN J.U., MAVLIGIT G.M., McBRIDE C.M., FREI E., FREIREICH E.J. and HERSH E.M., *Active immunotherapy with BCG for recurrent malignant melanoma.* « Lancet », *1*, 1208-1212 (1973).

[2] GUTTERMAN J.U., MAVLIGIT G.M., BURGESS M.A., CARDINOS J.D., BLU-MENSCHEIN G.R., GOTTLIEB J.A., McBRIDE C.M., McCREDIE K.B., BODEY G.P., RODRIQUEZ V., FREIREICH E.J. and HERSH E.M., *Immunotherapy of human solid tumors and acute leukemia with BCG: Prolongation of disease free interval and survival.* « Cancer Immunol. Immunother. », *1*, 99-107 (1976).

[3] GEHAN E.A., *A generalized Wilcoxon test for comparing arbitrarily singly-censored samples.* « Biometrika », *52*, 203-223 (1965).

[4] KAPLAN E.L. and MEIER P., *Nonparametric estimation from incomplete observations.* « J. Am. Stat. Assoc. », *53*, 457-481 (1958).

[5] BLUMING A.Z., VOGEL C.L. and ZIEGLER J.L., *Immunological effects of BCG in malignant melanoma: Two modes of administration compared.* « Ann. Intern. Med. », *76*, 405-411 (1972).

[6] MORTON D.L., EILBER F.R., HOLMES E.C., HUNT J.S., KETCHAM A.S., SILVER-STEIN M.J. and SPARKS F.C., *BCG immunotherapy of malignant melanoma: Summary of a seven year experience.* « Ann. Surg. », *180*, 635-643 (1974).

[7] EILBER F.R., MORTON D.L., HOLMES E.C., SPARKS F.C. and RAMMING K.P., *Adjuvant immunotherapy with BCG in treatment of regional lymph node metastases from malignant melanoma.* « N. Engl. J. Med. », *294*, 237-240 (1976).

[8] BERETTA A., *Controlled study for prolonged chemotherapy, immunotherapy, and chemotherapy plus immunotherapy as adjuvant to surgery.* « Immunotherapy of Cancer: Present Status of Trials in Man », Terry, W.D., and Windhorst, D. (eds), New York, Raven Press, 1978.

DISCUSSION

MATHÉ

Do you monitor the immune functions of the patient when you compare immunotherapy and chemoimmunotherapy?

GUTTERMAN

Well, the stem cell work is just beginning. Now we have seen some increase in CFU by *Pseudomonas* as well as with BCG. We have a variety of assays which virtually every laboratory probably does — needle skin tests to recall antigens, *in vitro* assays to mitogens, nonspecific antigens as well as the putative tumor antigens. None of these have been very useful, either as a group in terms of predicting benefits from immunotherapy or in terms of guiding us thus far in terms of immunotherapy. Now we have seen individual patients for example become immunologically suppressed on immune therapy, and when we have stopped, in some of these patients we have seen a recovery. But this is a small group of patients. When we take the entire battery of tests that we use — MIF, lymphocyte stimulation, etc. — thus far we have been very disappointed in terms of using these as correlates of immunotherapy. So, it is possible we have not looked at the data correctly, but they have not been of use to us. Now there are certain assays we are just beginning to use; for example, the natural killer assays and others, but the ones we used thus far, including cytotoxicity against established lines of melanoma, have not been very much help. We have a lot of data and maybe you would like to help us analyze it — but it has not been useful.

CHEDID

Cord factor has been extensively studied on animal models by Dr. Bekierkunst and by Dr. Rapp. In these experiments cord factor was solubilized in mineral oil. Since we have been told that non-degradable mineral oil could constitute a problem in clinical assays, we would like to ask what preparation was used. I find these results very encouraging. I would also like to suggest that since synthetic analogues have become easy to prepare and some of them which have been shown to be active in murine tumor systems are now available, they should be assayed also in such trials. Finally I would also like to ask you to comment a bit further on the incidents you mentioned and if fever is an important parameter in immunotherapy.

GUTTERMAN

First of all, in terms of toxicity BCG is beautifully tolerated in patients by scarification; we have treated hundreds, but we have never had a single incidence of disseminated BCG disease in these patients and it is well tolerated. However, when you do intralesional therapy, as was pointed out earlier today, there *is* a risk of disseminated disease. You are really giving an embolus and I think that there have been even two reported deaths — I think that the way it was administered in those patients who died was incorrect. I think the dose was much too high. Certainly for intralesional therapy one would prefer using nonviable materials, but as regards toxicity by scarification, that is not a reason not to use BCG. The other aspect is of course intravenous. Intravenous BCG is not an ideal way of administering it. Now as for the cord factor P-3 combination, this was certainly less toxic than intralesional BCG. We do get ulcerations, we do get a mild degree of fever, but the toleration compared with BCG is tremendously better. I know that Tubiana working with rabies has used synthetic P-3, I think with carbon added. I think that one of the exciting areas will be to use synthetic microbacterial subcomponents. I think that they are first of all being characterized and the number of carbon atom ions required for antitumor effect is quite interesting.

What the biologic significance of the temperature is, I am not certain. We have found that by giving MER intravenously — which we are now beginning to do — the kinetics of fever is quite different. Patients who are tuberculin positive, who get a dose of MER intravenously, will maintain a temperature for 3 to 4 days. They tolerate the MER much better than *C. parvum*. With *C. parvum* you get a very brisk rise of fever when you get a fever, tremendous chilling, the patients are relatively sick, there must be a tremendous outpouring of steroids and so forth. With MER the fever is slower to develop in the tuberculin positive patients and much more prolonged, such that these patients got *C. parvum* daily for two weeks; if one were to give MER one could not give it daily and I think one dose may be handled much differently and may last for several days to two weeks. With the cell wall skeleton, or cell wall material, with oil, we have not given this intravenously but I think this would be another interesting approach, because I suspect, particularly with the oil, the kinetics will be different and might stay around for a long time. We are going to extend this again — as to the true meaning of the fever and of the subsequent response to drugs I am not clear, but we are rather interested in this at this time.

WOLFF

I would like to make a couple of comments about the fever. Have you looked into using other pyrogenic agents to induce fever, such as etiocholanolone? Secondly, since you described decreasing fever with your *C. parvum* therapy, it suggests that they are developing hyposensitivity, or pyrogenic tolerance. If you will, you could overcome that by increasing the dose and see whether the fever is related to the clinical effects. Thirdly, if you give the cell wall skeleton in oil, you may have trouble, since Dr. Ribi had problems with monkeys. If you give this intravenously to people, wouldn't one anticipate that in fact you might get into serious trouble with that?

RAPP

I think you are referring to the fact that when Ribi used the BCG cell wall preparation in oil in monkeys, they developed granulomas. I do not know whether these granulomas produced any serious pathological effects. Granulomas produced by BCG in other animals seem to be harmless. So I am not sure that is a major problem.

WOLFF

I would think that unless it was, as Dr. Chedid described it, a heroic situation, developing granulomas in the lungs of people would mitigate against clinical use of these materials.

RAPP

No, I think they eventually go away and the organ returns to its normal architecture. They do in the animals that receive injections by routes other than intravenous.

I would like to make a comment about cell wall and cell wall skeleton. It may turn out to have been a mistake to use cell wall skeleton because of the following consideration. As I recall, Dr. Ribi developed the cell wall skeleton in the hope that this would give him an inactive preparation, so that then he could add back defined fractions and get activity to return. BCG cell wall skeleton is made by proteolytic enzyme digestion of the cell wall and by organic solvent extraction. This in itself adds a complication. But now the concept behind it turns out to be wrong, at least for the guinea pig model. Dr. Ribi expected that the cell wall skeleton by itself in oil would be inactive, and that is why cord factor was added. Using the guinea pig model, we have found no difference in the anti-tumor efficacy of whole cell walls and cell wall skeletons. So there is no need to add cord factor, which in itself may be toxic. I think needless complications are introduced by enzymatic digestion, organic solvent extraction and the addition of another potentially toxic factor.

GUTTERMAN

Dr. Rapp, I am not sure I agree with you, because the whole cell wall contains a considerable greater amount of protein than the skeleton cord factor P-3 combination.

RAPP

Yes, it does, but it does not seem to be a problem.

GUTTERMAN

We gave two patients whole cell wall and we rarely back off because of toxicity. We only gave, I think, 150 — and the most was 300 mi-

[4] *Gutterman* - p. 12

crograms — which is not as high as you have gone — that was just two patients — but we had tremendous hypersensitivity reaction.

RAPP

Had those patients already been treated with living BCG and did they have multiple injections?

GUTTERMAN

I suspect they had but I cannot recall.

RAPP

So you are asking for a hypersensitivity reaction. I have been talking about a single intralesional injection.

GUTTERMAN

Well, if a single injection works in man, then that is the way to do it.

RAPP

Yes, and I believe that it will work in stage I carcinoma.

GUTTERMAN

The question is: could you use, for example, in France, whole cell wall for a patient that you have in your schedule — a primary cancer of for example, anus, or melanoma? In France you would have, I would think, a lot more hypersensitivity reaction than you would using, for example, skeleton P-3 or endotoxin — as you know he is going on with the endotoxin.

RAPP

We have tested that in the guinea pig and it turns out that the cell wall skeleton is immunogenic in terms of inducing skin reactivity and a strong elicitor of delayed skin reactivity. The way to minimize allergic reactions to BCG is to give only a single injection. Patients with tuberculin reactivity might have an allergic reaction to BCG vaccines, but I do not think that will be prevented by using cell wall skeleton instead of cell wall. The addition of P-3 will add more potential complications.

GUTTERMAN

Yes, but P-3 is in the whole cell wall. Is there any less P-3 when you are injecting it as cell wall skeleton?

RAPP

I do not know.

WESTPHAL

I wonder whether any method is known to produce *long*-term *artificial* fever without overheating the patient physically. And of course we like to know in what respect the pyrogen-induced fever is different from the physically induced fever. We know that Greisman in Baltimore, for instance, infused endotoxin into rabbits and that it does not work because you run into tolerance very soon. So with endotoxin one cannot produce a long-lasting fever, due to the quick establishment of tolerance. You have just by change your long-lasting fever. You have selected your patients according to whether they reacted with fever or not. You are probably not able to predict whether a patient will react with this kind of fever or not.

GUTTERMAN

Yes, it is possible that this was selective for the patients, as you say. There are physical means however, to give temperature and they are being evaluated. You can do it with warm gasses and you can have a hot box where the patients get up to about 42°. There are several ways of doing it and there are reports now of individual patients having some degree of tumor regression with just physical heating, up to a certain critical temperature. So that is being evaluated, at least in the United States and in Scotland, I believe, by the anesthesiologists.

WESTPHAL

Is that whole body heating, or local?

GUTTERMAN

No, whole body. There are both approaches.

WOLFF

Let me call your attention to the experiences of the twenties when they tried to treat central nervous system syphilis with whole body heating and they lost a number of patients from hepatic failure. Thus, one must be extremely careful. The other thing to question here is about repeated injections. There is a circumstance that fascinates us — we took monkeys and gave them repeated injections of leucocytic pyrogen and then after about the sixth or seventh injection, instead of becoming tolerant, they suddenly became very sensitive and developed very high fevers. The other comment I would make about your MER response concerns the delay in fever. That suggests to me the sort of delayed fever that we see in hypersensitivity states, where guinea pigs are immunized with HSA BCG and then challenged with PPO, or we give them HSA and challenge. Since we see delayed fever in these situations I would be very careful. And I would like to ask whether you ever see anaphylaxis after these injections.

WEISS

Specifically, in responses to Wolff's question, in animals I do not think I have ever seen it. I now of three documented cases in patients, but those are three out of many thousands in which there was a suggestion, an appearance of something strongly suggestive, of a strong anaphylactoid reaction. All three of these patients had previously received intensive living BCG treatment, but the three out of quite a large number — there may be more — those are the only ones I know. If I just may take the opportunity in less than a minute to make a comment about intravenous injection of MER, I must say I worked with it for nearly twenty years before I even dared to give it to a mouse by the intravenous via, being quite sure that this mouse would die. The fact is that in fairly extensive studies done in Jerusalem, we find that we can give as large amounts as we can give interperitoneally with surprisingly little gross toxicity.

SOME ASPECTS OF THE INDUCTION
OF NON-SPECIFIC RESISTANCE TO INFECTION

SHELDON M. WOLFF and RONALD J. ELIN

National Institutes of Health
Bethesda, Maryland
Tufts University School of Medicine
Boston, Massachusetts

In patients with certain forms of cancer, for example, leukemia, infectious diseases remain the single most important cause of death. The types of infection that occur vary according to the underlying disease. For example, in Hodgkin's lymphoma where the patients manifest a deficiency in the cell mediated arm of the immune response, granulomatous diseases such as tuberculosis, systemic mycoses, etc., predominate. Of more importance is the fact that the various forms of cancer therapy employed so severely limit the normal host defense mechanisms (both immune and non-immune) that patients are at great risk for developing a severe infectious process.

Although the development and use of a wide range of antimicrobial agents, such as the aminoglycoside antibiotics, has had major effects on the morbidity and mortality of certain types of infectious diseases, we are still faced with a serious problem. Similarly, modern technology has made available replacement therapy such as granulocytes for transfusion and they have helped, but patients still die of infection. Large sums of money have been expended on such things as laminar flow rooms and they have had little, if any, impact on the problem. Although much hope was placed in the development of vaccines, they likewise have made little difference in the problem. For example, a pseudomonas vaccine which has proven to be of value in patients with burns has not had a similar effect in patients with leukemia. Further vaccine development should be pursued, but the likelihood of such efforts providing an overall answer to the problems of infection in cancer patients is unlikely.

For more than 80 years studies have been carried out attempting to induce non-specific resistance to infection. Unfortunately, most of the agents employed have been too toxic to even test in human beings. However, with the newer technology now available, we believe that renewed efforts in this area may provide information that will eventually be applicable to the problems of human disease.

Some of the agents employed to induce resistance to infections are listed in Table 1. As can be seen many of these agents are of microbial origin. In addition, many are also immunoadjuvants. Unfortunately, most are toxic at the doses employed. Resistance has been demonstrated to a wide range of microorganisms including bacteria [1-3], fungi [4], parasites [5] and viruses [6]. We have done a large number of studies in our laboratory on non-specific resistance to infection to *Candida albicans* induced by either bacterial endotoxin or a water soluble adjuvant derived from *Mycobacterium smegmatis* [4, 5, 7, 8, 9, 10, 11]. This work will be summarized below.

In the first series of experiments [4], we were able to show that as little as 100 µg. of endotoxin could significantly delay mortality in adult mice challenged with a lethal dose of *C. albicans*. A period of *increased* susceptibility ("negative phase") occurred if the endotoxin was given 1 hour before challenge with the fungi. However, when the endotoxin was given 24 hours, and as long as 9 days before the candida organisms, a significant delay in mortality developed. This resistance appeared to be bimodal, with maximum protection occurring when endotoxin was given 1 and 6 days before the fungi were administered. The endotoxin was effective whether given intravenously or by the intraperitoneal route (the fungi were administered intravenously). During these same experiments it was found that sterile sera obtained from mice which had received endotoxin 24 hours previously, could passively transfer protection to normal mice. Surprisingly, sera obtained from mice that had received endotoxin 6 days previously did not passively transfer resistance

[5] *Wolff, Elin* - p. 2

to infection.   The discrepancy between the effects seen in mice that had received endotoxin 1 and 6 days previously, as compared to the passive transfer experiments, was not readily explained.   Further studies indicated that gel fractionation (on Sephadex) did not allow isolation of the transferable factor from sera obtained from mice one day after endotoxin had been administered.   In addition, spleen cells obtained from inbred mice 6 days after endotoxin administration did not passively protect litter mates from challenge to candida organisms.

Subsequent studies employed injections of the same endotoxin to mice subsequently challenged with *Plasmodium berghei* [5]. These investigations showed that endotoxin induced protection in this experimental malaria model.   However, this protection was not transferable.   Furthermore, although reticuloendothelial system clearance was markedly enhanced by endotoxin, similar enhancement induced by zymosan or stilbesterol did not induce protection to infection.   Thus, enhanced reticuloendothelial function is not the mechanism for endotoxin-induced protection from infection with malaria. Since repeated injections of endotoxin ("endotoxin tolerance") not only abolished the toxic effects of endotoxin, but also negated the non-specific resistance inducing properties of endotoxin, one must assume that at least in the case of endotoxin, toxicity was required for protection.

Further studies attempted to further delineate the factors responsible for endotoxin non-specific resistance [7].   Mice given endotoxin 24 hours prior to challenge with *Candida albicans* demonstrated a significant enhancement of the clearance of these organisms from their blood stream.   Both *in vivo* and *in vitro* experiments were performed and neither supported the concept that serum opsonins played a significant role in the protection.   Organ localization studies showed that proliferation of the candida in the kidneys (the primary target organ for these infectious organisms in mice) was markedly decreased in animals pretreated 6 days before with endotoxin.   Another serum factor was discovered in these animals (in addition to the passive transferable factor) when serum taken 6 days after endotoxin was shown to significantly inhibit growth of *C. albicans in vitro*.

Additional studies done in our laboratory [9] shed considerable light on the mechanisms involved in non-specific resistance to candida infection induced by endotoxin. Since endotoxin markedly affects serum iron concentration in many species, and, in addition, iron is a growth requirement factor for candida, we investigated the role of iron in endotoxin-induced non-specific resistance. It was demonstrated that a significant correlation existed between the growth of *C. albicans* in serum obtained on a daily basis from mice challenged for up to 10 days previously and the percentage iron saturation of serum. Furthermore, the injection *in vivo* of iron at the time of infection with *C. albicans* led to a significant correlation between serum iron concentration and the mortality rate. The induction of resistance to infection by endotoxin could be reversed by the administration of iron. Thus, we postulate that in the experimental model employed, changes in iron metabolism were directly related to the resistance induced.

Since bacterial endotoxins are toxic and human beings are so exquisitely sensitive to these lipopolysaccharides, it is unlikely that they will ever find a clinically useful role to play. Therefore, the development of other materials with immunoadjuvant properties led us to study some of these. In experiments very similar to those employing endotoxin we studied the ability of a water soluble adjuvant (Neo-WSA) obtained from digestion of delipidated *Mycobacterium smegmatis* [11]. We chose to study this agent because other adjuvants had been shown to induce non-specific resistance to infection (Table 1) and because Neo-WSA had been shown to be essentially non-toxic.

Neo-WSA (1 mg.) was given intravenously to groups of mice 24 hours prior to infection with *Candida albicans* or *Klebsiella pneumoniae* or *Streptococcus pneumoniae*. In these experiments, Neo-WSA was shown to significantly enhance resistance to these various infectious microorganisms. Interestingly, no such protection was demonstrable when Neo-WSA was given prior to challenge with *P. berghei*. Of further interest was the fact that there was no "negative phase" with Neo-WSA since administration of Neo-WSA at or near the same time as the infections challenge still led to the induction of resistance. Furthermore, Neo-WSA did not affect serum iron concentrations in the mice. Thus, the mechanism of

TABLE 1 — *Agents reported to induce non-specific resistance to infection.*

Bacteria and bacterial products
    Endotoxin (lipopolysaccharide)
    Lipid A
    BCG
    Protodyne
    Staphylococcal ribosomes
    Neo-WSA

Materials of host origin
    Splenic RNA
    Leukocytic endogenous mediator

Synthetic materials
    Poly I - poly C
    Synthetic immunoadjuvants (MDP)
    Levamisole

Miscellaneous
    Vitamin A
    Fever
    Intracellular infections

action of Neo-WSA in the induction of non-specific resistance is different from that produced by bacterial endotoxin.

An ideal agent for potential clinical use as an inducer of non-specific resistance in cancer patients about to undergo chemotherapy should theoretically be non-toxic, non-antigenic, and if possible be active when administered by the oral route. The recent production of a whole family of synthetic immunoadjuvants (see CHEDID, this symposium) which are structural analogs of part of the mycobacterial peptidoglycan monomer offers great promise for study and even potential clinical trials. The analog which has been most widely studied is N-acetyl-muramyl-L-alanine D-isoglutamine (MDP). In an exciting series of studies Chedid and his colleagues [12] have given MDP to mice and subsequently challenged them with *Klebsiella pneumoniae* organisms. These studies demonstrated that MDP and some other petidoglycan monomers induced resistance to a lethal challenge dose of bacteria. Again, these compounds had properties distinctive from endotoxin. For example, MDP could even be administered after the infectious challenge rather than prior to it. Of real potential importance, however, is the fact that MDP was also effective when given by the oral route.

Since it is to be expected that anticancer regimens will continue to put the host at risk and that opportunistic infections will continue to be present, we must explore any possibility of protecting our patients from these risks. With the development of synthetic agents that are non-antigenic and effective in inducing resistance by the oral route, we may assume that we may be near to consideration of use of these agents in patients at risk. However, one must first ascertain that these agents are non-toxic in the human host. If so, then careful clinical testing may be applicable. If not, then other derivatives must be sought which are non-toxic, yet retain the ability to induce non-specific resistance. When that quest is successful, and it will be, then trials in the appropriate human situation should be forthcoming.

[5] *Wolff, Elin* - p. 6

BIBLIOGRAPHY

[1] ROWLEY D., *Stimulation of natural immunity to* Escherichia coli *infections.* « Lancet », *1*, 232 (1955).

[2] BERGER F. M. and FUKUI G. M., *Endotoxin induced resistance to infections and tolerance.* « Proc. Soc. Exp. Biol. Med. », *114*, 780 (1963).

[3] SULTZER B. M., *Endotoxin-induced resistance to a staphylococcal infection: cellular and humoral responses compared in two mouse strains.* « J. Infec. Dis. », *118*, 340 (1968).

[4] KIMBALL H. R., WILLIAMS T. W. and WOLFF S. M., *Effect of bacterial endotoxin on experimental fungal infections.* « J. Immunol. », *100*, 24 (1968).

[5] MACGREGOR R. R., SHEAGREN J. N. and WOLFF S. M., *Endotoxin induced modification of* Plasmodium berghei *infection in mice.* « J. Immunol. », *102*, 131 (1969).

[6] WAGNER R. R., SNYDER R. M., HOOK E. W. and LUTTERLL C. N., *Effect of bacterial endotoxin on resistance of mice to viral encephalitides.* « J. Immunol. », *83*, 87 (1959).

[7] WRIGHT L. J., KIMBALL H. R. and WOLFF S. M., *Alterations in host responses to experimental* Candida albicans *infections by bacterial endotoxin.* « J. Immunol. », *103*, 1276 (1969).

[8] ELIN R. J. and WOLFF S. M., *Effect of endotoxin administration on the growth of* Candida albicans *in sera from various species.* « Can. J. Microbiol. », *19*, 639-641 (1973).

[9] ELIN R. J. and WOLFF S. M., *The role of iron in non-specific resistance to infection induced by endotoxin.* « J. Immunol. », *112*, 737-745 (1974).

[10] ELIN R. J. and WOLFF S. M., *Endotoxin-induced non-specific resistance to infection - a possible mechanism.* In Braun, W. and Ungar, J. (Eds.): « Non-Specific » Factors Influencing Host Resistance. Basel, Switzerland, S. Karger (1973), 371-381.

[11] ELIN R. J., WOLFF S. M. and CHEDID L., *Non-specific resistance to infection induced in mice by a water-soluble adjuvant derived from* Mycobacterium smegmatis. « J. Infec. Dis. », *133*, 500-505 (1966).

[12] CHEDID L., PARANT M., PARANT F., LEFRANCIER P., CHOAY J. and LEDERER E., *Enhancement of non-specific immunity to* Klebsiella pneumoniae *infection by a synthetic immunoadjuvant (N-acetyl muramyl-L-alanine-D-isoglutamine) and several analogs.* « Proc. Natl. Acad. Sci. (USA) », *74*, 2089-2093 (1977).

DISCUSSION

ROSENBERG

Did you say that passage transfer of serum in the endotoxin model was capable of protecting?

WOLFF

Yes.

ROSENBERG

Are you implying that the serum contains some iron-binding protein?

WOLFF

Yes, I am.

ROSENBERG

I see; so you think that just reduction of the circulating serum iron was sufficient to cause protection? That should certainly be easy enough to control; one could use dialized serum and just be sure that dialized serum would accomplish the same thing.

WOLFF

I did not mention all the experiments since these were all old and published. We put animals on iron-deficient diets and challenged them with Candida and the animals were protected. And when we took animals we had given endotoxin to and then gave them iron back, we could completely reverse the protection. I am not saying it is the only cause, but certainly in the Candida model I think it plays a very important role.

NOSSAL

I wonder how you would react to a naive suggestion for a possible mode of action of at least some of these substances. A good few years ago, Dr. D. Metcalf at our Institute showed that one of the signal effects of endotoxin was the stimulation of the production of various colony-stimulating factors which could act not only *in vitro* but also *in vivo* to raise the number of granulocyte-macrophage colony-forming cells in the blood and the spleen. As these infections are largely dealt with by the process of phagocytosis, I wonder whether this stimulation might not be a factor in the protection.

WOLFF

I think that is potentially one of the mechanisms and I think it is not naive, I think it is reasonable.

OETTGEN

Could you explain again the difference in optimal timing between endotoxin and muramyldipeptide?

WOLFF

Muramyldipeptide is effective both in one hour and 24 hours and then loses its effectiveness within a matter of a few days. Endotoxin has the reverse effect — at one hour it is much more likely to produce increased susceptibility but at about 12 to 18 hours it begins to increase resistance, which is maximal at 24 hours in 5 or 6 days and then loses its effect by about the tenth day. So the major difference between the two is that if you give muramyldipeptide in about one hour you can protect the animal, whereas with endotoxin you markedly reduce its chances to survive.

OETTGEN

These are hours prior to infection?

[5] *Wolff, Elin* · p. 10

WOLFF

Prior to infection, that is right. If you give the endotoxin one day after you give the infection, you do not do very much.

CLERICI

Endotoxins are initiating factors for the alternative pathway of complement activation. Is it possible that the mechanism of action of endotoxins has something to do with the alternative pathway of complement activation? This is the first question. My second question is: you ascribe to iron deficiency the protective effect against Candida infection. If this is so, would it not be enough to feed mice on iron deficient diet instead of giving them endotoxins?

WOLFF

First, we had animals on iron deficiency diets and they got iron-deficient, and they were protected. Regarding the first part of your question, it is true that endotoxin does activate the alternative complement pathway and it is true that this is responsible for — for example — Candida phagocitosis. On the other hand, when we give it for 6 days, we have never measured the alternative complement pathway activation. I think, although we have not looked at that, that at six days the alternative complement pathway probably is no longer operative while at that time the animals are still being protected.

WESTPHAL

You certainly know that injections of endotoxin (LPS) in mice, in contrast to rabbit or man, will always cause a fall in body temperature - hypothermia, no fever. In our Institute, Dr. Ernst Th. Rietschel investigated this type of reaction [1]. Repeated injections of LPS in mice induce phases of tolerance (early and late) as well as increased reactivity to the hypothermic effect, depending on the time of challenge (Fig. We 1).

---

[1] GREER G.G. and RIETSCHEL E. Th.: *Lipid A-induced Tolerance and Hyperreactivity to Hypothermia in Mice*. « Infect. Immun. », *19*, 357-67 (1978).

RESPONSE TO DAILY INJECTIONS OF S. minnesota Re LPS

PREPARATION INJECTED (i.v.)	DOSE/MOUSE (µg)	DAY	MAXIMUM HYPOTHERMIC RESPONSE ΔT (°C)
Re LPS	10	0	(29) 2h
Re LPS	10	1	(19) 2h
Re LPS	10	2	(9) 3h
Re LPS	10	3	(19) 3h
Re LPS	10	4	(19) 3h
Re LPS	10	5	(9) 3h
Re LPS	10	6	(12) 3h
Re LPS	10	7	(12) 3h
Re LPS	10	8	(5) 2h

Figure We 1 (from (¹)).
Response to Daily Injections of S.minnesota Re LPS.

So, the whole dynamics of repeated endotoxin application in mice and the changes of their reactivity is different from those in rabbits and man.   Therefore, one must be careful in drawing conclusions with regard to the clinical application of endotoxin in man.

The second point I want to make is this: endotoxin exerts many typical reactions, the basic mechanisms of which may be quite different. Therefore, for a long time many investigators have tried to *partially* modify their original endotoxic preparation in order to reduce (or even eliminate) some unwanted, but retain some desired biological activities. Many efforts have been published to "detoxify" endotoxin in the sense that the acute toxicity of the preparation could selectively be reduced. But if one tests such (by the way: hitherto ill-defined) preparations, practically *all* their biological activities are more or less reduced.   I mentioned the phthalylation of LPS by which the polysaccharide component is being phthalylated.   The final compound is much less toxic compared to the

[5] *Wolff, Elin* - p. 12

original LPS, but is a very good adjuvant. This is interpreted by some workers to mean that the toxic properties were markedly reduced, but the immuno-stimulating activity is retained. On the other hand, phthalylation makes the nearly neutral LPS a *poly-anionic* compound, and it is well known that many poly-acidic macromolecules are good adjuvants. Thus, phthalylated dextran was shown to be an adjuvant (²). Phthalylated LPS or phthalylated de-O-acylated LPS, however, are significantly more active. By conversion of LPS to the poly-phthalyl-LPS, we may thus have introduced new additional structures conferring adjuvanticity. Would you agree?

WOLFF

I agree with that. As regards the first point, I would only say that we have done experiments in rabbits with endotoxin showing at least protection at 24 hours.

CHEDID

Following Dr. McIntire's original publication concerning detoxification of endotoxins by acylation, we also found that phthalylation reduced toxicity very markedly (about 30,000 fold) whereas adjuvant activity was maintained. However, certain other biological effects disappeared, such as non-specific resistance against a *Klebsiella* challenge. Although these results are very encouraging, in agreement with what Dr. Westphal said previously, I believe that the physical change produced by phthalylation is extremely important and that the new compound may no longer be related to the skeleton of lipopolysaccharide. I would like to ask Dr. Wolff to make some further comments on previous studies which were made in his laboratory on the effect of LPS on malaria in humans.

(²) McINTIRE F.C., HARGIE M.P., SCHENCK J.R., FINLEY R.A., SIEWERT H.W., RIETSCHEL E. Th. and ROSENSTREICH D.L.: *Biological Properties of Nontoxic Derivatives of a Lipopolysaccharide from* Escherichia coli K235. « J. Immunol. », *117*, 674-678.

WOLFF

We gave endotoxins to a group of volunteers before they were given malaria, twelve years ago, when malaria was a problem for our Armed Forces, but the doses of endotoxin that we used in human beings, were too small. In the 50's I think Jay Sanford and Maurice Landy gave some of his S. typin endotoxin to some Hodgkins disease patients; the first one they gave it to went into shock, and they stopped at that point saying that cancer patients had an increased sensitivity to endotoxin. I can assure you they do not, because we have given lots of endotoxin to cancer patients without untoward effects.

GUTTERMAN

I would like to make a small comment and ask Dr. Weiss if they have additional information. In a recent trial we carried out on acute leukemia, we added BCG only during remission, but in a subsequent trial we added it during the remission induction period, and in that trial, which was not a randomized trial, we did note a 50% reduction in the incidence of fatal infections which in general are due to gram-negative bacteria. I would like to know if Dr. Weiss knows of any data with MER? Perhaps Dr. Oettgen could also comment on the *Pseudomonas* work at Sloan-Kettering to see if there is any additional data regarding the possible decrease of infections.

WEISS

In answer to Dr. Gutterman's question, the data that I can cite was given me by Dr. Janet Cuttner of Mt. Sinai Hospital in New York a little over a month ago. It deals with a controlled clinical trial of the therapeutic efficacy of the MER tubercle bacillus fraction in Acute Myelocytic Leukemia (AML) patients; I understand that over 800 patients are now included in this cooperative study, which involves more than 30 hospitals. The patients are randomized into several different chemotherapy treatment groups, each one of which is subdivided into groups in which MER is or is not added as an additional therapeutic intervention. Where MER is administered, treatment is effected either both during remission induction and ongoing maintenance chemotherapy, or after onset of remis-

[5] *Wolff, Elin* - p. 14

sion only, as part of the maintenance schedule. This is by far the largest clinical immunotherapy trial based on concurrent, randomized control comparison that has been conducted so far in leukemia, and one of the largest for any neoplastic disease.

The trial is still in progress, and the data that are emerging are still only interim. It does appear already, however, that addition of MER to induction and maintenance chemotherapy is of value. Here, I wish to cite only one of the observations made so far: The incidence of severe infections in patients receiving a second cycle of induction treatment is reduced by nearly half when MER is added to the induction therapy. This result of MER treatment is of importance in its own right, infectious episodes during remission induction representing a major threat to the life of the patient. I believe that Dr. Cuttner will be presenting this information at the forthcoming leukemia meetings in Rome.

One other clinical finding with MER that may be pertinent to this discussion is the following: in another current clinical trial of MER, children with neuroblastoma are being randomized into two treatment groups, both receiving identical chemotherapy and one also receiving periodic injections of MER. At the last meetings, in the spring, of the Cancer Acute Leukemia Group-B, the cooperative clinical trials organizations, Dr. Thomas Necheles of Boston reported that the children given MER responded appreciably better to influenza vaccination than did those in the control arm. Although these observations of a heightened resistance to microbial and viral pathogens in subjects receiving MER are still tentative and incomplete, they are fully in line with a wealth of data from animal experiments which show the pronounced capacity of this agent to bestow heightened resistance against a variety of infectious diseases.

WOLFF

They may have had a higher antibody response, but they did not get infection because there were no controls, there were no infections last year.

DAVIES

The studies on endotoxins have mainly been confined to Enterobacteria of course and carried out by Otto Westphal's group. Now I recall

[5] *Wolff, Elin* - p. 15

that many years back we studied Chromobacteria and the lipid A fraction is rather different because it contains no phosphorous. We used it in the lab for many years as an adjuvant — it is a magnificent adjuvant — unfortunately we never published anything about that or compared it in detail with other adjuvants, but I think it is much less toxic than lipid A from Enterobacteria. It occurs to me that there is a variety of gram-negative organisms which would contain this kind of fraction and it might differ significantly and usefully in the context of the properties we have been discussing.

WESTPHAL

Dr. Rietschel in our Institute performed comparative studies on the structure of the lipid A component in lipopolysaccharides from bacteria of quite remote genera, including your *Chromobacteria*. The LPS from *Salmonella* or *Coli* does not induce cross-tolerance to LPS from *Chromobacterium violaceum* ([3]). Since tolerance to endotoxin is dependent on an immune response to the lipid A component ([4]), one could conceive that the Chromo-Lipid A differs from the widely occurring Salmonella or Coli-Lipid A. In fact, they are chemically different ([5]); (see Figure We 2).

This led us to the idea that patients could be screened for their relative sensitivity to endotoxin (LPS) without, at the same time, inducing tolerogenic effects which would inevitably also change this very reactivity. One could use the *Salmonella*-Lipid A type for screening and the Chromo-Lipid A type for clinical treatment.

([3]) WATSON D. and KIM Y.B.: *Modification of host response to bacterial Endotoxins. I. Specificity of pyrogenic Tolerance and Role of Hypersensitivity in Pyrogenicity, Lethality and Skin Reactivity.* « J. Exp. Med. », 118, 425-46 (1963).

([4]) RIETSCHEL E. Th. and GALANOS C.: *Lipid A Antiserum Mediated Protection against Lipopolysaccharide- and Lipid A-induced Fever and Skin Necrosis.* « Infect. Immun. », 15, 34-49 (1977).

([5]) HASE S. and RIETSCHEL E. Th.: *The Chemical Structure of the Lipid A Component of Lipopolysaccharides from* Chromobacterium violaceum NCTC 9694. « Europ. J. Biochem. », 75, 23-34 (1977).

[5] *Wolff, Elin* - p. 16

Salmonella

Chromobacterium violaceum

Figure We 2: *Chemical Structure of the Lipid A Component of Lipopolysaccharides from* Salmonella *and* Chromobacterium violaceum . ([5]).

DAVIES

Do you find that they differ in their acute toxicity?

WESTPHAL

No, both *Salmonella* and *Chromobacterium* LPS and free Lipid A are of comparable toxicity and pyrogenicity.

[5] *Wolff, Elin* - p. 17

WOLFF

Dr. Oettgen, Dr. Gutterman asked you a question before; I am sorry I did not give you a chance to answer.

OETTGEN

The question was whether the Pseudomonas vaccine altered the frequency or severity of infections in patients with acute myeloblastic leukemia? It did not, including infections with Pseudomonas itself.

WOLFF

That has been the experience at the NIH too, I think, in general.

RAPP

Dr. Ribi at the Rocky Mountain Lab in Montana has been using endotoxins from the so-called RE mutants of Salmonellae in combination with cord factor and mineral oil with some success against the line 10 guinea pig hepatoma. Do you think it might be possible to use such endotoxins in the treatment of human cancer?

WOLFF

I know of no trials.

WESTPHAL

Speaking of acute toxicity of different endotoxic preparations, derived from smooth or rough forms, it matters in what physicochemical state the preparations are tested and compared. Relative water solubility and degree of dispersion plays a significant role. Dr. Chris Galanos in our Institute was the first to point to the importance of the *salt form* of LPS. The lipid A component of LPS from the usual Enterobacteriaceae is a diphospho-ester of a glucosaminyl-β-1.6-glucosamine backbone (see Figure We 2), in other words an acidic compound which — in the bacterial cell wall or in the pure LPS — is neutralized by various naturally occurring kations (Na^+, K^+, Mg^{++}, Ca^{++}, organic bases etc.). By electrodialysis

[5] *Wolff, Elin* - p. 18

Galanos prepared the *pure* acidic form of LPS, which was then neutralized with known kations, such as Na^+, K^+ etc., or organic bases like triethylamine (TEA), to give the various *uniform salt forms* of LPS ([6]). Although the kations in these preparations account for only a few percent of the whole macromolecule, these different salt forms show very different biological activities! Thus, *one and the same* LPS preparation, depending on the kation(s) present, will differ markedly in particle size in water as demonstrated by their sedimentation coefficient ([6]) as well as in toxicity, pyrogenicity, interactivity with complement, etc. ([7, 8]). The pure Ca^{++} or Mg^{++} salts are almost insoluble and of little toxicity, while the TEA salt gives water-clear solutions, even in high concentrations, and is the most active typical endotoxin preparation we have been able to produce. Consequently, as long as LPS preparations are not investigated under such standardized conditions, comparison of biological activities — of any LPS preparations — will not tell us too much. Discrepancies between results of various research groups, dealing with the same bacterial LPS, may partly be explained along these lines.

OETTGEN

I am still intrigued by the protection which serum from endotoxin-treated mice affords against Candida. Is serum from nutritionally iron-deficient animals as protective as serum from endotoxin-injected animals?

WOLFF

I would have to go and look it up — all I can say is that it is significantly protective.

([6]) GALANOS C. and LÜDERITZ O.: *Electrodialysis of Lipopolysaccharides and their Conversion to uniform Salt Forms.* « Europ. J. Biochem. », *54*, 603-10 (1975).

([7]) GALANOS C. and LÜDERITZ O.: *The Role of the Physical State of Lipopolysaccharides in the Interaction with Complement.* « Europ. J. Biochem. », *65*, 403-08 (1976).

([8]) GALANOS C., LÜDERITZ O., RIETSCHEL E. Th. and WESTPHAL O.: *Newer Aspects of the Chemistry and Biology of Bacterial Lipopolysaccharides with Special Reference to their Lipid A Component.* Internat. Rev. Biochem., Biochemistry of Lipids II, Vol. *14*, 239-335. Edit. by T.W. GOODWIN, Univ. Park Press, Baltimore (1977).

SEROLOGIC STUDIES OF MURINE
AND HUMAN SARCOMAS

STEVEN A. ROSENBERG, GEORGE PARKER and WILLIAM P. THORPE

Surgery Branch, National Cancer Institute,
National Institutes of Health
Bethesda - Maryland 20014

INTRODUCTION

The demonstration of tumor antigens on most animal tumors has depended largely on the ability to immunize and subsequently challenge animals with these tumors. The inability to perform these maneuvers in humans has prevented the clear demonstration of tumor antigens on most human solid tumors. In vitro serologic studies provide an opportunity to analyze and dissect tumor antigens in both experimental animals and in humans. In this review, our studies of the serologic analysis of murine sarcoma antigens as well as antigens on human osteogenic sarcomas will be presented.

Serologic studies in the mouse have identified an antigen cross-reactive among tumors as well as an antigen specific for each tumor [1, 2, 3]. Similar antigens have also been identified on human osteogenic sarcomas [4, 5, 6].

METHODS

Murine Tumors. Murine sarcomas were induced in C57BL/6N female mice by the injection of 0.1 ml of 1% 3-methylcholanthrene in sesame oil into the right hind leg. These tumors have been transferred serially in syngeneic mice and have been used in the

6-21st transplant generations. Mice used in these studies were from 8-16 weeks old and were obtained from the Animal Production Unit, Division of Resource Service, National Institutes of Health, Bethesda, Maryland.

Human Tumors. Osteogenic sarcoma tissue was obtained from patients undergoing amputation as part of the treatment for this disease. Normal skin was obtained from these same patients at a site as far from the tumor as possible.

Tissue Culture of Murine and Human Tumors. Murine tumors, normal murine fibroblasts from muscle and lung, human skin, and human osteogenic sarcomas were placed in tissue culture by techniques previously described [1-7]. These cells were grown as monolayer cultures and were serially passaged when confluent in tissue culture. All tissue culture lines were cryopreserved at most passage generations and were used in the first 20 tissue culture passages for the experiments described in this review.

Microcytotoxicity Tests. The microcytotoxicity test we used was adapted from that of BLOOM [8] and has been described in detail previously [7]. In brief, on the day prior to assay, tissue culture tumor cells were harvested from confluent cultures and plated into micro test plates (Falcon 3034, Falcon Plastics, Oxnard, Calif.) so that approximately 100 cells were plated and attached to the surface of each well by the following day. Test sera were added to each well and incubated for two hours at 37°. The plates were then thoroughly washed and rabbit serum complement was added to appropriate wells. Following incubation for an additional one to two hours the plate was again washed. The plates were then fixed and stained and the number of residual cells in each well was counted. All tests were run in sextuplicate. Every plate contained controls consisting of wells incubated with only medium or complement. All serum samples were also tested for lytic activity in the absence of complement.

The % cytotoxicity was calculated as:

$$\frac{\text{Cells in control well} - \text{cells in experimental well}}{\text{Cells in control well}} \times 100$$

Cytotoxicity of 15% or greater in experimental wells was generally statistically significantly different from controls ($p < .05$,

[6] *Rosenberg, Parker, Thorpe* - p. 2

Student's t test) but was tested individually in each experiment with the data from that experiment.

Absorptions. All absorptions were performed in plastic test tubes. An appropriate number of cells was counted and serum added for one hour at 4°C. After one hour, cells were pelleted and the serum was collected. All serum used in these experiments were stored at $-15°$ and thawed immediately prior to use. All sera were heat inactivated at 56° for 30 minutes prior to use.

RESULTS

Murine Sarcomas Contain Unique Tumor Specific Transplantation Antigens [1]. Two separate methylcholanthrene induced murine sarcomas in C57BL/6N female mice were designated MCA-2 and MCA-3. In vivo immunogenicity of these tumors was tested by standard amputation challenge techniques. The tumors were injected in the right hind limb and allowed to grow to a size of 1 cm diameter. The tumor-bearing limb was then amputated and 13 days later the amputated mice were then challenged with the original tumor, as well as a second murine sarcoma. At the same time, control amputated mice were also challenged with each tumor. As can be seen in Table 1, mice were resistant to challenge of 10^5 cells of the previously amputated tumor but not resistant to chal-

TABLE 1 — *Immunogenicity of MCA-2 and MCA-3 tumor in vivo.*

	MCA-2 *	MCA-3 *
	(No. Tumors/Total Number Mice Challenged)	
Untreated Mice	10/10	10/10
MCA-3 Amputated **	10/10	0/10
MCA-2 Amputated	0/10	10/10

* Mice were challenged with 10^5 viable cells.
** 13 days after amputation.

lenge with a different sarcoma. For example, the MCA-2 tumor grew in 10 of 10 control amputated mice as well as in 10 of 10 mice that previously had amputations of a limb bearing the MCA-3 tumor. However, tumor did not grow in any mouse that previously had the MCA-2 tumor. This experiment demonstrated that the MCA-2 and MCA-3 tumors contained individually distinct tumor antigens.

Tumor-bearing Mice Contain Antibodies Cross-reactive between the MCA-2 and MCA-3 Tumors [1]. Using the microcytotoxicity assay, sera from tumor-bearing mice were tested against tissue culture cells of each tumor. As can be seen in Figure 1, serum from a mouse bearing the MCA-3 tumor was capable of lysing cells from both the MCA-2 and MCA-3 tumor. This lytic activity was complement dependent and was present in both tumor-bearing as well as post-amputated mice. Similarly sera from mice bearing the MCA-2 tumor reacted with cells from both the MCA-2 and MCA-3 tumor. Following hyper-immunization of syngeneic animals with

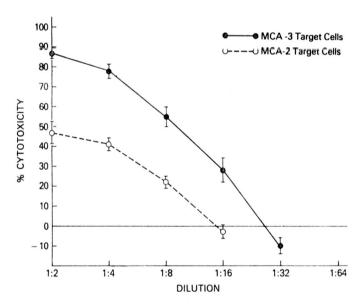

Fig. 1 — Cytotoxicity of serum obtained one day after amputation of MCA-3 tumor tested against MCA-3 and MCA-2 tumor cells.

[6] *Rosenberg, Parker, Thorpe* - p. 4

these tumors, approximately 10-20 fold increase in titres could be obtained.

Absorption with the Opposite Tumor Reveals Antibody Against Unique Tumor-Specific Antigens [1]. Sera from mice either bearing or hyperimmunized to the MCA-3 tumor were absorbed with MCA-2 tumor cells. As a control, these sera were simultaneously absorbed with normal syngeneic splenic lymphocytes as well as with MCA-3 tumor cells. Absorption of these sera with normal splenic lymphocytes did not change reactivity against either the MCA-3 or MCA-2 tumor (Table 2). Absorption of these anti-MCA-2 sera with MCA-3 tumor cells removed all reactivity against both the MCA-3 and MCA-2 tumor. However, absorption of these sera with MCA-2 tumor cells removed all reactivity against the MCA-2 tumor but left persistent reactivity against MCA-3 tumor that could not be further removed despite exhaustive absorptions. This experiment demonstrated that antibodies were present against at least two tumor associated antigens. One antigen cross-reacted between the MCA-2 and MCA-3 tumor and could be absorbed from the serum leaving residual reactivity against the unique tumor-specific antigen.

Cross-reactive Murine Antigen is Present on Fetal Tissue [3]. In an attempt to determine the biologic nature of these serologically detected tumor antigens, sera from mice bearing the MCA-3 tumor were absorbed with third trimester murine fetal tissue. Unabsorbed as well as serially absorbed sera were then tested against both the MCA-2 and MCA-3 tumor. As can be seen in Figure 2, absorption of the MCA-3 tumor-bearing serum with murine fetal tissue completely removed the reactivity against the MCA-2 tumor but did not alter reactivity against the MCA-3 tumor. Similarly, absorption of sera hyperimmune to the MCA-3 tumor with murine fetal tissue completely removed reactivity against the MCA-2 tumor but left residual reactivity against the MCA-3 tumor that could not be removed despite exhaustive absorptions. These experiments demonstrated that the serologically detected cross-reactive tumor antigen is present on fetal tissue. The unique tumor-specific antigen does not appear to be expressed on the third trimester mouse fetus.

[6] *Rosenberg, Parker, Thorpe* - p. 5

7

TABLE 2 — Absorptions of MCA-3HI[d] and MCA-3-28[e] sera.

Number of Absorptions	MCA-3HI Absorbed with						MCA-3-28 Absorbed with			
	MCA-3 Cells		MCA-2 Cells (Tested Against)		Splenic Lymphocytes		MCA-2 Cells (Tested Against)		Splenic Lymphocytes	
	MCA-3	MCA-2	MCA-3	MCA-2	MCA-3	MCA-2	MCA-2	MCA-3	MCA-2	MCA-3
0[a]	320[b]	80	320	80	320	80	8	16	8	16
1	80	80	80	30	160	60	2	16	8	16
2	40	40	40	0	320	80	2	16	8	16
3	60	15	60	0	320	80	0	16	8	16
4	20	30	60	0	320	160				
5	0	0								

[a] Unabsorbed sera.
[b] All data are reciprocals of 50% cytotoxic titers.
[c] Absorptions were performed with $1\text{-}3\times10^7$ viable tumor cells or $1\cdot4\times10^8$ viable splenic lymphocytes per ml serum.
[d] Sera from mice hyperimmunized to MCA-3.
[e] Sera from tumor bearing mice 28 days after tumor inoculation.

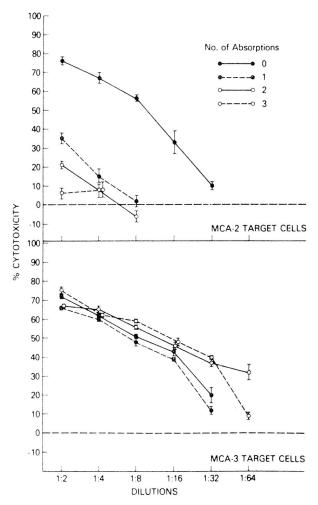

FIG. 2 — Effect of sequential absorptions with embryo cells on the cytotoxicity of MCA-3 tumor-bearer serum toward MCA-2 and MCA-3 cells.

Normal Mouse Cells in Tissue Culture also Express the Tumor Associated Fetal Antigen [2]. During the course of the above experiments normal sera as well as sera from tumor-bearing mice were tested for reactivity against normal murine cells in tissue culture. Surprisingly (Fig. 3), tumor-bearing sera, but not normal

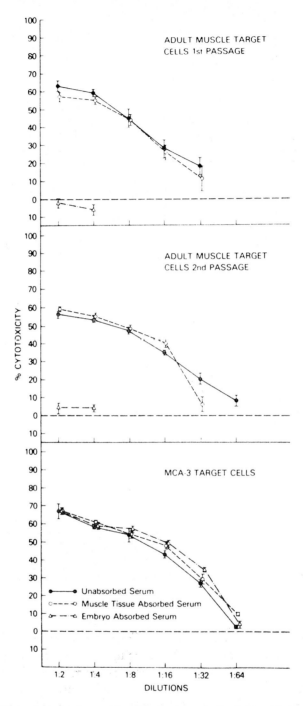

FIG. 3 — Effect of absorptions with adult murine muscle tissue and murine embryo cells on the cytotoxicity of MCA-3 tumor bearer serum toward normal adult muscle tissue culture cells in the first and second in vitro passage and MCA-3 tumor tissue culture cells in the 13th in vitro passage. Absorptions were performed with 2.9×10^8 viable 12- to 14-day-old embryo cells or an equal volume of adult muscle tissue per ml of serum.

sera, were capable of lysing murine muscle fibroblast cells in tissue culture. The titer of this reactivity was approximately the same as that directed against the tumor cells in tissue culture. Absorption with third trimester mouse fetus was capable of removing all reactivity against the normal muscle fibroblast cells in tissue culture. Though no loss of reactivity was seen against the specific MCA-3 tumor target cell (Fig. 3), absorption with adult muscle tissue was not capable of removing reactivity against the muscle cells grown in tissue culture. This experiment demonstrates that normal muscle fibroblasts in tissue culture contain fetal antigens that are reactive with sera from tumor-bearing mice. This fetal antigen on normal cells in tissue culture appears to be the same as that on the murine tumor in vivo since absorption with fresh mouse tumor is also capable of removing reactivity from tumor-bearing sera against normal adult muscle cells in tissue culture.

Normal Human Sera Contains Antibodies Reactive with Normal and Sarcoma Cells in Tissue Culture [4]. At the outset of our experiments with human sera and normal and malignant human tissue culture lines, we observed that sera from sarcoma patients was capable of lysing autologous skin fibroblasts in tissue culture. No difference was seen in the ability of these sera to lyse normal and sarcoma cells. We thus tested 155 normal human sera for reactivity against normal cells in tissue culture. As is seen in Table 3, the great majority of human sera contain complement dependent reactivity against normal cells in tissue culture. Similar reactivity is seen against sarcoma cells in culture. The presence of these antibodies against neoantigens expressed on normal and sarcoma cells in tissue culture obscures the presence of any tumor-specific reactivity present on tissue culture cells from sarcomas.

Normal Human Cells in Tissue Culture Express Fetal Antigens [5]. Normal human sera reactive against normal and sarcoma cells in culture was absorbed with first trimester human fetal tissue obtained from therapeutic absorptions. As can be seen in Figure 4, absorption with human fetal tissue completely removed reactivity from normal sera directed against normal cells in culture. Absorption with adult lymphocytes or maternal decidual tissue was not capable on removing this reactivity. Similarly, (data not shown) absorption with adult skin and muscle also could not remove this

[6] *Rosenberg, Parker, Thorpe* - p. 9

TABLE 3 — *Lysis of normal skin in tissue culture by normal human sera.*[a]

Patient Age, Yr.	No. of sera	Lysis at serum dilution of:			
		1:1		1:2	
		No. Positive [b]	% Positive	No. Positive	% Positive
6-10	16	14	88	9	56
11-20	23	22	96	8	35
21-30	37	32	86	5	14
31-40	29	14	48	6	21
41-50	32	11	33	4	13
51-60	18	10	56	4	22
Total	155	103	66	36	23

[a] Normal skin from a patient with osteogenic sarcoma was used.
[b] Greater than 50% lysis. All sera were simultaneously tested in the absence of complement and only one exhibited significant lysis.

reactivity. Similarly, fetal absorption removed reactivity from both normal and sarcoma patient sera directed against normal cells in tissue culture. It thus appears that normal human cells in culture express a fetal antigen against which many humans have naturally occurring circulating antibodies.

Identification of a Sarcoma-Specific Antigen in a Patient with Osteogenic Sarcoma [6]. As was demonstrated in the previous section, absorption with fetal tissue is capable of removing reactivity from normal serum directed against both normal and sarcoma cells. Similar absorption of serum from a sarcoma patient is shown in Figure 5. As can be seen, absorption of serum from a patient, J. B., with fetal cells removed all reactivity against autologous normal cells in culture. Despite exhaustive absorption, however, residual reactivity against autologous sarcoma cells in culture remained. This experiment was repeated many times and the same result obtained. Sera from patient J. B. is capable of recognizing

[6] *Rosenberg, Parker, Thorpe* - p. 10

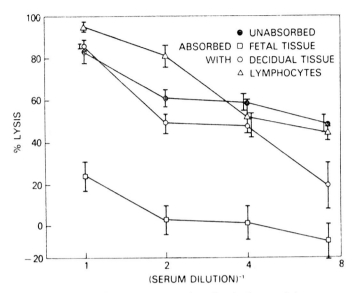

FIG. 4 — Comparison of the cytotoxicity of unabsorbed normal human serum with serum individually absorbed with 6.6×10^7 fresh first trimester fetal tissue cells, adult decidual tissue cells or adult lymphocytes per 0.5 ml of individual serum. The target cells in each case were normal human skin cells in tissue culture.

an antigen present on J. B. sarcoma cells but not J. B. normal cells in culture. A variety of normal sera have been studied and none have contained this reactivity. A summary of the results of the absorption of a normal sera and J. B. sera titred against J. B. normal and sarcoma cells in culture is presented in Figure 6.

Similar studies in four additional patients have revealed an antibody reactive with autologous sarcoma cells but not autologous normal cells in one patient and not in three other patients.

DISCUSSION

Many published reports have described serologic reactivity in cancer patients that have been attributed to tumor-specific reactivity [9-23]. Some of these reports have described antibodies widely cross-reactive among tumors of similar histology. The pres-

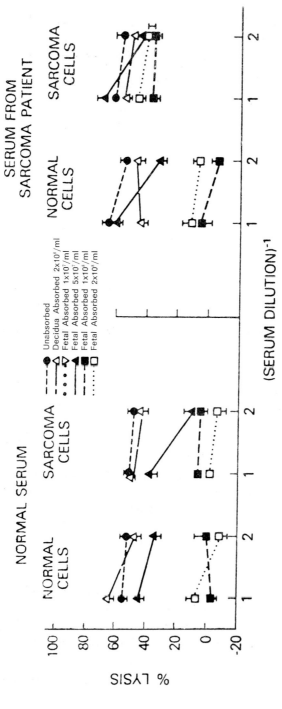

Fig. 5 — Reactivity of serum from a sarcoma-bearing patient (J.B.) with autologous normal and sarcoma cells in tissue culture. Serum from J.B. and a normal serum from a patient with no history of cancer were absorbed with fresh human fetal cells ranging from 1×10^7 per ml to 2×10^8 per ml and with adult maternal decidual cells at 2×10^8 per ml of serum. Absorptions were performed simultaneoulsy at 4°C for one hour. Absorption with adult maternal decidual cells did not remove reactivity from either normal serum or serum from a sarcoma-bearing patient against either normal or sarcoma cells in tissue culture. Absorption with fetal cells removed reactivity from a normal serum against both allogeneic normal and sarcoma cells in tissue culture and serum from a sarcoma-bearing patient against normal autologous cells in culture but failed to remove reactivity from this serum against autologous sarcoma cells in culture.

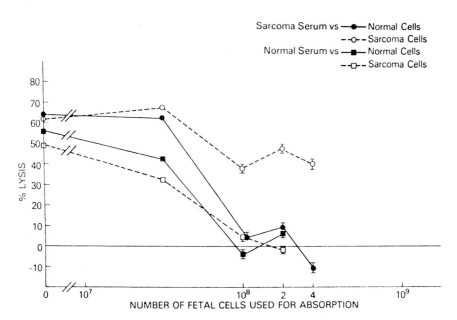

FIG. 6 — Detection of sarcoma-specific antigen. Data in this figure are from an experiment performed identically to that in Figure 5 except that further absorption of the serum from J. B. was performed. Even if 4×10^8 cells/ml were used — 4 times that required for complete removal of reactivity of that serum against autologous normal skin cells in tissue culture — reactivity against only autologous sarcoma cells in tissue culture remained. All reactivity from a normal serum against either a normal or sarcoma cells in tissue culture was removed at levels of 10^8 cells/ml or greater.

ence of anti-tumor antibodies in relatives or close acquaintances of cancer patients has also been reported. Recent information concerning the expression of neoantigens by cells in tissue culture [4] as well as the recognition of the possibility that tissue cultured cells may express a variety of environmental factors such as heterologous serum components [24], infecting viruses, etc. has led to a re-evaluation of previous serologic studies.

Our serologic studies in a murine sarcoma system [1-3] have parallelled our serologic studies in the human [4-6]. In the mouse sarcoma system both cross-reactive and tumor-specific antigens have been identified. The cross-reactive antigen is expressed on third trimester mouse fetal tissue, and only by removing reactivity against it by absorption with fetal tissue can the unique tumor antigen be identified. Of interest was the finding that serum from tumor-bearing mice was reactive with normal mouse cells in culture. This reactivity was also due to reaction with fetal antigen and could be completely removed by fetal absorption without affecting the reactivity to the tumor-specific murine antigen.

Our attempts to identify human sarcoma antigens were originally confounded by the presence in most normal humans of natural antibodies directed against neoantigens expressed on normal cells in tissue culture. Absorption of these normal sera with first trimester human fetal tissue have helped identify this neoantigen in tissue culture as a fetal antigen. Absorption of normal sera as well as sera from sarcoma patients with fetal tissue completely removed this reactivity against normal cells. It was then possible to identify an antibody in the serum of a sarcoma patient, J. B., that was reactive against autologous sarcoma cells but not with autologous normal cells.

These studies represent only the beginning of an attempt to serologically analyze the tumor antigens of human osteogenic sarcoma. The recognition that natural antibodies exist to neoantigens present on tissue culture cells has led to the development of techniques to avoid confusing such reactivity with tumor-specific reactivity. Studies of additional patients as well as possible cross-reactivities between these patients are in progress.

[6] *Rosenberg, Parker, Thorpe* - p. 14

REFERENCES

[1] PARKER G.A. and ROSENBERG S.A., *Serologic identification of multiple tumor-associated antigens on murine sarcomas.* « J. Natl. Cancer Inst. », in press.

[2] PARKER G.A., HYATT C. and ROSENBERG S.A., *Normal adult murine cells in tissue culture express fetal antigens.* « Transplantation », *23*, 161-163 (1977).

[3] PARKER G.A. and ROSENBERG S.A., *Cross-reacting antigens in chemically induced sarcomas are fetal determinants.* « Jour. Immun. », *118*, 1590-1594 (1977).

[4] ROSENBERG S.A., *Lysis of human normal and sarcoma cells in tissue culture by normal human serum: Implications for experiments in human tumor immunology.* « J. Natl. Cancer Inst. », *58*, 1233-1238 (1977).

[5] THORPE W.P., PARKER G.A. and ROSENBERG S.A., *Expression of fetal antigens by normal human skin cells grown in tissue culture.* « Jour. Immun. », *119*, 818-823 (1977).

[6] THORPE W.P. and ROSENBERG S.A., *Serologic analysis of human tumor antigens. I. Identification of a tumor-specific antigen in human osteogenic sarcoma.* « Jour Natl. Cancer Inst. », May, 1979.

[7] ROSENBERG S.A., SCHARZ S., ANDING H., HYATT C. and WILLIAMS G.M., *Comparison of multiple assays for detecting human antibodies directed against surface antigens on normal and malignant human tissue culture cells.* « Jour. Immunol. Meth. », *17*, 225-239 (1977).

[8] BLOOM E.T., *Quantitative detection of cytotoxic antibodies against tumor-specific antigens of murine sarcomas induced by 3-methylcholanthrene.* « J. Natl. Cancer Inst. », *45*, 443-453 (1970).

[9] BALDWIN R.W., EMBLETON M.J. and ROBINS R.A., *Cellular and humoral immunity to rat hepatoma-specific antigens correlated with tumour status.* « Int. J. Cancer », *11*, 1-10 (1973).

[10] MORTON D.L., MALMGREN R.A., *Human osteosarcomas: Immunologic evidence suggesting an associated infectious agent.* « Science », *162*, 1279-1281 (1968).

[11] WOOD W.C., MORTON D.L., *Microcytotoxicity test: Detection in sarcoma patients of antibody cytotoxic to human sarcoma cells.* « Science », *170*, 1318-1320 (1970).

[12] WOOD W.C. and MORTON D.L., *Host immune response to a common cell-surface antigen in human sarcomas: Detection by cytotoxicity tests.* « N. Engl. J. Med. », *284*, 569-572 (1971).

[13] EILBER F.R., MORTON D.L., *Demonstration in sarcoma patients of anti-tumour antibodies which fix only human complement.* « Nature », *225*, 1137-1138 (1970).

[14] EILBER F.R., *Sarcoma-specific antigens: Detection by complement fixation with serum from sarcoma patients.* « J. Natl. Cancer Inst. », *44*, 651-656 (1970).

[15] GIRALDO G., BETH E. and HIRSHAUT Y., *Human sarcomas in culture: Foci of altered cells and a common antigen: Induction of foci and antigen in human fibroblast cultures by filtrates.* « J. Exp. Med. », *133*, 454-478 (1971).

[16] PRIORI E.S. and WILBUR D.L. Jr., *Immunofluorescence tests on sera of patients with osteogenic sarcoma.* « J. Natl. Cancer Inst. », *46*, 1299-1308 (1971).

[17] BLOOM E.T., *Further definition by cytotoxicity tests of cell surface antigens of human sarcomas in culture.* « Cancer Res. », *32*, 960-967 (1972).

[18] MOORE M., WITHEROW P.H., PRICE C.H., *et al.*, *Detection by immunofluorescence of intracytoplasmic antigens in cell lines derived from human sarcomas.* « Int. J. Cancer », *12*, 428-437 (1973).

[19] MOORE M. and HUGHES L.A., *Circulating antibodies in human connective tissue malignancy.* « Br. J. Cancer », *28*, 175-184 (1973).

[20] MUKHERJI B. and HIRSHAUT Y., *Evidence for fetal antigen in human sarcoma* « Science », *181*, 440-442 (1973).

[21] HIRSHAUT Y., PEI D.T., MARCOVE R.C., *et al.*, *Seroepidemiology of human sarcoma antigen* (S_1). « N. Engl. J. Med. », *291*, 1103-1107 (1974).

[22] BYERS V.S., LEVIN A.S., JOHNSTON J.O., *et al.*, *Quantitative immunofluorescence studies of the tumor antigen-bearing cell in giant cell tumor of bone and osteogenic sarcoma.* « Cancer Res. », *35*, 2520-2531 (1976).

[23] BURK K.H., DREWINKO B., LIGHTIGER B., *et al.*, *Cell cycle dependency of human sarcoma-associated tumor antigen expression.* « Cancer Res. », *36*, 1278-1283 (1976).

[24] IRIE R.F., IRIE K. and MORTON D.L., *Natural antibody in human serum to a neoantigen in human cultured cells grown in fetal bovine serum.* « J. Natl. Cancer Inst. », *52*, 1051-1057 (1974).

DISCUSSION

G. KLEIN

Concerning the human system, I was wondering, did you test any lymphoid lines? Do they also express this fetal antigen?

ROSENBERG

We are testing the RAJI lymphoid line but have no results yet. It would be very nice to have a ready source of large amounts of tissue-cultured cells.

G. KLEIN

We have always been given to understand by Coggin and Anderson that the age of the fetus was extremely critical for the expression of fetal antigens. Did you find a similar age dependence in your system?

ROSENBERG

In the mouse, only last trimester fetuses appear to express this reactivity. In the human, as you can well imagine, last trimester human tissue is very difficult to obtain, and it appears that at least very large numbers of first trimester human fetal tissue work.

SELA

You state that normal sera do contain antibodies to these fetal antigens, but that the fetal antigens are expressed only on tissue cultured cells but not on fresh adult tissue. In other words, there must be some kind of regulation which prevents the antigens from being reflected on normal cells. Is it possible that the presence of this immune reactivity against such fetal antigens plays a role in the immunological surveillance? and that such antigens would be present maybe even in an adult fresh tissue on cancerous cells but not on normal cells, and that this is a way of surveillance?

ROSENBERG

I think that is an excellent point. I did not have time to present the data today but in fact, as in the mouse, in the human the only adult tissue that is capable of removing this reactivity from normal sera against normal tissue cultured cells is tumor tissue. We have looked primarily at sarcomas and all eight sarcomas that we have used for absorption are capable of removing this reactivity. So this fetal antigen, whatever it is, that is expressed on normal human cells in culture is also expressed on human sarcomas. We have also looked at human melanomas, and only about half of human melanomas that we have looked at are capable of removing this reactivity. Whether or not that antigen might be involved in surveillance with these antibodies I think is an intriguing idea. We do not have any direct evidence that it is.

NOSSAL

I also want to say how much I enjoyed the talk, presented with such great clarity, and I hope that it is introducing a note of excellence into what has been a controversial field. Because the results are so important I wanted to ask a few technical questions. First of all, how solid are the controls which speak against fetal calf serum antigens? When we had occasion to reinvestigate the phenomenon of autoreactivity in mouse spleen cell cultures, we reached the conclusion that the alleged auto-reactivity was all due to the absorption of fetal calf serum antigens to cultured mouse cells, and in fact the only satisfactory way to beat that criticism is to grow your cells in horse serum, or in albumin, or in some other protein source. Have you any control of that nature? — that would be my first question.

ROSENBERG

Yes, we have done exactly what you suggest; it was published in

[6] *Rosenberg, Parker, Thorpe* - p. 18

the JNCI about four months ago. If one grows these identical lines in human AB serum, identical results are obtained: that is, one still sees the reactivity of these natural antibodies. This is probably fairly conclusive that we are not dealing with fetal calf serum determinants. Secondly, the fetal tissue used for absorption has never been in tissue culture, nor has it ever been in contact with fetal calf serum.

NOSSAL

I think that is a very satisfactory explanation. My second question relates to the residual activity after the fetal absorptions. When one looks at your graphs very carefully, one notes that 100 cells have been used in cytotoxicity, and undiluted serum is added to achieve a final concentration of one in ten. You showed us 37% residual cytotoxicity. Now am I to take it then that in the vast bulk of the studies where specific antibodies are being claimed an investigator is comparing, let us say, 95 viable cells found in the bottom of the dish (that will be the control) with presumably 5% non-specific lysis with something like 70 or 65 viable cells left? It would appear to me that possibility of observer error is still considerable with such a marginal assay. In particular I would like to ask: have you any evidence that the lytic activity observed is in fact an antibody other than the fact that it only works with autologous sarcoma? Has any attempt been made to remove immunoglobulin and remove the activity? or any attempt to purify immunoglobulin and retain the activity? and have extensive attempts been made to eliminate any last vestige of observer error in such a delicate titration?

ROSENBERG

I think that is a good point and we have addressed ourselves to it in great detail, because in virtually all studies in tumor immunology and especially those in human tumor immunology, it is the lack of good assays that has prevented progress. We explored a variety of other kinds of assays that might be more objective and less subject to observer error than the counting assay itself — and they just were not sensitive enough in our hands to detect any of these antibodies. The studies are all blinded, as I have mentioned and run in sextuplicate; the investigator does not know the serum being used, and, because the lines look virtually identical, would

[6] *Rosenberg, Parker, Thorpe* - p. 19

not know whether the line that the serum is being tested against represents the sarcoma or the normal skin. And so, to the extent that it can be blinded, it has been, and the results I have shown have been obtained.

WEISS

One brief comment, and one brief question.

With regard to the observation of antibodies in normal sera against « fetal » antigens (and it must be emphasized that such antigens may continue to be expressed throughout life on some cells, perhaps on certain stem or precursor cells!), the interesting experiments of Triplett in the early 1960's should be noted (Triplett, E.L., J. Immunol. *89*: 505-510, 1962). This investigator found that the adult frog is immunologically capable against antigens which characterize some of his tadpole-stage tissues. The ability of adult organisms to react against antigens which appear in appreciable amounts only in early stages of ontogeny and then either eclipse totally or remain expressed only in very limited amounts and in a very restricted range of cells should not be surprising; certainly, the termination of a state of specific immunological unresponsiveness some time after disappearance of the inducing antigen, or after its diminution to very low concentrations, is not an unexpected occurrence.

My question is: what is known of any cross-reactivity of fetal antigens between species, i.e., across species barriers? Would antigenic markers distinguishing a certain tissue at a certain stage of embryonic or neonatal development be cross reactive over a spectrum of different species?

ROSENBERG

We have not looked. All of the fetal absorptions that we have done have been within the species of origin of the tumor, but I think that is a very reasonable thing to attempt. I should mention that this phenomenon of expression of fetal antigens that are not expressed on adult tissues does have precedent in a variety of other systems; for example, there are fetal hemoglobins that are expressed in the fetus which early after birth slowly disappear and give way to an adult form of hemoglobin, which is in fact re-expressed in some pathologic conditions in the adult.

[6] *Rosenberg, Parker, Thorpe* - p. 20

OETTGEN

I would like to add my compliments to what others have already said. I would also like to comment briefly on the study of malignant melanoma which our serology group under Lloyd Old's leadership has conducted over the last several years. We have come to believe that work which is based on serological reactions with allogeneic human cancer cells, with the exception of the Burkitt system, has been entirely unrewarding. The usual finding has been that sera from patients with a given cancer react more frequently with target cells derived from that type of cancer than serum from other individuals, but critical analysis of the specificity of these reactions has usually led nowhere. This is why we started several years ago to restrict our serological analysis of malignant melanoma to autologous reactions. We used only established cell lines as target cells so that the reproducibility of observed reactions could be tested, and patients could be followed over a long period of time. For analysis of specificity, extensive use was made of absorption tests. The two assay techniques that we have used most frequently are immune adherence and mixed hemadsorption. With these two methods we have been able to detect antibody in the serum of some 50% of the patients tested in autologous serum-target cell combinations. High-titered positive sera were subjected to extensive absorption analysis. So far, we have defined three types of melanoma antigens: (1) individually specific antigens, (2) shared antigens which are present on some but not all melanoma cells and on no other cell tested, and (3) antigens with a rather wide distribution including autologous melanoma cells, allogeneic melanoma cells and other tissue, and even xenogeneic tissue. These systems of antigens could not have been detected reliably had we used only autologous lymphocytes for absorption as is frequently done — or if we had relied on direct tests rather than absorption. One question I have for Dr. Rosenberg concerns the work in the mouse. The cross-reacting antibody, I believe, was obtained from hyperimmunized mice. Have you also tested transplantation resistance in hyperimmunized mice, or were these mice immunized much less vigorously than the mice from which the antibody was obtained?

ROSENBERG

Studies with the cross-reactive antibody and the absorption studies

[6] *Rosenberg, Parker, Thorpe* - p. 21

8

give the same results in a tumor-bearing serum as well as in a hyperim-munization serum. I might add, incidentally, and I am very glad you mentioned your very important work, that one of the things I have not done is review the other serologic work which has been done in this field, which is quite extensive, and in fact we have many other pioneers of this work right in this room. Dr. George Klein performed pioneering work with serologic analysis of Burkitt lymphoma antigens. Analysis of fetal antigens in the rat have been described very elegantly by Dr. Baldwin.

DAVIES

We have a phenomenon in mice, which is a synergism between drugs and antibodies; several clinical pilot studies are now under way to see if the phenomenon also exists in man. The sera are prepared individually against each patient's tumor. Especially we have studied post lung-resection bronchial carcinoma. The absorption was mostly done with spleen. That is rather difficult logistically and we transferred to placenta, which is more satisfactory. I am pleased to hear your absorption results. We have not absorbed with fetal tissue. We do not have as good a serological picture as you have and we depend largely on immuno-fluore-scence. By this means we can test each patient's goat antiserum against his own tumor. There is a degree of cross-reactivity, something like 70%, with other patients' antisera. While this trial is on the basis of an indi-vidual serum for each patient raised against his own tumor, and because of the cross-reactivity we see by fluorescence, I am under pressure to use a pool of antisera; however we cannot be sure that the fluorescence shows the relevant antigen. I have this question: have you any immuno-fluorescence data that reflects what you describe, which would pick up the cross-reactive antigen or distinguish it from the specific antigen?

ROSENBERG

We did not use fluorescence tests. Perhaps Dr. Klein might want to comment on that.

G. KLEIN

I am afraid I cannot comment on this since we have not studied

[6] *Rosenberg, Parker, Thorpe* - p. 22

this type of system. However, may I ask another question? One of the most interesting claims in the early work of Morton concerning the serology of human osteosarcoma concerned the relatives of sarcoma patients. It was claimed that the sera of the relatives gave frequently positive reactions, in contrast to normal donors. Now, with your improved distinction of the fetal and sarcoma associated antigens, can you confirm that finding?

ROSENBERG

There is a certain perversity of nature here, that probably gave rise to the results that he obtained. He did not check normal sera very extensively. When he did check normal serum, my guess is they were probably in adults, and adults tend to have a lower incidence of this natural reactivity than is present in younger people. Sarcomas tend to occur in younger people and if one therefore looked in the sera of sarcoma patients that tended to be younger, one would indeed find a much higher incidence of this antibody than in a comparable control population that was older, even though this antibody was due not to the tumor antigen but to the cross-reactive fetal antigen. Now, again, as he looked at relatives of these patients, my suspicion is that he did detect this reactivity in the sera of relatives because he was looking at this natural antibody that is present in many people. Now, we have not yet taken positive sera from relatives and performed the fetal absorption to see whether or not any residual reactivity is left in their serum. That would be quite interesting to do, although in every normal serum that we have looked at we have been able to completely remove that reactivity with fetal absorption. It is possible that sera of relatives will not give that result.

BALDWIN

I would just like to take up the point that I think Herb Oettgen was raising. I think the implication from his comments was: can you manipulate the response to fetal antigens in rejection response? Following our work on demonstrating fetal antigen on chemically induced tumors, we have tried heroically to use these fetal antigens in immune rejection. We have tried by immunizing both with fetal extracts and with intact fetal cells, by multiparity, and we have tried challenging to doses of cells given subcutaneously interperitoneally, interpleurally. In none of those situations can we really demonstrate the tumor rejection response, except in one situation, i.e. when we do the tumor cell challenge by giving tumor cells intravenously and animals are presensitized to fetal antigens. The question of course now is: what mediates the rejection? And that is the difficulty at the moment. In none of those systems, where you can get immunity to challenging tumor cells, can we demonstrate immunity to the tumor at another site; and that worriers me.

ROSENBERG

In our studies one does not see any protection due to these fetal antigens.

BALDWIN

In that respect I wanted to ask: have you actually started to see whether you can demonstrate an organ specific fetal reactivity? I mean certainly in the rat adenocarcinomas we can demonstrate a fetal antigen which shows organ specificity which would then match with the type of responses one sees to human breast cancer. I think one has got now to look into the specificities of these fetal antigens.

ROSENBERG

We are really just beginning the cell-mediated immune studies now.

WOLFF

Steve, I was just curious — on the slide where you showed the eight patients with the lysis-free in post-op, one patient JA was clearly different from all the rest. Is there anything about that patient?

ROSENBERG

We occasionally run into a patient that does not have reactivity against sarcoma or even normal cells in culture. That particular patient had a fairly extensive local problem but I cannot think of anything unusual

[6] *Rosenberg, Parker, Thorpe* - p. 24

about him. It will of course now be interesting to follow sera sequentially through the course of patients to see whether or not the specific antibody appears or disappears as a reflection of presence of tumor, but we have not done that yet.

WESTPHAL

I refer to the same slide. You remember that Roy WALFORD, based his immunologic theory of aging ([1]) on the appearance of auto-antibodies in adult life. Such antibodies against various organs are increasing with age; but the trend of antibodies which you described seems to be inverse. Did I understand this correctly? (ROSENBERG: that is correct). And my second point: are fetal antigenic structures not really disappearing, but rather becoming cryptic during growth? So they are still there and if they would be uncovered, for example by enzymic bloc in biosynthesis, they could come immunologically into play. A model of such kind is George F. Springer's finding about the disappearance of M and N blood group specificity on the surface of human mamma carcinoma cells and the appearance of the (normally cryptic) T-antigen structure ([2, 3]). What is your aspect about that?

ROSENBERG

That is entirely possible — we could be seeing genetic derepression and expression of a new protein, or we could be seeing the unmasking in the tumor system of a protein that is always present.

([1]) WALFORD R. L., *Auto-Immunity and Aging*. « J. Gerontology », 17, 281-85 1962). - WALFORD R. L., *The Immunologic Theory of Aging*. E. Munksgaard, Copenhagen 1965.

([2]) SPRINGER G. F., DESAI P. R., and SCALON E. F., *Blood Group MN Precursors as Human Breast Cancer-Associated Antigens and « Naturally » Occurring Human Cytotoxins Against them*. In Cellular Membranes and Tumor Cell Behavior. The William and Wilkins Comp. (1975).

([3]) SPRINGER G. F., DESAI P. R., YANG R. J., SCHACHTER H. and NARA SIMHAN S., *Interrelations of Blood Group M and Precursor Specificities and Their Significance in Human Carcinoma*. In Human Blood Groups, 5th Convocation Immunol., Buffalo, N. Y. 1976, pg. 179-87 (1977). Karger, Basle.

RAPP

Steve, how do you rule out the possibility that your sarcoma specific reactivity is due to auto-immune reactivity? You may be detecting antigens unique to each person.

ROSENBERG

What I have done really is bring you up to the last month or so of the work we are doing, and this is clearly in progress. I think it will be crucial to show that the residual reactivity that is left following all of the fetal absorptions is then capable of being removed by that same patient's fresh tumor. We have not yet done that. All we can say is that when we do the absorptions with fetal tissue, we end up with a reactivity against that autologous sarcoma that is not present against many other sarcomas.

G. KLEIN

Another question: do you have any data on successful surgical extirpation or chemotherapeutic management of osteogenic sarcoma? And what happens to the tumor specific antibodies in those patients?

ROSENBERG

I think we have the sequential sera at hand from all these patients to answer the question, but we have not done it.

CLERICI

I was not surprised that normal and tumor cells in tissue cultures express fetal antigens which cross react with fetal antigens in tumors, since the dedifferentiation of cells in tissue cultures is a *sine qua non* condition for their continuous growth, but I am wondering about the nature of fetal antigens in your tumors. In other words, I did not hear any comment on the viral situation of the MCA tumors that you have used. Are you sure that they were virus-free? Otherwise, I believe that it is possible that they were contaminated and, as is well known, a viral contamination *in vivo* and in tissue cultures may bring about the expression of fetal antigens.

[6] *Rosenberg, Parker, Thorpe* - p. 26

ROSENBERG

I think that is a good point. We have not tested these tumors for the presence of murine viruses — they might well contain them. They are all grown in tissue culture in the same incubators and the animals are housed together and so certainly anything that one has the others have. We can therefore say that it is perhaps possible that the cross-reactive reactivity is on the basis of some infectious particle — that is conceivable. I think it unlikely, however, that the specific reactivity is on that basis since we have identical reactivity just with autologous and not with other cross-reactive tumors, and they must all be contaminated with the same materials.

EFFECTS OF ENDOTOXIN
AND ENDOTOXIN-INDUCED MEDIATORS
ON CANCER AND ON THE IMMUNE SYSTEM

HERBERT F. OETTGEN, MICHAEL K. HOFFMANN, BAYARD D. CLARKSON
and LLOYD J. OLD

Memorial Sloan-Kettering Cancer Center
1275 York Avenue, New York, N.Y. 10021

One of the most striking phenomena of tumor biology is the hemorrhagic necrosis induced in certain experimental tumors by gram negative bacteria or by endotoxin (lipopolysaccharide, LPS) derived from their cell wall [1-5]. Within a few hours of intravenous LPS injection the subcutaneous tumor begins to show progressive darkening in color indicative of tumor cell death and hemorrhage, leading in many instances to complete tumor regression (figure 1). This reaction has long been viewed as the experimental counterpart of Coley's clinical observations of tumor regression in human patients following acute bacterial infection or administration of mixed bacterial vaccines [6].

Although extensively investigated over the past 40 years, the way LPS causes tumor destruction is not known. Direct action is ruled out by the fact that endotoxin lacks toxicity for tumor cells *in vitro*. A favored mechanism following ALGIRE's work in 1952 [7] is that endotoxin-induced systemic hypotension leads to collapse of the tumor vasculature with resulting tumor cell anoxia and death. In contrast to this view, the work of our group has led

Supported by grants from the National Cancer Institute - CA 08748, CA 17673 and CA 05826 - and the American Cancer Society - IM 82 and IM 87.

[7] *Oettgen, Hoffmann, Clarkson, Old* - p. 1

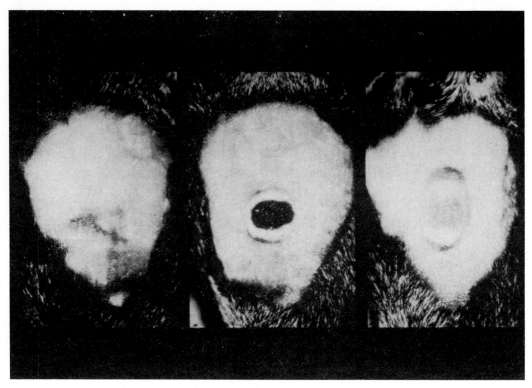

Fig. 1 — The classic effect of LPS on a mouse tumor. *a*) Transplanted BALB/c sarcoma Meth A growing in an untreated (BALB/c × C57BL/6)F₁ mouse. *b*) The same sarcoma showing extensive hemorrhagic necrosis within a few hours of intravenous injection of LPS. *c*) Total tumor regression occurring several days later. [From 1].

to the conclusion that endotoxin causes the release of a mediator, possibly of macrophage origin, which is directly responsible for killing the tumor cells. Apart from COLEY's fascinating clinical observations at the turn of this century, and the challenge posed by the striking phenomenon in the mouse, our own interest in LPS was greatly stimulated by the results of a therapeutic trial in patients with acute myeloblastic leukemia which was conducted by our leukemia group at the Memorial Hospital from 1970 to 1972.

At that time, a vaccine prepared from 7 strains of *Pseudomonas*

[7] *Oettgen, Hoffmann, Clarkson, Old* - p. 2

aeruginosa became available, designed to prevent or ameliorate Pseudomonas infections which pose a serious threat particularly to patients with severe burns or acute leukemia. The vaccine was a soluble extract which contained large amounts of LPS [8].

Adult patients with acute myeloblastic leukemia (AML) were treated according to the so-called L-6 chemotherapy protocol. Complete remission was first induced and consolidated with arabinosylcytosine and thioguanine, and then maintained with a multiple-drug regimen which included Vincristine, Methotrexate, BCNU, thioguanine, Cytoxan, hydroxyurea and Daunorubicin (figure 2). While all patients received the same chemotherapy, they were randomized to receive or not receive the Pseudomonas vaccine. The vaccine was administered by subcutaneous injection at a dose of

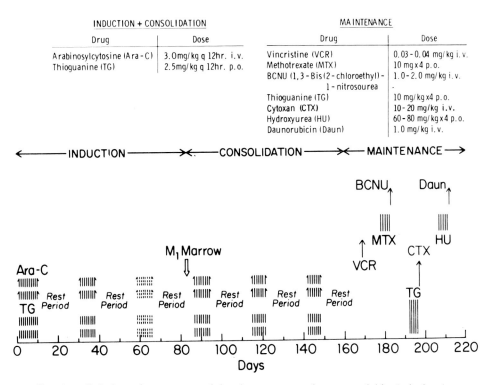

INDUCTION + CONSOLIDATION	
Drug	Dose
Arabinosylcytosine (Ara-C)	3.0mg/kg q 12hr. i.v.
Thioguanine (TG)	2.5mg/kg q 12hr. p.o.

MAINTENANCE	
Drug	Dose
Vincristine (VCR)	0.03 - 0.04 mg/kg i.v.
Methotrexate (MTX)	10 mg x 4 p.o.
BCNU (1,3 - Bis(2 - chloroethyl) - 1 - nitrosourea	1.0 - 2.0 mg/kg i.v.
Thioguanine (TG)	10 mg/kg x4 p.o.
Cytoxan (CTX)	10 - 20 mg/kg i.v.
Hydroxyurea (HU)	60 - 80 mg/kg x4 p.o.
Daunorubicin (Daun)	1.0 mg/kg i.v.

FIG. 2 — L-6 chemotherapy protocol for the treatment of acute myeloblastic leukemia.

[7] *Oettgen, Hoffmann, Clarkson, Old* - p. 3

0.1 to 1.0 ml (depending on individual tolerance) approximately twice a week, beginning during remission induction and extending well into the period of complete remission. This was not easily accomplished because the side effects — an inflammatory response at the site of the injection, as well as fever and general malaise — sometimes caused reluctance on the part of the patients and also the physicians. Thus, the schedule of vaccine administration was not always uniform. It does not appear, however, that the time required to induce complete remissions, or the duration of the remissions, was affected by these variations in the schedule of vaccine injections (figure 3). The frequency and severity of Pseudo-

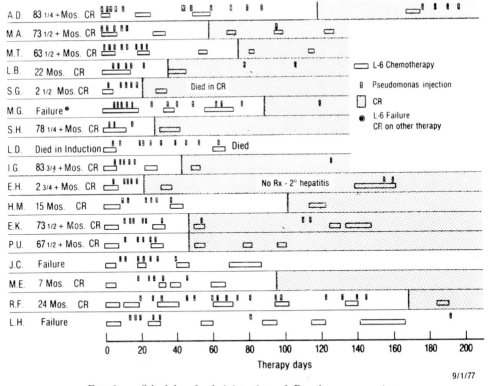

FIG. 3 — Schedule of administration of Pseudomonas vaccine.

[7] *Oettgen, Hoffmann, Clarkson, Old* - p. 4

monas infections was not significantly affected by the vaccine [9, 10].

Now, more than 5 years later, the results of the trial are as shown in table 1. While the Pseudomonas vaccine did not affect the frequency of complete remission, it caused a marked increase in its duration in some patients, the median being now more than five years for the group that received the vaccine, and only 9 months for the patients who did not receive the vaccine. An interesting point is that during the first 12 months of complete remission, the rate of relapse was identical in the two groups. From then on, most patients who had received the vaccine and were still in remission stayed in remission, while most patients who had not been treated with the vaccine continued to relapse (figure 4). Evidently, only half the patients responded to treatment with the Pseudomonas vaccine. So far, we have been unable to define any other criteria by which they can be distinguished.

Understandably, these results have contributed to a resurgence of our interest in the treatment of cancer patients with LPS, and we have started similar therapeutic trials in patients with AML, diffuse histiocytic lymphoma, other non-Hodgkin's lymphomas, and malignant melanoma. None of these trials have been underway for

TABLE 1 — *Results of treatment with L-6 chemotherapy, with or without Pseudomonas vaccine, in adult patients with acute myeloblastic leukemia.*

| | Randomization | |
	Pseudomonas vaccine	No Pseudomonas vaccine
Number of patients	17	27
Complete remissions	13	17
Duration of remission (months):		
median	$63\text{-}1/2^+$	9
mean	46.1	15.8
Still in complete remission (duration in months)	$6\ (64^+\text{-}84^+)$	$1\ (70^+)$

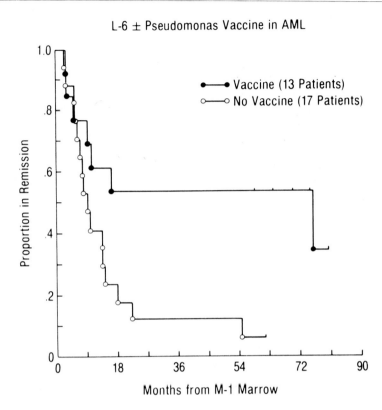

FIG. 4 — Duration of complete remission, induced and maintained by L-6 chemotherapy, in patients who received or did not receive Pseudomonas vaccine.

more than 1-1/2 years, and it would be unrewarding to discuss their
current state. One difficulty has been that the dose which causes
a "desirable" local and systemic reaction may vary by a factor of
more than 10 for different patients. The usual procedure, proceeding
from a safe dose to an effective dose in small increments, is complicated in the case of LPS by the development of tolerance. Impurities and lack of stability are other factors which have caused
problems. Now that highly purified and stable preparations are
becoming available through the efforts of Professor Westphal's

[7] *Oettgen, Hoffmann, Clarkson, Old* - p. 6

group, we look forward to resuming the study of LPS in human patients, including combinations with agents which abrogate some of its toxicity but need not be assumed a priori to interfere also with its action on tumors. The notion that the anti-tumor effect of LPS can be separated from some of its limiting toxic effects is in fact supported by results of recent research in the laboratory.

It began several years ago with the observation that acute tumor necrosis could be induced in mice not only with LPS, but also with serum obtained from BCG-infected mice after injecting them with LPS. The serum thus produced has been called tumor necrosis serum (TNS), although the term "serum" is not really applicable because blood with tumor-necrotizing activity so induced does not clot. The tumor-necrotizing activity (tumor necrosis factor, TNF) is found in a glycoprotein fraction with a molecular weight of about 150,000. Several lines of evidence (pyrogenicity, Limulus testing and chemical analysis for moieties of LPS) indicate that TNF activity cannot be ascribed to residual LPS. A further distinction between LPS and TNF is that TNF is directly cytotoxic for tumor cells *in vitro*; cultured cells from normal embryos are not injured [11, 12].

Conditions of TNF release have been well established. The criterion adopted as a standard for assaying TNF has been the visual observation of necrosis in subcutaneous transplants of the methyl-cholanthrene-induced BALB/c sarcoma Meth A. Figure 5 illustrates the grades of response elicited in individual (BALB/c × C57 BL/6)F_1 mice by administration of serum containing TNF. In the maximum (+ + +) response, the major part of the tumor mass is destroyed, leaving only a peripheral rim of apparently viable tumor tissue. In about 25% of mice treated with 0.5 ml of TNF-positive serum, the tumor regresses completely. Mice receiving TNF-positive serum show no marked signs of toxicity [11]. C. parvum and Zymosan are also effective priming agents for TNF release by LPS (table 2). These agents have in common the capacity to produce marked hyperplasia of the reticuloendothelial system. The best way to produce the tumor-necrotizing serum is to inject mice first with the priming agent and one to two weeks later with LPS, and to bleed them two hours after the LPS injection. Sensitivity to LPS is con-

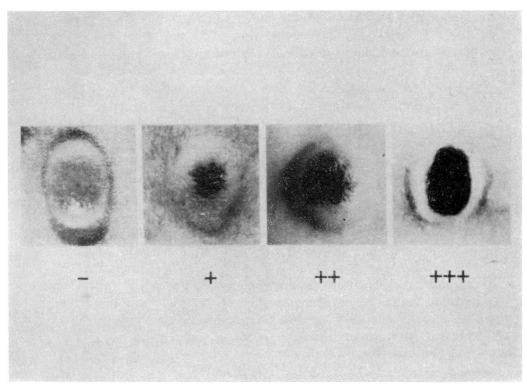

Fig. 5 — Grading of the necrotic response of BALB/c sarcoma Meth A (7-day subcutaneous transplants) 24 hr after intravenous injection of 0.5 ml of TNF-positive serum. [From 11].

siderably increased by pretreatment with the priming agent so that most of the mice would die if they were not bled.

Other factors that influence production of TNF are now being investigated, and several clues have emerged from these studies: 1) Although athymic nude mice (nu/nu) respond well to C. parvum in terms of macrophage hyperplasia in spleen and liver, TNF cannot be elicited by LPS in such mice. This suggests participation of T cells in the process of TNF-release. 2) Two substrains of C3H mice are known to differ in their response to LPS as measured by B cell mitogenesis and resistance to endotoxin lethality. A transplanted

[7] *Oettgen, Hoffmann, Clarkson, Old - p. 8*

TABLE 2 — *Assays for TNF in the serum of mice treated with various priming agents* [11].

Treatment of serum donors *		TNF assay: Necrotic response **			
		+++	++	+	—
Priming agent	Eliciting agent	Number of mice			
—	LPS 25 μg				9
BCG 2 × 10⁷ viable org.	—			2	7
BCG 2 × 10⁷ viable org.	LPS 25 μg	171	109		
C. parvum 1000 μg	⎪	24	7		
Zymosan 2000 μg	↓	4			

* CD-1 Swiss mice received the eliciting agent 14 days after the priming agent (both IV) and were exsanguinated 2 hr later.
** For scoring of the necrotic response, see Fig. 5.

C3H sarcoma, BP8, capable of progressive growth in both substrains, showed LPS-induced necrosis when passaged in the LPS-responsive C3H/An strain, but not when growing in LPS-resistant C3H/HeJ mice. In contrast, injection of TNF bypasses this genetic block, producing necrosis of BP8 tumors in both lines of C3H mice [11].

As we consider therapeutic application of TNF in man, and thus production in xenogeneic donors, the question of species specificity arises. Both rats and rabbits produced TNF which caused necrosis of the BALB/c sarcoma Meth A in syngeneic mice. As in the mouse, both BCG and endotoxin were required to induce appreciable amounts of TNF. Because rabbits are particularly sensitive to LPS, the dose was adjusted accordingly (table 3) [11].

Activity of TNF against cells in culture was tested on mouse embryo fibroblasts, Meth A sarcoma cells and L cells. The L cells proved most sensitive, Meth A sarcoma cells somewhat less so, and mouse embryo fibroblasts were virtually insensitive. The criterion employed was the count of viable cells after 48 hour exposure. Judging by proportional viability counts, the effect of TNF on Meth A sarcoma cells appeared primarily cytostatic, whereas L cells

[7] *Oettgen, Hoffmann, Clarkson, Old* - p. 9

TABLE 3 — *TNF release in rats and rabbits* [11].

Treatment of serum donors *		Serum donors							
		CD rat				NZW rabbit			
		TNF assay: Necrotic response **							
BCG	LPS	+++	++	+	−	+++	++	+	−
		Number of mice							
−	−				8			2	6
+	−				8			1	7
−	+			1	7			1	7
+	+	5	6	1	2	11	23	10	7

* BCG (7 × 10^7 viable organisms IV per rat or 3 × 10^8 IV per rabbit) was given 14 days before LPS (250 µg IV per rat or 100 µg IV per rabbit) was given 2 hr before exsanguination.

** For scoring of Meth A necrotic response, see Fig. 5. Heat-inactivated sera from 17 different rabbits assayed in three mice each. Each mouse was injected with 0.5 ml of rat serum or 1 ml of rabbit serum.

died within the 48 hour test period. The toxicity was delayed; no effect of TNF was demonstrable in the first 16 hours of exposure. Measurable toxicity for L cells was demonstrable with dilutions of TNF-positive serum as high as 1:10^4. Toxicity was not abolished by heating the TNF serum to 56° for 30 minutes. Sera from normal mice, or mice treated with either BCG or LPS alone, showed no cytotoxicity. LPS itself, in concentrations as high as 500 µg/ml, was not toxic for L cells. Rabbit and rat TNF sera showed the same pattern of cytotoxicity as mouse TNF, being highly toxic for L cells but not for mouse embryo fibroblasts (figure 6) [11].

The cytotoxic action of murine TNF is not restricted to mouse tumors. TNF was found strongly inhibitory for an established cell line derived from human melanoma but not for normal fibroblasts [13]. An extensive series of human tumor cells is now being screened to determine how frequently human tumors exhibit sensitivity to TNF.

In addition to inhibiting tumors, serum containing TNF as

[7] *Oettgen, Hoffmann, Clarkson, Old* · p. 10

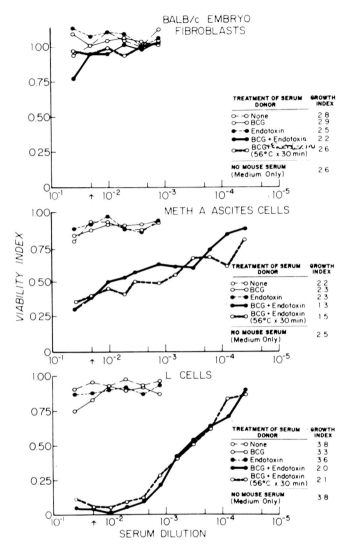

FIG. 6 — Inhibition of growth of cultured cell lines by TNF-positive serum. L cells (NCTC Clone 929) and BALB/c embryo fibroblasts (MEF) were grown as monolayers, and Meth A cells in suspension. Culture medium: Eagle's minimum essential medium plus nonessential amino acids, 10% heat-inactivated fetal calf serum, penicillin (100 U/ml), and streptomycin (100 µg/ml). One milliliter of cell suspension (2×10^5 MEF or L cells per ml; 2.5×10^5 Meth A cells per ml) was plated with 1 ml of the mouse serum to be tested, in serial dilution (abscissa), or 1 ml of culture medium (standard). Incubation: 48 hr in 5% CO_2 in air at 37°. Viability index = number of viable cells present in culture with test serum, divided by number in culture with medium alone. Insets: growth index = total number of cells (viable and dead) after 48 hr in culture in 1/50 mouse serum (↑) divided by number of cells plated. (Replicate plates; duplicate readings). [From 11].

well as the TNF fraction have striking effects on immunologic reactions, some similar to the effects of LPS, and others distinct. Our immunologic studies have focused on the production of antibody *in vitro*, as tested in the MISHELL-DUTTON culture system [14]. Briefly, mouse spleen cells are incubated with red blood cell antigen for several days and then mixed with agar containing the same red blood cell antigen and exposed to complement. Spleen cells which secrete antibody cause lysis of the red blood cells in their immediate vicinity.   The number of lytic plaques represents the number of antibody-secreting cells (plaque-forming cells or PFC). One advantage of the system is that it permits removal of selected cell populations — T cells, B cells, their subsets, and macrophages — and subsequent exploration of manipulations which can replace their function in the cooperation that is necessary for the production of antibody.

Initial experiments showed that the production of antibody to sheep red blood cells (SRBC) by spleen cells was accelerated and augmented by addition of TNS or TNF to the culture medium. Table 4 shows the number of PFC after 3 or 4 days of culture, with various additions to the culture medium. TNS and TNF produced an increase in PFC, serum from untreated mice or mice treated with

TABLE 4 — *Effects of TNS and TNF on the production of antibody to SRBC* in vitro [15].

Addition to culture	Anti-SRBC PFC per culture	
	Day 3	Day 4
None	65	3,900
TNS 2%	1,850	13,000
TNF 0.13 mg ml^{-1}	1,280	10,200
Normal mouse serum	28	4,000
LPS serum *	108	6,500
BCG serum **	78	4,000

* Serum from mice given LPS only.
** Serum from mice given BCG only.

[7] *Oettgen, Hoffmann, Clarkson, Old* - p. 12

LPS or BCG alone did not [15]. This observation led to the question of whether TNF acted directly on B cells, or indirectly through macrophages or T cells. When macrophages were removed by filtration through Sephadex G-10, spleen cells failed to produce antibody to SRBC (figure 7). Responsiveness was restored by 2-mercaptoethanol, but not by adding TNS. In the presence of 2-mercaptoethanol, however, addition of TNS increased antibody production by macrophage-depleted spleen cell cultures. To determine whether this effect reflected action on T cells or B cells, T cells were eliminated by treatment with anti-Thy-1 serum and complement. Addition of TNS completely restored antibody production in these T cell-depleted cultures (figure 7) [15].

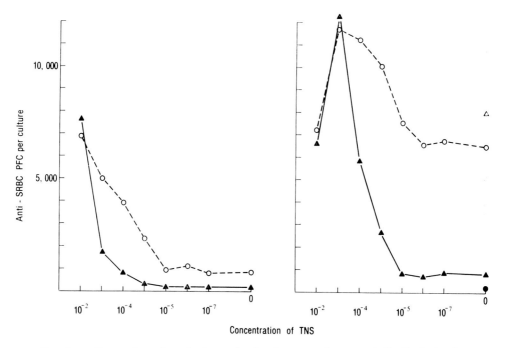

FIG. 7 — Restoration of antibody production by macrophage-, and T-cell- depleted spleen cell cultures with TNS. PFC response on days 3 (a) and 4 (b). Each point is the average of 2 cultures. ● 2-ME not added; ○ 2-ME added; ▲ 2-ME added, T cells removed by treatment with anti-Thy-1 and rabbit complement; △ 2-ME added, cells treated with rabbit complement (control). [From 15].

Similar results were obtained with cultures of spleen cells from congenitally athymic nu/nu mice. Since they lack helper T cells, spleen cells from these mice do not produce antibody to red blood cells *in vitro*. Addition of TNS to the culture medium permitted a response of the same magnitude as that of spleen cells from littermate nu/+ mice which do not lack T cells (figure 8). Addition of

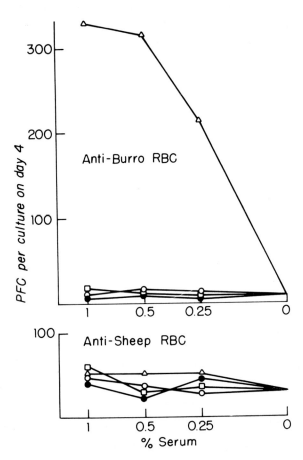

FIG. 8 — Restoration of antibody production by spleen cells from nu/nu mice with TNS. Cultures (in MEM + 5% FCS) were immunized with BRBC. Anti BRBC (a) and anti-SRBC PFC (b) were assayed on day 4. △ TNS; ● normal mouse serum; ○ serum from mice treated with BCG only; □ serum from mice treated with LPS only. [From 15].

[7] *Oettgen, Hoffmann, Clarkson, Old* - p. 14

TNS supported the production of antibody only to the antigen to which the spleen cells had been sensitized — in this case burro red blood cells — but not to an unrelated antigen — in this experiment sheep red blood cells (figure 8). Addition of TNS was effective even if delayed as long as two days, and this was also true for TNF [15].

While 2-mercaptoethanol can substitute for some aspects of macrophage function, and cannot be replaced by TNS in this respect, we have described another macrophage function for which 2-mercaptoethanol is not a substitute. Macrophages are essential for the cooperation between primed helper T cells and B cells which have been depleted of the subpopulation that carries receptors for complement. To determine if TNF can replace macrophages in that respect, two spleen cell preparations were used — cells depleted only of macrophages by passage through uncoated Sephadex G-10 columns and cells depleted of macrophages and complement receptor bearing (CR-positive) cells by passage through Sephadex G-10 columns coated with complement-reacted antigen-antibody complexes. Production of antibody to trinitrophenyl-conjugated SRBC (TNP-SRBC) was tested without and with addition of SRBC-primed helper T cells (figure 9). CR-negative spleen cells not only generated less antibody than CR-positive spleen cells, but also failed to cooperate with primed helper T cells. TNS induced CR-negative cells to produce antibody, and also enabled them to cooperate with primed helper T cells in the absence of macrophages [15]. This effect may be due to maturation of CR-negative cells to CR-positive cells which, as we have shown, can be induced by macrophages which have been activated by BCG or helper T cells [16].

TNS does in fact support various steps in B cell differentiation, as shown in figure 10. Bone marrow cells (for induction of Ig, Ia and Thy-1) or spleen cells (for induction of CR) were separated on a discontinuous bovine serum albumin gradient and the cells of the C layer (the 23-26% interface) were cultured with or without TNS, LPS or thymopoietin. LPS at a standard concentration of 30 μg/ml induced all three B cell markers as well as the T cell marker thy-1. TNS induced Ig, Ia and CR, but not Thy-1. Conversely, both calf thymopoietin and synthetic thymopoietin induced Thy-1 but not any of the B cell markers [17]. The selective support of phenotypic and

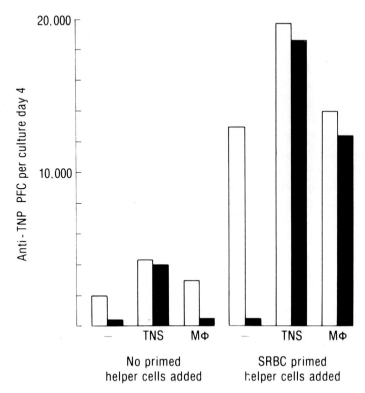

Fig. 9 — Induction of antibody production in cultures of CR⁻ spleen cells by TNS. Spleen cells were passed through Sephadex G-10 columns coated with complement-reacted antigen-antibody complexes (CR⁻ spleen cells, black bars) or uncoated Sephadex G-10 columns (CR⁺ spleen cells, open bars). TNS was added at 1% final concentration. As source of macrophages (MØ), 5×10^4 peritoneal cells were added to the cultures. Average of 2 cultures. [From 15].

functional B cell differentiation by TNF was found to extend to C3H/HeJ B cells which are genetically unresponsive to LPS [18].

The findings discussed so far led to the notion that macrophages play a critical role in the LPS-induced augmentation of the B cell response, and that TNS contains B cell-directed mediators elaborated by macrophages. That notion was pursued in experiments whose essential features were the use of the LPS-unresponsive mouse strain C3H/HeJ and its histocompatible LPS-responsive counterpart

[7] *Oettgen, Hoffmann, Clarkson, Old* - p. 16

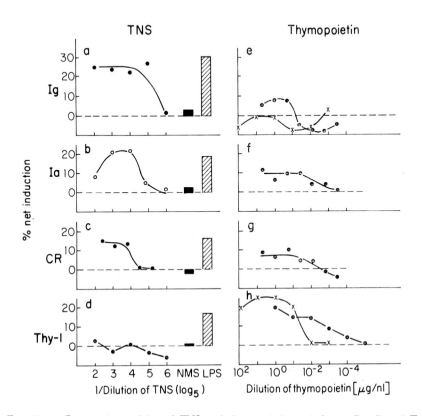

FIG. 10 — Comparative activity of TNS and thymopoietin in inducing B cell and T cell markers. Bone marrow cells or spleen cells of (C57BL/6 × A)F₁ mice, 3-4 weeks of age, were fractionated on a discontinuous bovine serum albumin gradient. Cells from the 23 to 26% interface were cultured at a density of 5×10⁶ cells per ml in the presence of different dilutions of TNS (left panels), 1:25 diluted normal mouse serum (NMS) (solid bar), LPS at 30 μg/hl (shaded bar), thymopoietin (right panels, ●—●) or synthetic thymopoietin (right panels, x—x), or with no addition (control cultures, broken line). The percentage of cells expressing Ig (panels a and e), Ia (panels b and f), CR (panels c and g), and Thy-1 (panels d and h) was determined by standard cytotoxicity or rosette-formation techniques. The percent net induction represents the difference of cytotoxicity indices or rosette-forming cells between cultures with inducing agent and control cultures without agent. Cytotoxicity indices were computed according to the formula $(a-b)/c \times 100$ where a = percent of non-viable cells in antiserum and complement, b = percent of nonviable cells in complement, and c = percent of viable cells in complement. [From 17].

C3HeB/FeJ, and of an antigen, TNP-conjugated mouse erythrocytes
(TNP-MRBC), which is not itself immunogenic in the mouse but
becomes immunogenic when given with LPS [19].

First, the effects of TNS and LPS on the production of anti-
hapten antibody by spleen cell cultures immunized with TNP-MRBC
were compared (figure 11). In the absence of TNS or LPS, no antibody response was seen on day 4. Addition of LPS caused a response
in cultures of C3HeB/FeJ spleen cells but not C3H/HeJ spleen cells.
Addition of TNS, on the other hand, facilitated antibody production

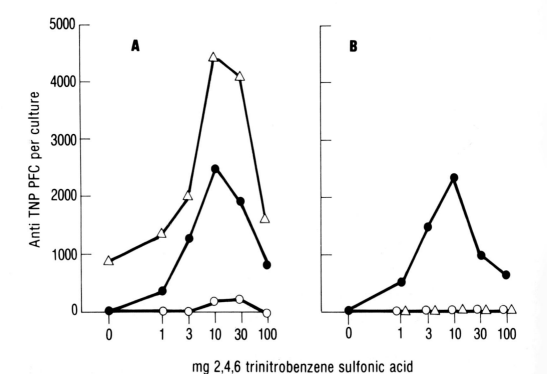

mg 2,4,6 trinitrobenzene sulfonic acid

Fig. 11 — Facilitation of anti-TNP response by LPS or by TNS. 10^7 spleen cells
from C3HeB/FeJ mice (A) or C3H/HeJ mice (B) were immunized with 10^6 mouse
red blood cells conjugated with TNP at different densities. Amount of 2, 4, 6-trini-
trobenzene sulfonic acid per 10 ml buffer containing 10^8 mouse erythrocytes is indicated
on the abscissa. Additions to cultures: ○ — ○ none, ●—● TNS 1%, △—△ LPS
10γ/ml. [From 20].

[7] *Oettgen, Hoffmann, Clarkson, Old* · p. 18

by cultures of spleen cells from both the LPS-responsive and the LPS-unresponsive substrain [20].

To determine the role of macrophages in the LPS-dependent production of antibody, we removed them by passing the spleen cells through Sephadex G-10 columns. Table 5 shows results obtained with C3HeB/FeJ or C3H/HeJ cells, cultured without addition or with TNS or LPS added, depleted or not depleted of macrophages, and exposed or not exposed to antigen. LPS did not support the antigen-dependent production of antibody in macrophage-depleted C3HeB/FeJ cultures, but continued to induce the antigen-independent polyclonal response. TNS, on the other hand, did not support the polyclonal response, but supported the antigen-dependent production of antibody even in the absence of macrophages [20].

Facilitation of the antigen-dependent production of antibody by LPS was fully restored by adding purified peritoneal C3HeB/FeJ macrophages to the macrophage-depleted spleen cell cultures (figure 12). Addition of C3H/HeJ macrophages had no effect. On the other hand, C3HeB/FeJ macrophages failed completely to support the mitotic response of C3H/HeJ spleen cells to LPS [20].

To recapitulate (table 6), TNS confers responsiveness, in terms of LPS-dependent antibody production but not LPS-dependent mi-

TABLE 5 — *Role of macrophages in the LPS-induced production of antibody to MRBC-TNP* [20].

Source of spleen cells (5×10^6/culture)	Addition to culture	Unfractionated spleen cells		Macrophage-depleted spleen cells (Sephadex G-10)	
		No antigen added	Antigen added	No antigen added	Antigen added
C3HeB/FeJ	—	92	79	65	63
	TNS 1%	83	890	75	1230
	LPS 10 μg/ml	910	6200	2050	2130
C3H/HeJ	—	40	38	80	75
	TNS 1%	45	620	45	750
	LPS 10 μg/ml	42	44	95	88

[7] *Oettgen, Hoffmann, Clarkson, Old* - p. 19

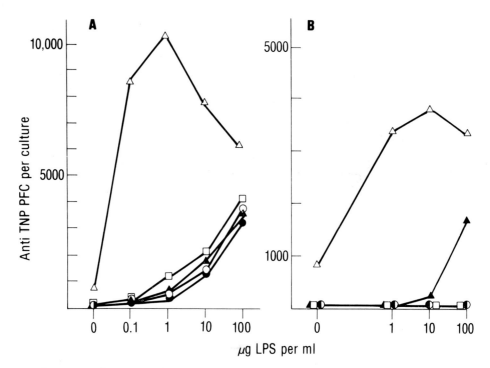

FIG. 12 — Facilitation of antigen-dependent and polyclonal antibody production, in the presence of LPS, by macrophages from an LPS-responsive mouse strain. (A) response of macrophage-depleted C3HeB/FeJ spleen cells. (B) response of macrophage-depleted C3H/HeJ spleen cells. Additions to cultures: ●—● none, ○—○ MRBC-TNP, ▲—▲ 6×10⁴ C3HeB/FeJ macrophages, △—△ 6×10⁴ C3HeB/FeJ macrophages + MRBC-TNP, □—□ 10⁵ C3H/HeJ macrophages + MRBC-TNP. [From 20].

tosis, to unfractionated LPS-unresponsive spleen cells. It confers the same type of responsiveness — antibody production but not mitosis — to macrophage-depleted spleen cells from non-responder as well as responder strains (the latter also unresponsive to LPS when depleted of macrophages). TNS thus replaces a product which is generated by LPS-responsive macrophages in response to LPS.

In summary, the spectrum of immunological activities of LPS-induced TNF presents itself as shown in table 7. Similar to LPS, TNF induces maturation of B cells and substitutes for helper T cells. Unlike LPS, TNF inhibits the proliferative response of T and B

[7] Oettgen, Hoffmann, Clarkson, Old - p. 20

TABLE 6 — *Different requirements for induction of antibody production or B cell mitosis by LPS* [20].

	Antigen-dependent production of antibody	Mitosis
Unfractionated spleen cells		
Responder + LPS	+	+
Non-responder + LPS	—	—
Responder + TNS	+	—
Non-responder + TNS	+	—
Macrophage-depleted spleen cells		
Responder + LPS	—	+
Non-responder + LPS	—	—
Responder + TNS	+	—
Non-responder + TNS	+	—
Non-responder spleen cells plus responder macrophages and LPS	+	—
Responder macrophage-depleted spleen cells plus non-responder macrophages and LPS	—	+

TABLE 7 — *Biological effects of LPS-induced Tumor Necrosis Factor (TNF).*

Effect	TNF	LPS
Tumor necrosis in vivo	+	+
Tumor necrosis in vitro	+	—
Differentiation of T cells	—	+
Differentiation of B cells	+	+
Proliferation of B cells	—	+
Inhibition of T cell proliferation	+	—
Polyclonal Ab. production	—	+
T cell helper function	+	+
Reversal of Ab. suppression		
by Concanavalin A	+	—
by antibody	+	—
Replacement of macrophages in		
LPS-dependent Ab. production	+	—

[7] *Oettgen, Hoffmann, Clarkson, Old* - p. 21

cells to mitogens and reverses the suppression of antibody production *in vitro* induced by Concanavalin A or specific antibody (unpublished observation). TNF also differs from LPS in that it is not a mitogen for B cells, does not induce maturation of T cells and does not induce polyclonal production of antibodies. The immunological effects defined so far are consistent with the assumption that TNF is a macrophage product. The antitumor effects of TNF *in vivo* and *in vitro* and the effects on immunological functions have not been dissociated during the TNF purification steps taken thus far. Proof that these activities can be ascribed to the same molecule awaits the isolation of TNF. The dissection of SHEAR's phenomenon which is now well underway should clarify (and possibly link) the mechanisms involved in the initial necrotic response (which does not depend on the immune system) and the subsequent rejection response (which depends on the immune system), and guide us as we are beginning to take a new look at the potential of LPS in the treatment of patients with cancer.

[7] *Oettgen, Hoffmann, Clarkson, Old* - p. 22

REFERENCES

[1] OLD L. J. and BOYSE E. A., *Current enigmas in cancer research.* The Harvey Lectures, Series 67, 273-315, Academic Press, New York and London 1973.

[2] GRATIA A. and LINZ R., *Le phenomene de Shwartzman dans le sarcoma du Cobaye.* « C. R. Seances Biol. Ses. Fil. », *108*, 427-428 (1931).

[3] SHEAR M. J., *Chemical treatment of tumors. IX. Reactions of mice with primary subcutaneous tumors to injection of a hemorrhage-producing bacterial polysaccharide.* « J. Nat. Cancer Inst ». *4*, 461-476 (1944).

[4] NOWOTNY A., *Molecular aspects of endotoxin reactions.* « Bacteriol. Rev. », *33*, 72-98 (1969).

[5] PARR I., WHEELER E. and ALEXANDER P., *Similarities of the antitumor actions of endotoxin, lipid A and double-stranded RNA.* « Brit. J. Cancer », *27*, 370-389 (1973).

[6] NAUTS H. C., SWIFT W. E. and COLEY B. L., *The treatment of malignant tumors by bacterial toxins as developed by the late William B. Coley, M. D., reviewed in the light of modern research.* « Cancer Res. », *6*, 205-216 (1946).

[7] ALGIRE G. H., LEGALLAIS F. Y. and ANDERSON B. F., *Vascular reactions of normal and malignant tissues* in vivo. V. *Role of hypotension in action of bacterial polysaccharide on tumors.* « J. Nat. Cancer Inst. », *12*, 1279-1295 (1952).

[8] HANESSIAN S., REGAN W., WATSON D. and HASKELL T., *Isolation and characterization of antigenic components of a new heptavalent Pseudomonas vaccine.* « Nature New Biol », *229*, 209-210 (1971).

[9] CLARKSON B. D., DOWLING M. D., GEE T. S., CUNNINGHAM I. B. and BURCHENAL J. B., *Treatment of acute leukemia in adults.* « Cancer », *36*, 775-795 (1975).

[10] YOUNG L. S., MEYER R. D. and ARMSTRONG D., *Pseudomonas aeruginosa vaccine in cancer patients.* « Ann. Int. Med. », *79*, 518-527 (1973).

[11] CARSWELL E. A., OLD L. J., KASSEL R. L., GREEN S., FIORE N. and WILLIAMSON B., *An endotoxin-induced serum factor that causes necrosis of tumors.* « Proc. Nat. Acad. Sci. USA », *72*, 3666-3670 (1975).

[12] GREEN S., DOBRJANSKY A., CARSWELL E. A., KASSEL R. L., OLD L. J., FIORE N. C. and SCHWARTZ M. K., *Partial purification of a serum factor that causes necrosis of tumors.* « Proc. Nat. Acad. Sci. USA », *73*, 381-385 (1976).

[13] HELSON L., GREEN S., CARSWELL E. A. and OLD L. J., *Effect of tumor necrosis factor on cultured human melanoma cells.* « Nature », *258*, 731-732 (1975).

[14] MISHELL R. I. and DUTTON R. W., *Immunization of dissociated spleen cell cultures from normal mice.* « J. Epx. Med. », *126*, 423-442 (1967).

[15] HOFFMANN M. K., GREEN S., OLD L. J. and OETTGEN H. F., *Serum containing endotoxin-induced tumor necrosis factor substitutes for helper T cells.* « Nature », *263*, 416-417 (1976).

[16] HOFFMANN M. K., HAMMERLING U., SIMON M. and OETTGEN H. F., *Macrophage requirements of CR^- and CR^+ B lymphocytes for antibody production in vitro.* « J. Immunol. », *116*, 1447-1451 (1976).

[17] HOFFMANN M. K., OETTGEN II. F., OLD L. J., CHIN A. F. and HAMMERLING U., *Endotoxin-induced serum factor controlling differentiation of bone marrow-derived lymphocytes.* « Proc. Nat. Acad. Sci. USA », *74*, 1200-1203 (1977).

[18] KOENIG S., HOFFMANN M. K. and THOMAS L., *Induction of phenotypic lymphocyte differentiation in LPS-unresponsive mice by an LPS-induced serum factor and by lipid A-associated protein.* « J. Immunol. », *118*, 1910-1911 (1967).

[19] SCHMIDTKE J. P. and DIXON F., *Immune response to a hapten coupled to a nonimmunogenic carrier. Influence of lipopolysaccharide.* « J. Exp. Med. », *136*, 392-397 (1972).

[20] HOFFMANN M. K., GALANOS C., KOENIG S. and OETTGEN H. F., *B cell activitation by LPS: Distinct pathways for induction of mitosis and antibody production.* « J. Exp. Med. », in press 1977.

DISCUSSION

MATHÉ

About tolerance I would like to say that the injection of Pseudomonas aeruginosa as micro-organism is perfectly tolerated at the dose of
3.10^9 organisms, while the LPS induced noticeable side effects. My
question is: what about the effect of Pseudomonas LPS effect on delayed
skin hypersensitivity and its restoration in anergic patients?

OETTGEN

It is difficult to estimate what dose of Pseudomonas vaccine is correct for an individual patient, i.e., causes a definite but tolerable local
reaction and a definite but tolerable systemic reaction. The "desirable"
dose may vary considerably from patient to patient.

MATHÉ

Could you induce the tumor necrotizing factor with Pseudomonas
injected as a micro-organism 15 days after BCG or do you with its LPS?

OETTGEN

In the mouse we can induce tumor necrosis factor with Pseudomonas
extract as well as with endotoxin. In our patients with acute leukemia
there was no noticeable difference between the patients who received the
vaccine and other patients who did not receive it. But this is not a
patient population where this type of reactivity is easy to test, as you
know.

NORTH

Why has it not been recorded that tumor necrosis factor is produced

[7] *Oettgen, Hoffmann, Clarkson, Old* - p. 25

by the tumor bearer itself, when the tumor is regressing under the influence of endotoxin? Why is it necessary to always go to BCG or C. parvum-treated animals? In other words, why have you not looked in the animal that you should be analyzing?

OETTGEN

Pretreatment with BCG or C. parvum is the condition under which tumor necrosis factor is released best in response to lipopolysaccharide. This is why, in studies of various effects of tumor necrosis factor, we have obtained it from mice so treated. It is a question of obtaining the largest possible quantity.

NORTH

But if it is responsible for the regression of the tumor, then surely it should be in the tumor bearer. What I am asking is why do you have to go to C. parvum and BCG to show this?

OETTGEN

For all I know, it is simply a quantitative difference.

NORTH

I just had not seen it reported; that is why I ask you. But does the tumor-bearing mouse have more than a normal mouse?

OETTGEN

I do not know.

NOSSAL

I would like to go back to the beginning of your talk about TNF and its action and ask you a sort of speculative question of principle. It would appear that this TNF *in vitro* can kill a variety of different tumor cells, always with different efficiencies, and has no effect on normal cells.

[7] Oettgen, Hoffmann, Clarkson, Old - p. 26

Could you give us some kind of an idea on what feature of the cell the material may be exercising its discriminatory activity? You have told us that TNF is an alpha-globulin, i.e. not an antibody. So what feature of the tumorous cell might it be that this non-immunoglobulin material is recognizing, allowing it to kill the tumor cell but not the normal cell?

OETTGEN

We do not know the nature of the receptor. Of a spectrum of mouse tumors, some are, and some are not, susceptible to this material.

ROSENBERG

Two questions: first, you showed us intradermal tumor necrosis and you mentioned that subcutaneous tumor will also disappear. What about tumor in visceral organs, i.e. pulmonary metastases induced by intravenous injection?

OETTGEN

Animals with pulmonary metastases have not been tested. Mice with tumors growing in the peritoneal cavity have been treated with intra-peritoneal injections, and this treatment caused tumor regression. With the BALB/c sarcoma Meth A we can do this, as you know, because it grows well in the peritoneal cavity. A true systemic effect on tumors other than cutaneous transplants has not yet been tested.

ROSENBERG

I am intrigued by the effect on *in vitro cells*. The direct effect of TNF on tumor cells and not normal cells would appear to bypass all of the immunizing mechanism that you are describing *in vivo*. Do responsive cells have receptors for TNF, that is: can you absorb TNF with intact cells that are capable of being inhibited *in vitro* by TNF? and also, could you give us some feeling for how extensively those studies have been performed — what kinds of tumors have you looked at? — have you ever found a normal cell that is capable of being inhibited?

[7] Oettgen, Hoffmann, Clarkson, Old - p. 27

OETTGEN

The *in vitro* studies have not yet been extensive. We only know that a spectrum of sensitivity exists, ranging in the mouse from highly sensitive L cells to insensitive BALB/c embryo fibroblasts, BALB/c sarcoma Meth A being of intermediate sensitivity. Similar differences appear to exist for human tumor cells.

WOLFF

How about the first question: can responsive cells bind TNF?

OETTGEN

We do not know.

WOLFF

I have a few specific questions. One is that there is an intravenous Pseudomonas endotoxin commercially available — it is the only endotoxin commercially available in the United States — it has protein in it, it is not a very reproducible one but have you tried that?

OETTGEN

No, the only preparation we have used is the one produced by Parke, Davis and Co. We have never injected it intravenously.

WOLFF

Secondly, have you ever taken the serum from your patients that you have treated with BCG and liver endotoxin and seen *in vitro* what effects it exerts?

OETTGEN

We have done very few experiments of this sort. The serum of patients who were extensively treated with BCG, and later with endotoxin,

[7] *Oettgen, Hoffmann, Clarkson, Old* - p. 28

did not show tumor necrosis factor activity when tested on a mouse tumor. We have also not been able to detect tumor necrosis factor activity in the serum of a patient who developed a disseminated intravascular coagulation syndrome after endotoxin administration. You may remember I mentioned earlier that serum containing tumor necrosis factor that does not clot.

RAPP

As you know, so-called BCG-activated macrophages *in vitro* are more active against tumor cells than normal cells or embryo cells.

OETTGEN

Yes, BALB/c embryo fibroblasts were not susceptible.

WOLFF

Embryo cells?

OETTGEN

Yes.

BARCINSKI

I would like to know if you can substitute TNF activity by a supplement of macrophage culture supernatant?

OETTGEN

We have not done such experiments.

CHEDID

I congratulate you for this very exciting presentation and wish to ask the following questions. Since the BCG-sensitized mice received a high dosage of endotoxin in your experiments and since such mice can

[7] *Oettgen, Hoffmann, Clarkson, Old* - p. 29

be killed at the microgram level instead of the milligram level, I wonder if the toxicity parameter is not essential. More precisely could you tell us, for instance, if in adrenalectomized mice TNF is produced with much smaller dosages of endotoxin?

OETTGEN

When we give mice that have been pretreated with BCG 100 micrograms of endotoxin to produce tumor necrosis factor, the mice would die if we would not bleed them after two hours — they would be dead after four hours at the latest. But endotoxin toxicity is not all that is required for the production of tumor necrosis factor. Dr. Galanos in Professor Westphal's laboratory investigated another situation where mice are considerably more sensitive to endotoxin, even more so than after treatment with BCG. Adrenalectomized mice are exquisitely sensitive, but their blood does clot, and it does not contain tumor necrosis factor. Professor Westphal will now try to induce tumor necrosis factor in another species that is as resistant to LPS as the mouse. Perhaps he would like to comment.

WESTPHAL

Certain primates are remarkably insensitive to endotoxin. For example, the baboon (kg 10-25) stands intravenous injections of 100 milligrams (!) of pure endotoxin (LPS of *Salmonella*) with almost no signs of untoward effects, no significant change of the white blood count, no change of body temperature (as measured by a swallowed small emitter recording temperature) ([1]). The baboon is, thus, about a million-fold less sensitive compared to the human. We are now trying whether the baboon and other primates, such as the vervet, can produce the tumor-necrotizing factor (TNF) after priming with *C. parvum*. How much endotoxin will they stand after this "sensitizing" pretreatment and will TNF be released under such conditions?

----

[1] WESTPHAL O.: *Bacterial Endotoxins*. The 2nd Carl Prausnitz Memorial Lecture. « Internat. Arch. Allergy Appl. Immunol. », *49*, 1-43 (1975).

[7] *Oettgen, Hoffmann, Clarkson, Old* - p. 30

LEVI-MONTALCINI

I would like to ask Dr. Oettgen if anyone has tried to see whether the exclusion of the sympathetic system which can be achieved in neonatal animals by immunological or chemical procedures, does in some way influence the response to endotoxins. This possibility has been suggested by some investigator (unfortunately I do not remember his name) but I do not know if this line of studies has been pursued.

OETTGEN

An excellent suggestion, but we have not tested it.

CHEDID

Since so many pharmacological and biological activities can be elicited by LPS, have you tested whether TNF also produces these biological effects, such as pyrogenicity, abortion, protection against lethal irradiation, etc.?

OETTGEN

I can answer a few but not all of these questions. We have not yet compared tumor necrosis factor with Dr. Wolff's leukocyte pyrogen. That TNF induces abortion in the rabbit does not seem very likely for the following reasons. Treatment with corticosteroids protects the rabbit against endotoxin toxicity but does not prevent abortion, and mice treated with corticosteroids do not produce tumor necrosis factor.

CHEDID

In the experiments concerning protection against lethal irradiation, has TNF effects similar to CSF?

We have previously shown that C3H/HeJ mice which are unresponsive to phenol-water polysaccharide can respond, however, to other endotoxic preparations such as, for instance, a Boivin preparation. I would like to ask if such endotoxins which are mitogenic in LPS-low responder mice can still liberate TNF in these same sublines?

[7] Oettgen, Hoffmann, Clarkson, Old - p. 31

OETTGEN

I cannot answer this question directly, but I would like to add one word of caution. The C3H/HeJ mouse strain, although unresponsive to purified endotoxin, is as responsive as other mouse strains to the lipoprotein prepared from bacterial cell walls. The experiments which I reported depend on the use of highly purified LPS preparations.

CHEDID

It must be recalled that although a Boivin preparation is mitogenic for HeJ cells, it is still unable to enhance the resistance of this subline against a *Klebsiella* or a *Listeria* infection. Therefore HeJ mice have a genetic defect which is more important than what is measured by unresponsiveness to B mitogens.

OETTGEN

The data indicate that mitosis and antibody production are activated through different pathways. Clearly, nothing needs to be between LPS and the B cell to produce the mitotic response. By contrast, the macrophage is necessary between LPS and the B cell for induction of antibody production. In this respect the two pathways clearly differ.

DAVIES

Well, I am not sure whether my question has been answered or not — it was related to this point — the TC extract does have the protein fraction attached. That has some properties of its own, as shown by recent work. So I was wondering whether in fact all the features you describe are reproducible with LPS as you define it, or whether that protein component is a necessary constituent?

OETTGEN

We know that in the LPS-unresponsive C3H/HeJ mouse the lipoprotein as it is prepared by Morrison induces all effects which LPS itself induces in LPS-responsive mice.

[7] *Oettgen, Hoffmann, Clarkson, Old* - p. 32

NORTH

Dr. Oettgen, I would just like to return to the selective action of TNF and ask you the following question: if TNF directly kills tumor cells, why is it that it only acts against tumors of a certain critical size? in other words the Meth A tumor has to be about seven days old before this TNF causes regression. If it acts directly, why does it not kill tumors of a smaller size?

OETTGEN

We need more information on that point. Optimal tumor size for the phenomenon of acute necrosis has not been established as well for TNF as for LPS.

CLERICI

Maybe my question is a bit naive, but you stated that the TNS activity cannot be attributed to a residual LPS activity in the mice serum. Well, you inject about 100 μg of LPS into a 25 g mouse, that is 4 μg of LPS/g of body weight, and bleed them 2 hours later. As far as I know, all the bacterial polysaccharides are slowly metabolized, since they are retained for a long time in the cells of the reticuloendothelial system: may I remind you, in this connection, of the so-called Felton's paralysis? Therefore, it is possible that minimal amounts of LPS remaining in the TNF may bring about some kind of polyclonal stimulation of lymphoid cells and the ensuing production of anti-tumor antibodies. In conclusion, I would like to ask you how can you be sure that there is no more LPS in your serum? Did you try to detect LPS traces, if any, by means of the sensitive *Lymulus polyphemus* test?

OETTGEN

Three types of tests — pyrogenicity tests, *Lymulus* assays, and chemical analysis have failed to show residual LPS in TNF. More compelling is the evidence that TNS does not have some of the effects which LPS has in culture, and that it has other effects which LPS does not have. Taking all this into account, I think it unlikely that an undetectable minimal LPS residue is the active principle of TNF.

[7] *Oettgen, Hoffmann, Clarkson, Old* - p. 33

RAPP

Getting back to North's question, isn't the phenomenon that he referred to consistent with the possibility that endotoxin may be interfering with the development of a blood supply to the tumor?

OETTGEN

Histological examination of the sequence of events in tumors undergoing necrosis indicates almost immediate single cell necrosis, which is followed only later by hemorrhage. So it seems that circulatory changes occur after necrosis has already started.

RAPP

But it is my understanding that it will not work if you do not wait at least seven days.

OETTGEN

That is correct for endotoxin. As I said in response to Dr. North's question, I do not have sufficient information on this point for TNF.

CLERICI

May I ask, Dr. Oettgen, if there is any relationship between complement levels in the serum and the TNF?

OETTGEN

I am afraid I cannot answer your question. In relation to complement, the only statement I can make is that heat inactivation does not destroy the necrotizing activity of TNF.

CLERICI

Because with lipopolysaccharide you activate the alternative pathway.

OETTGEN

Yes.

[7] *Oettgen, Hoffmann, Clarkson, Old - p. 34*

IMMUNOLOGICAL ADJUVANTS
IN TUMOUR IMMUNOTHERAPY

R.W. BALDWIN

Cancer Research Campaign Laboratories, University of Nottingham
Nottingham, England

Immunotherapy is being considered as a component in the treatment of human malignant disease following studies indicating that immunity can be induced against transplanted animal tumours. Clinical evidence of host immunity to human cancer is still largely circumstantial, however, and there is no conclusive proof that human tumour associated antigens detected by *in vitro* assays of cell mediated or humoral immunity can, or do, function *in vivo* to mediate tumour rejection. Furthermore the mechanism of tumour rejection mediated by immune responses to tumour associated antigens in well defined animal systems is still inadequately understood. Because of these uncertainties, most clinical immunotherapy trials have adopted an empirical approach utilizing bacterial adjuvants such as bacillus Calmette Guérin (BCG) and certain species of the anaerobic Corynebacteria, notably C. parvum. The initial proposition was that non-specific immunostimulation with these bacterial adjuvants would also enhance tumour specific immune responses. Basically, however, several modes of treatment can be identified including:

a) Systemic immunostimulation, where the enhancement of immune responsiveness may also boost tumour specific immunity. Following recognition that cancer patients may frequently suffer a degree of immunosuppression, this form of treatment is also being given to restore immunocompetence.

b) *Active specific immunotherapy*, involving immunization with tumour antigen-containing vaccines, the objective being to stimulate specific immune responses to tumour associated antigens.

c) *Adjuvant contact therapy* where bacterial adjuvants such as BCG or C. parvum are administered so as to localize in tumour deposits. This initiates non-specific as well as, perhaps, specific host responses, including macrophage activation which can lead to local destruction of tumour cells.

Of these three approaches, attention is being given to adjuvant contact therapy since this has proved particularly versatile. It is frequently possible, for example, to suppress tumour growth by contact with BCG or C. parvum even with tumours displaying little or no immunogenicity as defined by the capacity to induce immunity to transplanted tumour in pre-immunized syngeneic recipients. Furthermore, bacterial adjuvants can be used to control metastatic tumour developing in different anatomical locations, when these agents are administered so as to localize at the site of tumour deposits.

Adjuvant Contact Suppression of Tumour Growth

Infiltration of bacterial adjuvants such as BCG and C. parvum into tumour deposits often will significantly inhibit tumour growth (BALDWIN and PIMM, 1977; MILAS and SCOTT, 1978). This form of treatment, which can be referred to as adjuvant contact therapy, was originally demonstrated in tests showing that intradermal injection of hepatoma line 10 cells admixed with BCG into syngeneic guinea pigs prevented growth of the tumour and also inhibited metastatic spread to the draining lymph nodes (ZBAR and TANAKA, 1971). This approach was subsequently extended to show that intralesional injection of BCG into intradermal tumour nodules in guinea pigs prevented the spread and development of lymph node metastases, although often without markedly influencing growth of the local tumour. (ZBAR et al., 1972). These effects on the guinea pig hepatoma are akin to the responses observed with human malignant melanoma where intralesional injection with agents such as

[8] *Baldwin* - p. 2

BCG or vaccinia virus induces regression of the injected lesion (MASTRANGELO et al., 1976). Furthermore, trials have now been established in carcinoma of breast and bladder to evaluate the therapeutic response to either BCG or C. parvum when directly infiltrated into the tumour.

The relative effectiveness of different bacterial preparations in adjuvant contact therapy has so far not been evaluated and the nature of the host responses is still poorly defined. Therefore, these two points have been investigated using transplanted rat tumours of different histological types and aetiologies. The responses observed with a series of transplanted rat tumours when tumour cells were injected in admixture with different adjuvants into normal syngeneic hosts, this being used as screening system for adjuvant contact therapy, are summarized in Table 1. In the initial studies a commercial BCG vaccine (Glaxo, percutaneous) was tested against 3-methylcholanthrene (MCA)-induced sarcomas and this was shown to be highly effective in suppressing growth of these tumours. These studies were then developed to show that BCG and the methanol extraction residue (MER) as well as C. parvum suppressed the growth of several types of tumour including carcinogen-induced and spontaneously arising sarcomas and mammary carcinomas. The main feature to be noted from these studies was that both immunogenic and non-immunogenic tumours could be suppressed when tumour cells were injected in admixture with bacterial vaccines. However, with the immunogenic tumours, e.g., MCA-induced sarcomas Mc7 and Mc40, rejection of tumour cells resulted in the development of systemic tumour immunity directed against the individually specific rejection antigens expressed upon these tumours (BALDWIN, 1973). Consequently, these animals were able to reject a subsequent challenge with cells of the same tumour as that suppressed by contact with the bacterial vaccine, but not other tumours (BALDWIN and PIMM, 1971). No such immunity could be demonstrated following adjuvant contact suppression of non-immunogenic tumours such as AAF-induced mammary carcinomas, further emphasizing that this form of treatment does not require recognition of a tumour-specific antigen.

One of the requirements in developing clinical trials of adjuvant contact immunotherapy is for suitable animal systems for comparing

TABLE 1 - *Adjuvant Contact Suppression of Transplanted Rat Tumours.*

Tumour	Immunogenicity Index [a]	No. Tumours BCG	Cells MER	Suppressed C. Parvum
SARCOMAS MCA-induced				
Mc7	5×10^6	1×10^6	1×10^6	2.5×10^5
Mc40A	5×10^6	5×10^6	NT	4×10^6
Mc57	5×10^6	5×10^6	1×10^6	1×10^6
Spontaneous				
Sp24	1×10^3	2×10^5	NT	2×10^4
Sp41	1×10^5	5×10^5	NT	NT
MAMMARY CARCINOMAS AAF-induced				
AAF57	None	2×10^4	2×10^4	5×10^3
Spontaneous				
Sp4	2×10^4	5×10^4	NT	NT
Sp15	1×10^3	1×10^3	NT	NT
Sp22	None	None	NT	NT

[a] Immunogenicity index is defined as maximum tumour cell challenge rejected in pre-immunized syngeneic rats.
[b] Tumour cells injected in admixture with bacterial vaccines into normal rats. (NT - not tested).

the relative potencies of bacterial preparations. Therefore, a screening system has been developed using two immunogenic MCA-induced sarcomas (Mc7 and Mc40A) which compares the effectiveness of adjuvants in suppressing tumour growth when injected in admixture with defined numbers of tumour cells. Data from tests with one sarcoma (Mc40A) and several BCG preparations from the Trudeau Mycobacterial collection obtained as suspensions of organisms (3 to

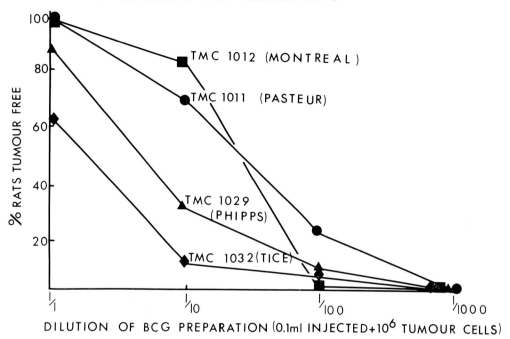

CONTACT SUPPRESSION OF SC GROWTH OF SARCOMA Mc 40A
BY DIFFERENT BCG PREPARATIONS

FIG. 1

4.5×10^8 units of single or clumped organisms/ml), are summarized
in Fig. 1. From these results, it is evident that all of the BCG preparations were effective at the highest concentration tested, although
the Montreal (TMC 1012) and Pasteur (TMC 1011) strains of BCG
were most potent. This is more clearly indicated by the data in
Table 2 comparing the dose of vaccine producing inhibition of tumour
growth in 50% of treated rats (MD.50). This shows that BCG/
TMC 1011 and TMC 1012 are 5 to 10 times more effective than the
other preparations, doses of the order of 1.2×10^6 bacterial units $/10^6$
tumour cells resulting in complete suppression of tumour growth in
50% of treated rats. The relative potencies of the various BCG preparations were similar when tested with another rat sarcoma Mc7, but

TABLE 2 - *Median Effective Dose (MD-50) of BCG for Adjuvant Contact Suppression of Sarcoma Mc40A.*

Preparation	MD-50 against sarcoma: Mc40A	
	No. units	No. organisms
BCG - TMC 1011 (Pasteur)	1.4×10^6	3×10^6
BCG - TMC 1032 (Tice)	2.0×10^7	6×10^7
BCG - TMC 1012 (Montreal)	1.2×10^6	4×10^6
BCG - TMC (1029 (Phipps)	6.3×10^6	1.9×10^7
BCG - Glaxo	6.0×10^6	2.2×10^7 *
C. parvum - Wellcome	2.3×10^7	2.3×10^7

* Count uncertain.

it has still to be established whether similar responses are obtained with other tumour types such as spontaneously arising rat sarcomas and mammary carcinomas. However, these approaches should identify, at least with rat tumours, the type and dose of bacterial vaccine which is most effective for adjuvant contact therapy, taking in consideration also the toxicity of the various preparations. Then, perhaps, by comparison with trials conducted in other species, it should be possible to develop a predictive screening programme for clinical trials. In this context it has been shown that human tumour cells growing in congenitally athymic (nude) mice can be suppressed by contact with BCG. This is illustrated in Fig. 2 showing suppression of growth of human bladder carcinoma cells (T24) in athymic mice following exposure to BCG. In this case, however, host cells, probably macrophages, from the athymic mouse are involved and the nature of the effector cells in humans remains to be identified.

Clearly there are many questions still to be resolved in adjuvant contact therapy, but if clinical trials continue to be developed, it is of paramount importance to establish screening systems for potent agents. At the present time many clinical studies simply use commercially available bacterial vaccines which often have not been

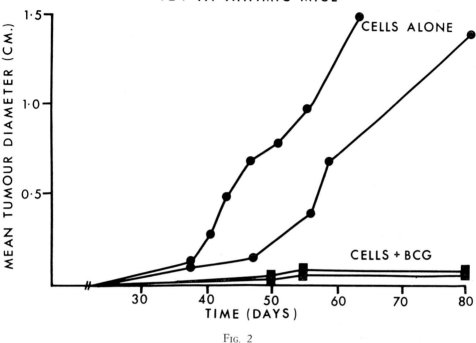

FIG. 2

evaluated in animal tumour systems and so it cannot be established that the maximum therapeutic response is produced.

Host Factors Involved in Adjuvant Contact Therapy

The host responses involved in adjuvant contact therapy are thought to involve both lymphocytes and macrophages, their relative importance varying with different tumours. In the rat tumour systems, there is evidence that lymphocyte-mediated reactions are less important, since it has been shown that BCG-mediated suppression of growth of MCA-induced sarcoma cells is just as effective in animals immunosuppressed by whole body irradiation (BALDWIN and

PIMM, 1977). Also, rat sarcomas and hepatomas in athymic (nude) mice can be completely suppressed when tumour cells are injected together with either BCG or C. parvum (PIMM and BALDWIN, 1975a, 1976a). On the other hand, there is evidence, albeit still inconclusive, implicating macrophages in adjuvant contact suppression of growth of transplanted rat tumours. Thus the growth inhibitory effect obtained when rat sarcoma or hepatoma cells are injected in admixture with either BCG or C. parvum is abrogated in recipients pretreated with a silica preparation which depletes host phagocytic cells (HOPPER et al., 1976; PIMM and BALDWIN, 1977). Also the therapeutic effect of BCG against rat tumour xenografts in athymic mice is abrogated by silica treatment of the mice (HOPPER et al., 1976). In keeping with these findings, tests with a range of rat tumours show that there is a direct correlation between the maximum number of tumour cells suppressed by contact with BCG and the degree of infiltration of the developing tumour by host macrophage (BALDWIN, 1976). For example, subcutaneous grafts of spontaneous mammary carcinoma Sp15 in syngeneic rats have relatively low degrees of infiltration of macrophages in the developing tumour, and it is not particularly susceptible to adjuvant contact therapy. Subcutaneous grafts of MCA-induced sarcomas, on the other hand, generally have a significant infiltrate of host macrophages, these cells often accounting for up to 30% of the total cellular content of the tumours, and these can be effectively controlled by contact with BCG or C. parvum (BALDWIN and PIMM, 1977). This requirement for host macrophage in adjuvant-mediated suppression of tumour growth is further illustrated by experiments showing the facilitation of BCG contact inhibition of a transplantable hepatoma D23 by syngeneic macrophages. This tumour generally shows a low infiltration of macrophages and a subcutaneous challenge with 2×10^5 tumour cells cannot be suppressed by contact with BCG. When, however, the tumour cell inoculum is supplemented by the addition of peritoneal exudate cells induced by paraffin oil injection, tumour growth was suppressed by contact with BCG. But it is notable that simply increasing the population of peritoneal cells in the tumour cell inoculum is not sufficient to inhibit tumour growth and the extra stimulus such as that provided by BCG is required.

Adjuvant Contact Therapy

Animal studies have indicated that adjuvant contact therapy can be used to treat metastatic tumour deposits as well as local tumours and this indicates, perhaps, its greatest clinical potential. Intralesional injection of bacterial vaccines may, for example, limit metastatic spread of tumours as well as retarding growth of the primary. This is illustrated by studies on a transplanted rat squamous cell carcinoma and an osteogenic sarcoma where growths of the subcutaneous tumour were only partially controlled by injecting tumour cells admixed with BCG, but nevertheless the development of lung, liver and lymph node metastases was restricted (BALDWIN and PIMM, 1973a; MOORE *et al.*, 1975). Also, with line 10 guinea pig hepatoma, injection of BCG into established intradermal tumours caused local regression and prevented the development of lymph node metastases (ZBAR *et al.*, 1972). In searching for clinically relevant animal models, a system has been developed in which tumour cells from transplanted lines of spontaneously arising mammary carcinomas are re-implanted into mammary pads of syngeneic normal female rats (GREAGER and BALDWIN, 1978). These tumours develop progressively over a period of 70 days to produce a local mammary tumour growth, which metastasizes to the regional lymph nodes and subsequently to lungs. Using this system, it has been shown that multiple intralesional injections of BCG commencing when the implanted tumour has developed to a substantial size, produced a marked inhibition of the local tumour although most of the rats still developed regional lymph node metastases (Fig. 3). An enhanced therapeutic response was obtained, however, when C. parvum was injected intralesionally and in this case, the number of rats developing regional lymph node metastases was markedly reduced.

Since bacterial vaccines contacted with tumour tissue can excite local host responses leading to tumour suppression, this approach has potential for treating metastatic foci, if the vaccines can be administered so as to localize at the site of tumour deposits. Experimentally, this type of treatment has been explored for controlling pulmonary tumours developing following intravenous injection of tumour cells and both BCG and C. parvum are effective (BALDWIN and PIMM, 1973b; BOMFORD and OLIVOTTO, 1974; PIMM and

INFLUENCE OF MULTIPLE INTRATUMOUR INJECTIONS OF BCG OR Cp ON THE GROWTH AND SPREAD OF RAT ADENOCARCINOMA SP4

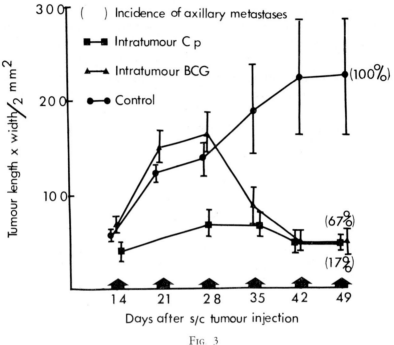

Fig. 3

BALDWIN, 1977). In the rat, for example, several types of tumour including sarcomas, mammary carcinomas and hepatomas developing in pulmonary tissue following intravenous injection of tumour cells can be completely inhibited following intravenous injection of BCG and C. parvum. Furthermore, intrapleural injection of BCG significantly modifies lung tumour growths. These findings are pertinent to current trials on the treatment of carcinoma of the lung by post-surgical instillation of BCG into the pleural space (MCKNEALLY et al., 1976. The rat tumour systems are therefore being developed essentially to compare the effectiveness of different bacterial adjuvants in this form of therapy for lung cancer and to evaluate the nature of the host responses involved.

[8] *Baldwin* - p. 10

In addition to the treatment of pulmonary metastases, intrapleural injection of bacterial vaccines might be used as an adjuvant to conventional therapy in the control of malignant effusions, particularly in the thorax and peritoneal cavity. There are, for example, several investigations showing that growth of tumour cells injected intraperitoneally can be suppressed by intraperitoneal injection of either BCG or C. parvum. (reviewed by MILAS and SCOTT, 1978). It has also been established with several rat tumours that tumour cell effusions as well as solid tumours in the pleural cavity can be controlled by intrapleural injection of BCG or the MER extract and C. parvum (PIMM and BALDWIN, 1975b; 1977). Furthermore, intrapleural BCG cell wall injections have proved effective in treating pleural sarcomas induced with 3-methylcholanthrene (YOSHIMOTO et al., 1975). These experimental investigations point to the possible value of injecting bacterial vaccines intrapleurally in treating malignant effusions. For example, phase I studies have demonstrated that intrapleural BCG can be effective against malignant effusions in primary mesothelioma of the pleura (PIMM and BALDWIN, 1976b). In this particular study, BCG preparations sterilized by γ-irradiation were used, since treatment was given as to patients with advanced disease and so where at risk for developing BCG infections. This approach was based upon experimental animal studies showing that non-viable BCG organisms were effective for suppressing pleural tumour growth (BALDWIN et al., 1974).

CONCLUSION

These studies using experimental rat tumours of defined immunological characteristics demonstrate that non-specific effects are produced by contacting bacterial adjuvants with tumour cells, leading to tumour rejection. These approaches are now being developed in a number of clinical situations, the most promising being the use of intrapleural BCG and C. parvum in the treatment of lung cancer. Future developments, particularly in the design of more effective agents with reduced toxicity, will establish whether this form of therapy has a significant place in the treatment of cancer.

REFERENCES

BALDWIN R.W., « Adv. Cancer Res. », *18*, 1 (1973).

BALDWIN R.W., « Transplant Rev. », *28*, 62 (1976).

BALDWIN R.W. and PIMM M.V., « Europ. J. Clin. Biol. Res. », *16*, 875 (1971).

BALDWIN R.W. and PIMM M.V., « Int. J. Cancer », *12*, 420 (1973a).

BALDWIN R.W. and PIMM M.V., « Brit. J. Cancer », *27*, 48 (1973b).

BALDWIN R.W. and PIMM M.V., *Immunopathology VIIth*. International Symposium, pp. 397-410. Ed. D.A. Miescher, Schwake & Co. Basel (1977).

BALDWIN R.W., COOK A.J., HOPPER D.G. and PIMM M.V., « Int. J. Cancer », *13*, 743 (1974).

BOMFORD R. and OLIVOTTO M., « Int. J. Cancer », *14*, 226 (1974).

GREAGER J.A. and BALDWIN R.W., « Cancer Res. », *38*, 69 (1978).

HOPPER D.G., PIMM M.V. and BALDWIN R.W., « Cancer Immunol. Immunother. », *1*, 143 (1976).

MASTRANGELO M.J., BERD D. and BELLET R.E., « Ann. N.Y. Acad. Sci. », *277*, 94 (1976).

MCKNEALLY M.F., MAVER C. and KAUSEL H.W., « Lancet », *i*, 377 (1976).

MILAS L. and SCOTT M.T., « Adv. Cancer Res. », In Press (1978).

MOORE M., LAWRENCE N. and NISBET N.W., « Int. J. Cancer », *15*, 897 (1975).

PIMM M.V. and BALDWIN R.W., « Nature », *254*, 77 (1975a).

PIMM M.V. and BALDWIN R.W., « Int. J. Cancer », *15*, 260 (1975b).

PIMM M.V. and BALDWIN R.W., « Brit. J. Cancer », *34*, 453 (1976a).

PIMM M.V. and BALDWIN R.W., « Clin. Oncol. », *2*, 300 (1976b).

PIMM M.V. and BALDWIN R.W., « Int. J. Cancer », In press (1977).

YOSHIMOTO T., AZUMA I., SAKATANI M., NISHIKAWA H., OGURA T., HIRGO F. and YAMAMURA Y., « Gann. », *64*, 441 (1975).

ZBAR B. and TANAKA T., « Science », *172*, 271 (1971).

ZBAR B., BERNSTEIN I.D., BARTLETT G.L., HANNA M.G. and RAPP H.J., « J. Nat. Cancer Inst. », *49*, 119 (1972).

ACKNOWLEDGEMENTS

These studies were supported by a grant from the Cancer Research Campaign and through Contract No. NO1-CB-64042 from the National Cancer Institute, National Institutes of Health, Bethesda, Maryland, U.S.A.

DISCUSSION

MATHÉ

I am very glad that you confirmed that a given preparation of BCG is not the same as another preparation of BCG, and one has to mention clearly the strain of BCG, the number of viable units and all known characteristics when publishing the results of an attempt at immunotherapy. And you confirm that Glaxo BCG is not the best. I would like to ask you if the 15 patients who had fever in your bronchus carcinoma trial did better than the patients who did not have fever. This is my first question. My second question concerns your inhibition effect by soluble antigens. Do you have the same inhibition whatever the modality of administration, or do you have it mainly by the intravenous route and would the subcutaneous route do differently?

BALDWIN

Most of the antigens have been given interperitoneally and we have monitored the distribution of antigen, and within about thirty minutes the interperitoneally injected antigen is in circulation — so that the main thing that you have got to do is to get that antigen into circulation. No, I have not looked at i.v.

ROSENBERG

You have presented a fair amount of evidence with your screen for testing BCG preparations, etc., but I did not follow whether or not that was reflecting immuno-therapeutic effects in models when the adjuvant was given after the tumor was established. Clearly it is important at this point to validate that the screen is really measuring what you want.

BALDWIN

I do not think we have got to that stage yet. We have not been doing the experiments of intralesional injection on the local tumor. I think we are mainly interested in getting tumor cells into the lung and giving the adjuvant so that it localizes in the lung.

EVA KLEIN

You have demonstrated cytotoxic lymphocytes and macrophages infiltrating the tumors, and these lymphocytes react with other tumors also. The target cells — were they cultured or could you use tumor cells from the tumor itself? Or did you have to use cultured target cells?

BALDWIN

Yes, we had to use cultured target cells. I presume you could just about generate the tumor cells as well. We could take cells from the tumor also.

KLEIN

And then the question is whether you still would have the cross-reactivity.

RAPP

I would like to reinforce Dr. Rosenberg's point. We are able to suppress tumor growths by putting in mixtures of tumor cells plus a variety of agents. We are usually injecting them in the skin, but very few of those agents will make established tumors go away. So I think we should be very cautious about extrapolating from suppression tests about the efficacy of different preparations of BCG. Did you or somebody in your lab determine the viability of each preparation?

BALDWIN

I have a slide — I did not show it to you. All these BCGs have viability counted on them — in our laboratory — we do all the viability counts — they are all compared on viable units.

RAPP

And these are all done just before you use them in the tests?

BALDWIN

That is right. I think your point, though, that — we have looked at it two ways: let's find out, comparative with BCG's, what will stop tumors from growing. The dilemma: that we are trying to get it to what I think is mimicking what the clinical protocols are asking.

TERRY

I have a comment and a question. The comment is that, in terms of your clinical interpleural trial, it would have been nice if you had elected to use the same BCG and the same dose, that McKneally used. If you had done that, we would have some very useful information for comparison as a result of your trial.

BALDWIN

I think this is the same as McKneally — that is our problem: the dose that we have given is that of McKneally's.

TERRY

Which BCG preparation have you used?

BALDWIN

We have used Glaxo BCG.

TERRY

Yes, but McKneally does not; he is using Tice BCG. That is quite different from Glaxo. Any differences you find in your trial might be due to the different BCG preparation and dose.

BALDWIN

You appreciate that there are ethical problems regarding different kinds of BCG. This is the problem.

TERRY

The question that I have concerns the apparent lack of immunogenicity of the spontaneous tumors. How far have you pushed these studies? Have you looked at other means of trying to immunize with these tumors, to determine whether or not they may be relatively poorly immunogenic but still immunogenic? Also, have you attempted to determine whether the apparent absence of immunogenicity may actually be due to the induction of suppression?

BALDWIN

Well, not the last part, but all the spontaneous tumors are evaluated by the capacity to induce immunity with repeatedly irradiated grafts, surgical resection of developing tumor, implantation of tumor cells admixed with BCG, and a whole stream of things.

TERRY

But you have not determined whether you are getting a suppressive type of response?

BALDWIN

Not in a specific sense. We have shown that animals immunized to these tumors where they do not produce immunity, will still be immunized to another tumor. But that does not quite answer the question.

OETTGEN

With reference to immune complexes in breast cancer patients, your general finding seems to be that the patients with more advanced cancer had higher levels of immune complexes than patients with early cancer. What I am not quite clear about is what good prognosis and poor prognosis mean as you use these terms. This cannot really be grouping of patients who are otherwise identical. More often than not, prognosis after surgery is determined by the extent of disease, notably the presence or lack of regional lymph node metastases. My question is whether an increase in the levels of immune complexes precedes or follows progression of the disease.

BALDWIN

These patients were all patients with primay breast cancer, and they were graded according to a number of factors, some immunological and as you say, some with a degree of lymph node involvement, hormone receptors, scanning, a whole battery of pre-clinical trials. Now, it is probably correct to say that the immune-complex level may be reflecting the extent of tumor at the time when the patients present — this will come out in the continuing of these trials — you appreciate this is a preliminary trial.

EDMUND KLEIN

In your interlesional administration, did you ever find the converse, an accentuation of metastasis? Did that ever occur?

BALDWIN

In all of the animal studies that we have carried out, interlesional injection has always slowed down metastatic spread.

KLEIN

This is of great significance for two reasons. First of all, of immediate practical importance would be to see whether this is applicable to the clinical situation and on the basis of our experience it most certainly would be, because the question of disseminating tumors during surgery

[8] *Baldwin* - p. 17

is a very real one and if what you have found is so, and people always
believe what you find in animals but they never believe what you find
in people — we found the same thing in people of course — then this
should be emphasized because this is the one practical application that so
far has come out of this meeting that is really useful for people. You can
cut down the metastasis of carcinoma of the breast, or whatever it is, by
interlesional administration of these agents. This is of enormous importance — I know it is of no importance to the laboratory, but it is of
tremendous importance to the clinic. That is number one. Number two:
there has been the hypothetical hullabaloo that if you disturb the environment of the tumor you somehow make the patient worse. Now we have
not found that, and evidently you have not found it in your animal
experiments. So I would suggest that we submit this to very thorough
dissection and discussion and if this is indeed the case, that you do not
disseminate and possibly reduce the dissemination of metastasis, that this
be projected into some sort of practical application.

BALDWIN

In fact, the very point that we are carrying out at the moment is
trial like that, because we are a little bit unhappy using transplanted
tumors. We have experiments in focus at the moment where chemically
induced sarcomas are getting interlesional injection of adjuvant prior to
surgery, to see exactly what happens to those animals.

KLEIN

I am aware of the fact that Herb Rapp and Steve Rosenberg have
a study in that area and I am sure he wishes to address himself to that.

RAPP

In the guinea pig line 10 hepatoma model, when there is a tumor
transplant in the skin and metastasis in the draining lymph nodes, a single
intralesional injection of BCG into the skin transplant reverses the growth
of the metastasis.

[8] *Baldwin* - p. 18

KLEIN

I am fully aware of that.

WEISS

Dr. Terry raises a point which I would like to support. Dr. David Naor of our laboratories in Jerusalem has been conducting studies in collaboration with Eva Klein on the immunogenicity of the YAC lymphoma in *A* mice, the strain of origin. It appears that a sensitizing exposure of YAC cells freshly obtained from a donor mouse does not afford the test animals a significant degree of heightened resistance against subsequent challenge with the corresponding tumor; in contrast, YAC cells passaged once or several times in culture are able to elicit a degree of acquired immunity when used for immunization. Analysis of this differential immunogenic behavior of YAC cells of immediate *in vivo* or *in vitro* origin has suggested that the former stimulate markedly suppressor cell activity in the host into which they are implanted, whereas the latter do not. It may be, then, that the seeming non-immunogenicity of the *in vivo*-grown tumor cells is not, in effect, a lack of immunogenic cell surface determinants, but rather a proclivity for the induction of suppressor function. This tendency may be due to the presence of added surface antigens not expressed on YAC cells grown in tissue culture, or to a unique arrangement of the same antigens, presented to the immunological apparatus in a manner conducive to the stimulation of suppressor activities; conversely, it could be that the *in vitro* cultured cells express antigen(s) sufficiently encouraging of cytotoxic immune responses to counteract or overshadow suppressor responses elicited by YAC cells regardless of their growth milieu. It is also conceivable that YAC cells grown *in vivo* and *in vitro* differ with regard to the production of modulating factors which direct responsiveness to the identical antigen(s). Whatever the explanation may be, the possibility exists that a variety of neoplasms may possess varying ability to incite suppressor cell reactions, and otherwise to modulate immunological responsiveness, as a function of the environment in which they have developed. By analogy, it is well known that the virulence and immunogenicity properties of many bacteria show large differences, depending on the immediate growth prehistory of the organisms, in the test tube or in the tissues of a host animal.

[8] *Baldwin* - p. 19

BALDWIN

In that respect many of these spontaneous tumors have been maintained in culture and have not changed their immunogenicity *in vivo.*

OETTGEN

I appreciate your recommendation that experiments with suitable tumors in animals should serve to develop guidelines for human chemoimmunotherapy trials. What disturbs me in this respect, however, is that we have had at least ten different types of BCG tested in animals for many years. Pronouncements have been made at times, on the basis of these experiments, that a particular type of BCG should be used in preference over other types. And yet the recommended BCG was either not available in sufficient amounts or, if it was available, there was no evidence in human trials that it was superior over other types. So we are still uncertain — are we not? — which BCG should be used.

BALDWIN

I think that we would like to compare BCGs in, say, one carcinoma trial, but there is no way, for local reasons, that we can do that. For example, we are limited by the responsiveness of the chest physician going into the patients and giving them the material that they are used to handling. It is a matter of confidence. These are all patients with advanced disease and we worked quite hard in the lab to show that intrapleural dead BCG was working as well as intrapleural viable BCG. And when we went to the Clinical Committee to get this approved — they were not going to have dead BCGs at any price because they were all chest physicians — they had all been used to handling BCGs, but irradiated BCG was something beyond their experience and so they were much happier administering viable organisms.

MATHÉ

An intrapleural BCG immunotherapy trial conducted in Great Britain has given negative results, contrary to McKneally's trial. This may be a clinical confirmation that some BCG preparations are effective while others are not.

[8] *Baldwin* - p. 20

BALDWIN

I would have thought that is the logical way to approach it. People are going to have local restrictions, but after a number of years there are going to be data from several trials and they should indicate which is the best of all BCG preparations.

RAPP

One way out of this dilemma might be to use BCG cell walls in oil droplets because certain Mycobacteria which are not active even when they are live, are active when dead and in combination with oil droplets. The use of such vaccines would eliminate the possibility of BCG infection.

BALDWIN

We have used the same preparation from Dr. Levy intrapleurally and it worked, and I am certain that we would have exactly the same local problems if we tried to substitute these preparations. Of course these are problems for private investigation, but this seems to be compounded at the moment by national clinical trials being set up by committees who are going to use the safest BCG.

OETTGEN

I would like to comment once more on the lung cancer trials. I do not think the non-clinicians around this table should be left with the impression that clinical trials are comparable to experiments with the same inbred strain of mice and the same tumor done in different laboratories. There are serious questions with regard to the comparability of the staging used by different groups, depending as it does on surgical technique and aggressiveness. It is not quite as easy as saying: Let us ask lung surgeons in the Unted States and in England and in France to treat Stage 1 lung cancer in a certain way and see what comes out. It is more complex than that.

APPROACHES TO «NONSPECIFIC» IMMUNOTHERAPY OF CANCER WITH MICROBIAL IMMUNOMODULATORS

DAVID W. WEISS

Lautenberg Center for General and Tumor Immunology, Hebrew University
Hadassah Medical School, Jerusalem

Rather than present a detailed account of our recent findings with the MER tubercle bacilli fraction, as was indicated in the program, I intend to devote a major part of this talk to a delineation of the areas of nonspecificity and specificity within which microbial immunomodulators exert their effects on host resistance against progressive neoplasia.

I take this occasion to classify and describe the domains of nonspecificity and specificity as such, not as an exercise in taxonomy for its own sake, but rather because I believe there is a substantive need for functional categorization of the phenomena which we attempt to master. Specific and nonspecific compartments of immunological responses interact, overlap, lead to one another sequentially, and bring into play as well a variety of nonimmunological reactions, peripherally and sometimes as the dominant elements. Unless we can define, or at least delimit, the distinct components of immunological defenses that participate in host-tumor associations and which we seek to direct towards therapeutic ends, we shall be

This manuscript was prepared while the author was aguest in the laboratories of Drs. JAMES HOLLAND and GEORGE BEKESI of Mt. Sinai Hospital and Medical School in New York City, as Visiting Professor of Neoplastic Diseases. The hospitality of his hosts is acknowledged with the greatest appreciation.

[9] *Weiss* - p. 1

likely to misinterpret events in which we intervene and to miss opportunities. I believe, therefore, that this conference should go not only to a review of old data and the tabling of new, but also to a grouping of the phenomena which will aid their eventual analysis. It is an inescapable caveat that the processes of ideation, including certainly the design of experiments and the reading of results, are set in a semantic matrix; if the placement and terminology of observed occurrences is casual, so may be both our comprehension and level of control.

What, then, are the loci of immunomodulator (or, simply, "modulator", or "adjuvant") action in the heightening of anti-tumor resistance?

Loci of action of microbial immunomodulators in anti-tumor immune responses

The following schema of effects is suggested; only a few selected references, largely to our prior work with MER, are cited to illustrate and document some of the arguments advanced:

1. *Nonspecific Potentiation of Specific Responsiveness to Tumor Associated Transplantation Antigens (TATA)*

This class of effects elicited by immunomodulators on host resistance to neoplastic cells is the one that has been considered the most commonly manifested and important, and it is the one that appears most closely related in mechanisms to classical adjuvant behavior. Ability to respond to specific antigenic stimulation by synthesis of antibodies or formation of sensitized effector cells is heightened, or skewed in one direction or another, by the modulating substance. The nature of the effects thus lies with a nonspecific magnification or deviation of specific immunological reactions; in many instances, these would have been possible, at least potentially, even in the absence of the excipient agent, but to a lesser extent or in other avenues. Several distinct possibilities of action can be entertained; these may take place simultaneously or consecutively in a given immunological response.

[9] *Weiss* - p. 2

For one, the immunomodulator may alter the structure and topography, and thereby the degree and kind of immunogenicity, of cell membrane antigens. A variety of eventualities can be envisaged: simple adsorption to, or chemical interaction with, antigenic sites, leading to true or pseudo-haptenization; insertion into complex macromolecular or polymolecular determinants; deletion and substitution of reactive groups; and others bringing about changes in the make-up, configuration, and charge of TATA. The altered antigenic entity may thus become a more potent immunogen, quantitatively, or one able to steer immunological responses in other pathways. New carrier-hapten and helper circumstances may have been created; tolerance may be broken towards the corresponding native configurations; and, new equilibria of activating and suppressing reactions may have been initiated. The common denominator of all these events is modification of the sensitizing antigen itself. Once triggered into being, the new or turned immunological reactions evoked may be perpetuated by, and expressed against, the unmodified antigen as well.

Second, modulators impinge on the maturation, differentiation, and replication of immunocytes and their precursors and affect the functionality of the mature end cells, directly [1] or via influence on other cell types. Many investigators have observed profound impacts by mycobacterial and other microbial adjuvants on antibody formation, the generation of cytotoxic lymphocytes, and a spectrum of macrophage functions even when the agents have been introduced *in vitro* to immunologically reactive tissue or to isolated immunocyte populations [2-4]. For at least some adjuvants, effects on lympho-reticular cells themselves appear to be the main modality of immunoregulation.

In certain instances, such central mechanisms of action can be explained largely or solely by a stimulated proliferation of reactive cells. The expansion of lymphocytes and macrophages may be general, providing the organism with an enlarged equipment of potentially responding units, including clones specifically programmed for the antigens in question. A more selective enlargement of the numbers of *specifically* responding cells can also be entertained, and is suggested by experiments in which modulators have been seen to potentiate the synthesis of specific antibodies and the generation of cytotoxic effector cells *in vitro* at dosages orders of magnitude below the threshold of polyclonal mitogenicity [2-6]. Discriminative clonal expansion could conceivably comprise both lymphocytes with the appropriate receptors for antigen, and macrophages carrying antibody or Ir gene products serving as specific receptors. Deletion of suppressor cells, generally reactive or specific for a given antigen, may accompany the positive stimulation of responding clones [3] and contribute to the increment in responsiveness.

Alternatively, the mode of action may involve *qualitative* changes in lymphoid and macrophage immunological functions — lymphoid cells altered in their receptivity to antigenic stimulation and in their faculties as helper, suppressor, and effector cells for specific humoral and cellular responses, macrophages in their participating roles in antibody formation and the development of lymphocyte-effected cellular immunity, and in their own capacity as specifically armed attacking cells. The alterations brought about by any one modulator in immunocyte morphology and physiology may involve more than one family of cells. The molecular bases of such qualitative alterations, and their relation to changed immunological function, remain to be clarified; different mechanisms have been postulated [viz., 7], and it seems probable that they are induced and expressed at different molecular loci in the affected cells. Thus, for example, the MER mycobacterial fraction raises markedly both the activity of macrophage lysozomal enzymes [8] and the responsiveness of lymphocytes to mitogenic stimuli [9]. Within the interlocking mesh of forward and reverse responses which makes up immunological function, departures from norms at one location are likely, moreover, to lead to chain-reactions of divergence.

Third, immunomodulators affect the circumstances of specific sensitization in a variety of ways. The one longest recognized and exploited in general immunology is the prolonged maintenance of antigen in tissues, the depot effect. Clearly one of the bases of action of such diverse modulators as Freund's adjuvant and alum (in precipitated bacterial toxoids, for instance), depot effects may also be entailed in heightened immunological reactivity to tumor cells. Even if introduced to the host at sites removed from neo-

[9] *Weiss* - p. 4

plastic foci, and before or after these develop or are implanted, modulators may eventually come into intimate contact with intact tumor cells or their antigenic moieties, and mediate storage effects. These can occasion delays in degradation and clearance of TATA from tissues, and facilitate an ongoing, immunologically opportune release of antigens and thereby a perpetuated responsiveness.

Depot action may subsume more than the creation of relatively inert barriers surrounding deposits of antigen, and delaying their disruption and breakdown by host factors. More complicated inter-actions between antigen, adjuvant, and host tissues have been pos-tulated, and these may pertain to deviant cells with new antigenicities as well as to soluble antigens. One example is the facilitated seques-tration, or "trapping", of antigenic entities by networks of lymphoid and macrophagic cells in lymph nodes or spleen [10], and perhaps also throughout the tissues where immunocytes accumulate and confront neoplastic invasion.

Other circumstances augmenting such mechanical effects may be brought into being in the course of depot establishment, and as additional, independent mechanisms. For instance, many adjuvants are irritants, and the inflammatory and other responses which they provoke can produce new microenvironments in which the handling of antigen is altered and to which immunocytes may be attracted, perhaps with a preference of cell types that can mount immunological reactions more felicitous for host resistance than would otherwise be the case. Where the modulator is itself immunogenic, immuno-logical responses directed against it may participate in the formation of novel tissue microenvironments.

2. Nonspecific "Spill-Over" of Potentiated Specific Responsiveness to TATA

Nonspecific magnification by immunomodulators of specific immunological reactivity to TATA is manifested both specifically, against the antigens which incited sensitization, and generally. Antigen-reactive lymphoid cells, both B and T, liberate an array of soluble substances upon interaction with the provoking antigen. These lymphokines amplify immunological responses and extend them nonspecifically. Target cells can be injured not only by contact with matching immunocytes, but also by the released substances; the mediators of cellular immunity indeed play a larger role at times as effectors of the reactions than do the sensitized cells themselves. The soluble agents have a diverse bearing on host resistance: They attract, immobilize, and nonspecifically activate immunocytes, and may also effect recruitment to specific reactivity; some are directly and nonselectively toxic for transformed cells; and, some cause changes in tissue microenvironment of immediate or secondary consequences for the afferent and efferent arcs of immunological reactivity, and for tumor cell survival. Lymphokine activity is thus expressed by an enlargement of initially specific immunological reactions, and also by an extension of these in directions wholly nonspecific, except for an apparent discrimination by activated cells and some of their products between normal and neoplastic targets.

Macrophages, too, liberate upon certain forms of stimulation soluble factors with activities similar to those of lymphokines [11]. Macrophages passively armed for specific reactivity against TATA may be especially apt to secrete such factors, as well as to undergo excitation to nonspecific anti-tumor cytotoxic behavior, at contact with the antigens for which they were armed at the outset [12, 13]. Certain lymphoid cells also take on nonspecific cytotoxic propensities for neoplastic variants following an initial interaction with TATA for which they were programmed and ensuing blast transformation.

These manifold activities are in effect a "spill-over", broadly, of the interactions between specifically sensitized or specifically armed immunocytes and their neoplastic targets. The classes of immunocytes involved in such an overflow from reactions initially specific may have to be broadened to include non-T lymphocytes which effect antibody-dependent cell-mediated cytotoxicity. These cells (and perhaps NK cells, too) may secrete soluble mediators upon reaction with their targets. In potentiating and shifting specific immunological responsiveness, immunomodulators thus also broaden appreciably the compartment of secondary, nonspecific effects which follow cell-mediated immunological events.

Nonspecific potentiation of the production of free TATA-specific antibodies is of significance not only with regard to the arming of otherwise quiescent immunocytes. It might perhaps also lead to a generalized amplification of defenses involving mediators of humoral hypersensitivity, released in consequence of antigen-antibody interactions and the direct impact on tissues of antigen-antibody complexes. Little attention has been given the possibility that this category of mediators, and complexes, can act positively in anti-tumor defenses, consideration having been focused on their immunopathological and blocking activities. It is not inconceivable, however, that changes in tissue environment caused by these factors in the vicinity of tumor foci, and even systemically, can also prove inimical to progressive tumor development [14].

The creation, in the wake of anti-TATA reactions and their potentiation, of tissue conditions affecting tumor growth has components patently non-immunological in nature. For instance, processes of containment and healing of inflammations that originated in immunological events have implications for the fate of neoplastic cells in the affected localities. Infiltration of fibroblasts and deposition of fibrin and other substances accompanying the repair of inflammation may serve to restrict mechanically the spread of invasive clones, or conversely, to provide nutrients for their growth and physical surfaces for their malignant deportment [15].

3. Nonspecific Potentiation of Specific Immunological Reactions Against Antigens Other than TATA

The production of some lymphokines and related substances, the creation of tumor-hostile tissue environs, and the transformation of specifically reactive immunocytes to nonspecific tumor cytotoxicity could all be heightened not only by the potentiation of anti-TATA responses, but also by magnified and broadened immunological reactivity in general. It is difficult to evaluate *in vivo* the relative importance to anti-tumor defenses of modulator-potentiated responsiveness to antigens other than TATA or, for that matter, of the nonspecific extension of magnified reactivity to TATA themselves. Both these classes of transaction could well play a larger role in resistance than may appear at first sight. A multitude of immunological reactions take place constantly in the tissues of every organism, against

a plethora of antigens (among which there are undoubtedly represented microbial moieties cross-reactive with TATA). Introduction
of extrinsic immuno-modulating agents to the animal can be an
antigenic stimulus in itself, as well as affect background reactions
and those which are the object of the intended intervention. It may
be the nonspecific consequences of the incidental immunological
events, now potentiated, which ultimately bring about heightened
refractoriness to a tumor, as much as the modulated specific responsiveness to TATA and consequent spill-over.

In a still wider context, it has been suggested that intact immunological functionality may be requisite for optimally effective chemotherapeutic intervention [16]. This condition may imply more
than a mere summation of different modalities of anti-tumor action.
For instance, immunological responses against haptenic drugs may
influence directly their distribution and maintenance in the organism
and the degree of their toxicity. Reactive immunocytes and their
soluble products may also alter the activities of microsomal and
other enzymes involved in drug metabolism. Other modes of interaction can be envisaged for the recorded additive, synergistic, and
antagonistic effects of cojoint treatment of malignant diseases by
chemotherapeutic and nonspecific immunological means [17, 18].

The consequences of immunopotentiation very likely find expression at many of the frontiers of host defense against neoplasia,
and enter into many aspects of the total management of malignant
disease. Not only chemoimmunotherapy, but also combined schedules
of radiation therapy and immunological intervention have been
shown to be of greater efficacy than either modality alone [19].
Healing after surgery and after exposure to ionizing irradiation is
probably facilitated by immunocyte activities, as may be resistance
to unrelated neoplastic variants appearing in body areas where local
immunological function has been compromised by radiation or concentrated chemotherapy. Immunological capability is clearly a decisive element in resistance to infections secondary to progressive
cancer and leukemia and their treatment, and the protection "incidentally" bestowed against threatening infectious episodes by immunomodulators may be of major import.

[9] *Weiss* - p. 8

4. *Antigenic Cross-Reactivity Between Microbial Immunomodulators and Tumor Cells*

Evidence has accrued in recent years for a prevalent cross-reactivity between a variety of microbial antigens and TATA [20, 21]. The phylogenetic and evolutionary implications of these findings may be large, but a cohesive picture of their meaning has not yet emerged. Of imminent interest to us is the eventuality that some of the activities of microbial "adjuvants" do not, in fact, originate with nonspecific modulation and potentiation of specific responsiveness, but rather with a *de facto* immunization and hyperimmunization against related antigens.

Whereas it is doubtful that cross-reactivites between supposed nonspecific modulator and specific target antigen can explain all or most of the activities of such microbial compounds, the degree of their contribution to immunological responsiveness is still to be ascertained. The possibility cannot be ignored that microbial materials are presented to the immunological apparatus in a uniquely immunogenic state, and that the specific immunization thus effected by determinants cross-reactive with TATA is far more powerful than for the same markers located on the tumor cell surface.

5. *Direct Nonspecific Activation of Immunocytes and its Nonspecific Consequences*

Substances with nonspecific immunomodulator properties may be capable not anly of abetting the development of specific immunological responses to TATA and other antigens, but also of bestowing on lymphoid and macrophagic cells directly and nonspecifically the capacity to inhibit or destroy neoplastic variants. All immunocytes may be so affected, including NK cells [22] and perhaps also lymphocytes with seemingly "promiscuous" cytotoxic tendencies [23].

Such effects must be considered apart from the potentiated participation of immunocytes in specific reactions triggered by antigen, and in their spill-over, although the responsible mechanisms may be related. Thus, the mitogenicity of modulators and their effects on membrane characteristics, enzymology, and other functions of immunologically competent cells may express themselves in new capabilities of the cells *both* to take part in specific immunological events [e.g., 24], *and* to cause damage straightforwardly to neoplastic tissue, with little limitation of specificity, by contact or by mediator release. A case in point is the nonspecific excitation of macrophages to tumor cytotoxicity by macrophage activating factors (MAF) liberated from lymphoid cells by various stimuli [13], among which direct exposure to modulators is one. For instance, recent work by RUTH GALLILY in our laboratories [25] suggests that the excitation by MER of nonspecific macrophage cytotoxicity for tumor cells, and of heightened capability to deal with bacterial pathogens [26], is mediated by soluble T-lymphocyte products released upon contact of the cells with the fraction. Other reported observations on immunomodulator activities lend themselves to similar interpretation: a mobilization of indifferent immunocytes to generalized antitumor contact reactivity and to the freeing of substances which affect tumor cell growth and survival diffusely, without the involvement of sensitizing antigen, antibody, or specific effector cell receptors.

Another, intriguing possibility of mechanism that has come under scrutiny is the production or release by immunocytes (upon stimulation?) of factors that can reverse the neoplastic characteristics of transformed cell variants, and in this manner impede the further progression of a neoplastic process [27].

6. *Non-Immunological Loci of Action of Substances with Immunomodulator Properties*

The unifying feature of the multifaceted activities of immunomodulators discussed so far is that the effects are exerted on immunocytes, or are mediated, amplified, and extended by them and their soluble products. The boundaries between "immunological" and "pharmacological" reactions are axceedingly uncertain, and it is obvious that the effector arms of many types of interaction between specifically sensitized effector cells and antibodies on the one hand, and their corresponding targets on the other, are truly pharmacological in nature, and may lack all specificity. Nonetheless, phenomena brought into being through influences *on immunocytes* or actions exerted *by immunocytes* may be termed, at least for the sake of convenient classification, as immunological. Many of the categories of immunomodulator action undoubtedly fall within the scope of such a liberal definition. It must be considered, however, that the same agents that are capable of acting via the pivot of immunologically reactive tissue may also elicit primary effects on cells and tissues wholly unrelated to the lymphoreticular system. Microsomal enzyme function of pertinence to drug metabolism, for example, may be modified not only indirectly by modulators hitting at lymphocytes and macrophages which then transmit effect to other cells, but also by the immediate action of the agents. Or, the irritant properties of many adjuvants can provoke inflammatory responses directly, and tumor cells may suffer injury as "innocent bystanders" of inflammatory and other developments that evolve with little or no dependence on potentiated immunocyte participation.

Non-immunological lines of action may be initiated even by modulators of defined structure and recognized influence on specified cellular and molecular loci of immunologically reactive cells; the same or similar alterations in cell morphology and physiology may be manifested by both immunocytes and by unrelated cell types. This is still more likely to be true for complex, undefined microbial moieties, whose distinct components may each cause separate effects, on different tissue systems. The fact that our attention is given to events played out on, or by, immunocytes must not obscure the simultaneous occurrence of profound changes in other cells and their ultimate translation into altered states of host resistance.

7. Summation

I have found it difficult to essay this classification of microbial immunomodulator activities, perhaps not surprisingly. The primary loci and molecular bases of their influence on immunological capacity and host resistance to neoplastic cells remain largely tenuous and speculative, and discrimination in the dark is an undertaking doomed to imprecision. The attempt seems to be obligatory, nonetheless. Clarification and management of the complex phenomena before us is dependent on recognition of at least the outlines of their diversity and distinctiveness, even though the distinguishing features are still hazy.   The ordering of effects in nature is often as much a condition as a corollary of their understanding.   Arragement and analysis are reciprocal undertakings, furthering each other, and each demanding even efforts that can only be partial at a given moment.

Several aspects of this tentative organization of modulator action are already apparent.

Reactions that are distinct in origin, scope, and prominence for host resistance nevertheless share common mechanisms.   The classification of effects must therefore take into account not only the modes of action, but also their orientation within the total scheme of host-tumor confrontations.

Some of the parameters and modalities of immunomodulator influence on host resistance to tumors are identical with those characteristic of classical adjuvant effects on immunological responsiveness; others are different, and it is necessary, accordingly, to consider independently the dimension of nonspecific modulation in different contexts.

Our discussion has been concerned largely with the positive effects of immunomodulators on host defenses against tumors. It is evident, however, that nonspecific manipulations can also have adverse results for immunological capability and states of resistance. Host defenses may be injured by the general diminution of immunological responsiveness which immunomodulators effect not infrequently, or by a steering of anti-TATA reactions away from the formation of cytotoxic elements, or by events otherwise inimical to resistance produced at one of the many loci of action of substances with modulator properties.   The negative impact of such agents may reflect distortions of the same mechanisms that, under optimal conditions, potentiate refractoriness to neoplastic development; or, it may be caused by distinct modalities unrelated to those of favorable consequence.   The numerous manifestations of modulator influence on the immunological apparatus must be viewed as a concatenation of immunological happenings of which some are beneficial, others indifferent, and still others potentially deleterious to the survival of a challenged organism.   Much further insight into immunological behavior and the potentialities of nonspecific immunomodulation is required before the complex and interlocking phenomena of immunological responsiveness can be sorted out, as to mechanism and as to import for host defenses. A step in this direction which *is* within our means is the quantification of immunological and immune responses which are affected by standardized agents in standardized test models and in carefully designed and controlled clinical trials [28, 29]. A major advantage of the MER mycobacterial fraction over other immunomodulators under scrutiny today is that this adjuvant lends itself to such standardization.

It must also be noted that much of what has been said here for the activities of immunomodulators of microbial origin also applies to other substances that enter nonspecifically into immunological and resistance functions. For all such agents, the qualification stands that not all their effect on host defenses are evoked via immunological pathways, but rather that their multifaceted influence is often mediated and realized by a variety of tissue systems.

ADVANTAGES INHERENT TO THE NONSPECIFIC APPROACH TO TUMOR IMMUNOTHERAPY

At this still preliminary stage in our efforts to develop immunological means of therapeutic intervention in malignant diseases, the data available, especially that coming from controlled clinical investigations, does not offer clear indication of whether specific or nonspecific approaches are likely to be most advantageous. Certainly, the clinical studies reported so far have been overwhelmingly with nonspecific immunomodulators, such as living BCG, MER, and *C. parvum*. As has emerged forcefully from this and from other recent meetings devoted to tumor immunotherapy [30], the clinical benefits attained have been very limited, however. This could be due more to unsatisfactory design and conduct of the studies than to intrinsic limitations of the agents employed [31], but the fact remains that there has been little solid ground for enthusiasm so far regarding the efficacy of nonspecific immunotherapy of cancer. On the other hand, some of the investigations conducted in patients in the realm of specific tumor immunization have yielded results no less impressive than the best obtained by nonspecific intervention.

D.A.L. Davies has presented some such data at this conference, and
as one other example, the work of Bekesi et al should be cited:
treatment of acute myelocytic leukemia (AML) patients with neuraminidase-modified AML blast cells seems to lead to a prolongation
of first remission and of patient survival at least as convincing as
anything achieved in this or other malignant disease by nonspecific
adjuvant treatment [32], and perhaps more so.

Animal experimentation, too, has been largely focused on the
nonspecific option, but some of the findings coming from various
programs of specific TATA hyperimmunization have been no less
striking than the accomplishments of nonspecific treatments. The
assumptions that underlie immunization of tumor hosts with chemically, enzymatically, or virally modified neoplastic cells have a
sober rooting in basic immunology, even in light of the probability
that the tumor-associated immunogenicity of spontaneously appearing neoplasms is minimal [33].

It is pertinent to question, therefore, whether emphasis should
now be given to further explorations along nonspecific or specific
avenues of immunological stimulation of tumor hosts. It may well
be that both types of modalities need be utilized to obtain maximum
therapeutic benefits in certain circumstances (*), and there is surely
reason to pursue research in both directions. Nontheless, a policy
assessment would be helpful at this time, and a conference dedicated
to a discussion of nonspecific immunity in the prevention and treatment of cancer should serve as an occasion for reflection of whether
this strategy holds inherent advantages. I personally believe that
it does, and I would like to summarize some of the arguments in
support of this belief.

1. Specific immunotherapy entails formidable technical difficulties that are not encountered by nonspecific approaches. Salient
among these obstacles are the ones encountered in the preparation
of TATA vaccines.

Tumor tissue is often unavailable from the autochthonous pa-

(*) The opposite eventuality, of negative consequences accruing from mixed
immunological intervention cannot be ignored; indications of such conflict have
been recorded [37].

tient, or available in amounts too small to permit the making of sufficient quantities of vaccine. Autochthonous tumor cells may be requisite, however, where cross-reactivity between TATA of histologically related neoplasms is weak or absent. Moreover, the relevant antigens may be unstable. Manipulations assuring complete inactivation of living tumor cells and of any oncogenic agents that may be present are also likely to degrade the antigens; introduction of vaccines not fully inactivated is a dubious procedure at best, for patients in remission, and is precluded for healthy individuals who might otherwise serve as donors of effector cells or antibodies in passive/adoptive intervention. And, even if inactivation can be accomplished without degeneration of TATA immunogenicity, the introduction of antigenic neoplastic tissue to the patient is accompanied by the dangers of receptor blocking of cytotoxic effector cells, formation of blocking antigen-antibody complexes, stimulation of specific suppressor cell reactivity, and induction of other deviations from immune competence.

The pitfalls of induced departure from optimal immune function exist for active nonspecific as well as for active specific immunotherapy, but they appear less predictable and less controllable in the case of the latter, where individualized vaccines may have to be used for each patient. It could also be argued that nonspecific immunomodulation has a margin of safety accruing from evolutionary circumstances: Higher organisms are in contact ubiquitously with immunomodulators of microbial derivation, and it is not unreasonable to assume that the immunological mechanism is so adapted to their presence that reactivity will not be compromised against threatening pathogens which, too, are encountered frequently — microorganisms and neoplastic variants — and will not be directed readily against normal self components.

It might be anticipated, indeed, that receptivity to microbial immunomodulators has evolved in such a manner as to assure ongoing protection against microbial disease and incipient neoplasia. Therapeutic employment of such agents may thus represent exploitation of a prevalent defense system in nature. That it is really possible to harm immunological and immune capacity by the artificial introduction of microbial adjuvants is common experience, and dosage, route, and other parameters of their administration demand careful titration. Nonetheless, there may well be an edge of advantage to nonspecific immunomodulation, residing in the natural circumstance, that does not exist for specific TATA immunization. Organisms do not usually have to cope with large numbers of neoplastic cells until late in life, and certainly not under conditions by which tumor tissue may have to be presented to evoke hypersensitization. It is improbable that there have developed evolutionary safeguards for the immunological handling of massive amounts of TATA characteristic of neoplasms that become apparent only late in ontogeny, or are infrequent in populations [33]. It cannot be taken for granted, therefore, that any evolutionary adaptations for dealing immunologically with microscopic, nascent tumor foci furnish as well assurances for "appropriate" immunological responses to specific tumor immunotherapy.

Furthermore, the availability of highly stable, standardized preparations of nonspecific immunomodulators not only affords a major technical advantage in its own right, but also opens manifold possibilities of "thematic variation". Isolation and identification of the active components will permit chemical manipulations designed to produce units whose activities may be far superior than those of the starting material. Elegant, albeit still limited, demonstrations of the feasibility of such overtures are seen in the recent studies of CHEDID, here reported, and of RIBI and coworkers [34].

2. The range of effects elicited by a nonspecific lifting of the baseline of immunological responsiveness is wide, and such breadth of activity may be indispensable for effective intervention in malignant disease. It has been shown that tumor cells in metastatic aggregates may express TATA differently than do cells in the original growth; and, such differences may be individual for each metastatic lesion [35, 36]. Immunological control of disseminated disease cannot be essayed, therefore, by specific hypervaccination with preparations of TATA indigenous to only some of many tumor masses Nonspecific immunostimulation, on the other hand, could provide a broad umbrella of heightened reactivity against many of the tumor associated antigenic configurations. The same protective umbrella could extend to elevation of resistance against multiple

primary neoplasms, and against the ever-present, life-threatening hazard of infection in patients debilitated by neoplastic disease and its treatment. Indeed, many of the nonspecific agents now under investigation for cancer immunotherapeutic potency have been shown capable of bestowing marked, nonspecific protection to experimental animals against microbial pathogens, and such activities are now also being recorded in cancer patients [37].

There is the hope, moreover, that combined stimulation of a tumor bearing organism with nonspecific immunomodulators and with the specific TATA, presented spontaneously in the course of the disease or administered as specific vaccine, may leave the host with greater specific resistance to recurrent growth of residual tumor foci than does stimulation by only specific or only nonspecific means. Such observations have been reported from animal models [38]. Nonspecific immunotherapy could thus be seen as providing, if nothing more, an increment in the state of immunity devolving on an animal that has managed to keep an initial outbreak of neoplastic proliferation in check.

3. Our attention has been given in this discussion to the therapeutic aspects of nonspecific immunomodulation. It is apparent that the potentialities of this approach exist also for the prevention of future neoplastic disease in still healthy individuals, and indeed the magnitude of nonspecific immunoprophylactic effects often attainable in many animal test models is generally greater than that achieved in the therapy of already established neoplasms [39, 40].

If some of the nonspecific immunomodulators now employed in tumor immunotherapy will be found moderately effective and safe, their eventual application to prophylaxis in normal individuals at a high risk of subsequent neoplastic disease becomes feasible [33]. A variety of circumstances — family history, age, habitual smoking, industrial exposure, and other variables — contribute to the designation of high risk. If the human organism responds to nonspecific immunomodulators in a manner analogous to that of a variety of experimental animals, intervention prior to the emergence of frank neoplasia might prove highly effective in delaying its eventual onset and in reducing its incidence. Such immunoprophylactic steps might be especially relevant in subjects with idiosyncrasies of immunological capacity indicative of inadequate native capacity to inhibit neoplastic variants, or of special receptivity to nonspecific immunopotentiation [33].

It is difficult, in contrast, to imagine the development of specific prophylactic intervention. Unless there can be established the existence of prevalently cross-reactive determinants expressed by many of the most common tumors, it is not given to offer specific immunization against an eventual neoplasm of unknown type. Moreover, the "minimal hypothesis" to which we must now retreat, that spontaneous neoplasms may be commonly of very poor or even inapparent immunogenicity, and that the task of the immunologist lies with the magnification of responses that would otherwise not be mounted or would remain below the threshhold of efficacy, prejudices strongly attempts at specific prophylatic intervention.

4. The host of a progressively developing neoplasm is evidently an organism that has failed to mount efficacious defenses against the challenging cells. Although this fact does not necessarily vitiate attempts to increase responsiveness by specific immunization with modified tumor tissue, to break states of tolerance, or to close escape routes of the tumor cells from immunological attack, all such efforts are undertaken against the gradient of demonstrated immune failure. Similarly, the normal individual standing at high risk of later neoplastic disease may also be one with smoldering immunological dyscrasia. It may be more opportune, therefore, to seek means of a basic rehabilitation of immunological strength, by nonspecific stimulation, than to try correction of the deficiencies by still more presentation of antigen, albeit in altered and more potent form.

OUR RECENT STUDIES WITH THE MER
MYCOBACTERIAL IMMUNOSTIMULATOR

The MER tubercle bacillus fraction is a nonliving, very stable, standardized entity whose profound differential influences on immunological function and on resistance have been studied and reported for nearly twenty-five years [41, 42]. Virtually every known arm of immunological responses comes under the influence of the agent, in a variety of test animals, and apparently also in patients [28, 40], and the immunoprophylactic and immunotherapeutic potency of MER is considerable [39, 40]. The agent has proven well tolerated at dosages at which it is efficacious, even when administered system- ically [43, 44]; and, in the many tumor immunotherapy models in which it has been investigated, enhancement of tumor growth has not been found to occur when treatment is in combination schedules with chemo- or radio-therapy. Although we have considered MER essentially as a model of immunomodulation with a nonliving mi- crobial derivative, it appears to be of interest in its own right in the therapy of human malignant disease [45, 46].

MER is, incontrovertibly, an agent from the "Dreckapotheke", as my colleagues Otto Westphal and Herbert Fischer have been quick to point out, and at a time when the emphasis in immunology is, very rightly, on analysis of the relations of structure to function, it may be an anachronism. Nonetheless, it seems that until the present moment none of the chemically characterized microbial fractions that have been obtained show equivalent activity in tumor protection systems. The sophistication of the chemist has not been matched so far by biological felicity, certainly not as yet on the clinical level. While I join my more sophisticated colleagues in the enthusiastic search for simpler, defined substances with powerful activity not only in the classical adjuvant sense but in the elicitation of protection against progressive neoplasia, I continue to view work with the crude MER moiety — and it is, after all, considerably less capricious a material than living BCG or intact C. parvum — as increasing our stock of information on the aptitudes of nonspecific immunotherapy and immunoprophylaxis.

In the verbal presentation of this topic, I described two new areas of work conducted in our laboratories with MER. These findings are now in press and will be published prior to appearance of this manuscript; accordingly, I shall here only summarize very briefly the data to which I referred in my talk.

1. *The Question of Local or Regional vs. Distal Immunotherapy with Microbial Immunomodulators*

Some investigators have, in the past, taken a rather doctrinaire position on the need of introducing microbial adjuvants directly into a tumor focus, or closely adjacent to it. An eloquent proponent of this persuasion, Herbert Rapp, is present at this conference, and has stated the credo with fervor. Other workers, including myself, have argued against the validity of this restricted view.

It is no doubt true that intralesional/regional adjuvant administration is the condition of efficacy for certain agents *against certain* tumors. It is equally apparent that the same and other agents are effective even when introduced at sites removed from the direct lymphatic drainage zone of a malignant growth; and, the ability to intervene with nonspecific immunodulators in disseminated neoplasia of hemopoietic tissue certainly contradicts the doctrine that by regional administration and regional administration alone is salvation of the organism achieved. Most disturbing to me in the creed of the regionalists is the implication that those animal tumors which can, in effect, be cured only by regional adjuvant administration are *the* models of neoplasia in man. The tenacity of the faith is astounding. The charismatic example of intralesional orthodoxy is the model of Line 10 hepatomas in Strain 2 guinea pigs, and one must ask: Can it really be held that a subcutaneous implant of a venerably ancient hepatoma, induced in the laboratory with a chemical carcinogen, having undergone hundreds of transplantation transmigrations, and now being tested in remote descendants of the line of animals in which the tumor first arose — that all this constitutes a reasonable fascimile of primary liver neoplasia in a human being?

Yet, I have no intention here to tempt the faithful with a phantasmagoria of monstrous cold reflection. Rather, I come in the spirit of ecumenicism, not as *defensor fides* but as *defensor pacis* of compromise. Not that I have embarked on the road to Canossa; the distance from Jerusalem to Rome is sufficient for me. But I do wish to bring glad tidings to Dr. Rapp and his disciples, by qualifying my own previous stand on the intralesional heresy.

I had held that MER, perhaps more than some other such

agents, tends to be effective, against tumors susceptible to any kind of nonspecific immunoprophylaxis or immunotherapy, when administered by routes other than intralesional or immediately adjacent to a malignant growth.   Even in the guinea pig - hepatoma model, prophylactic injection of the fraction as early as 180 days prior to challenge implantation, and at a site contralateral to that of the eventual tumor isograft, offers solid protection to approximately half the animals [47].   In inbred mice challenged with mammary carcinoma isografts, the limited help that could be bestowed with MER was greater when treatment was at subcutaneous sites far removed from the growing tumor implants than when it was regional [48]. These and similar observations persuaded me to a rather orthodox, or at least conservative, stance on the systemic side of the controversy.   Now, however, I must present data that indicates that the efficacy of MER in other circumstances is *in veritas* circumscribed to intralesional/regional introduction.

Unlike the situation of MER prophylaxis, *treatment* of established hepatoma isografts is, in fact, efficacious only when the material is brought into direct contact with the implanted tumor. The recently appearing work of MARK WAINBERG and colleagues can leave little room for skepticism on this point [49, 50].   The same principle has now emerged in an entirely different tumor model.   Young White Leghorn chickens infected with 10^6 focus-forming units of Rous Sarcoma Virus (RSV) invariably develop progressively growing sarcomas *in situ*.   When, however, the birds are treated with appropriate amounts of MER some days to weeks before viral challenge, a large proportion of the growing sarcomas regress and disappear permanently — but only when injection of the agent is into the same wing area as the subsequent RSV challenge [51]; injection into the contralateral wing effects, at best, a slight retardation of growth of the appearing tumors.   More recently, the same demand for regional treatment has been seen in the therapeutic situation, and with surprising punctiliousness. Single injection of MER directly into the developing sarcomas had little impact when the agent was suspended in a small volume of suspending fluid (0.05 cc or less).   When, however, the volume was increased by a factor of 10 or 20, and multiple injections were made, a majority of the birds were permanently cured (MARKSON Y.

and WEISS D. W., observations to be published); that success by this procedure cannot be accounted for, at least not entirely, by a mechanical disruption of the tumor is indicated by the failure to cure with similar multiple injections of the fluid vehicle only.

In truth, the dispute between the advocates of intralesional/regional and of systemic administration of nonspecific immuno-modulators is a pseudo-contention. The question cannot be posed in the abstract, and in the individual case, the facts speak for themselves. Moreover, there is need here for semantic precision. Adjuvant material may indeed have to come into intimate contact with tumor cells, and perhaps jointly with immunologically reactive tissue, but this probably occurs in many instances throughout the body, regardless of what the initial portals of entry of tumor and adjuvant were. The question to be asked of each individual tumor model must be, then, whether it is mandatory that treatment administration be into the tumor area, not whether contact between adjuvant, tumor cells, and immunocytes is requisite. It may be that repeated distal administrations of modulators, in larger amounts, can effect the same results as a single limited injection into a tumor mass. All possibilities should be entertained when the leap is made from animal models to clinical neoplasia of man. Where close proximity between neoplastic foci and immunomodulators may be required in human tumor immunotherapy, this might be attainable by intravenous application of the modulators, assuring wide distribution of the agents and hits on tumor aggregates as well as systemic activation of lymphoid centers. As has been emphasized above, the same immunomodulator may exert its protective effects by more than one distinct modality. Assurance of wide distribution of modulators in the tissues thus holds promise of covering more than one possibility of action, and circumvents the formidable clinical difficulties in many cases of reaching every major tumor focus by direct inoculation.

2. *The Employment of MER to Potentiate the Sensitization of Cytotoxic Effector Cells in Vitro, for Use in Passive/Adoptive Immunotherapy*

The nature of immunological responsiveness holds inherent, serious constraints on the evocation of effective immunization against TATA by active means. The ramifying network of positive and negative reactions which constitutes immunological responsiveness, and which is made more labyrinthine by the participation of diverse humoral as well as of cellular entities, may indeed reflect evolutionary necessity. It is not difficult to postulate a pressing need for multiple guarantees against autoimmune pathogenesis; the preservation of body economy may well require several modalities for terminating antibody production and effector cell generation beyond the point of utility; and, most basically, the fine discernment of non-self and deviant-self components on which the immunological contribution to vertebrate physiology and defense rests can only be executed by a multiplicity of mechanisms. Within this fluid immunological matrix, active stimulation of the concourse of events needed to effect selective tumor destruction is a fearfully intricate task of navigation. The obligatory pathways are likely to be enmeshed in bifurcating side-tracks, some leading to pathological consequences, to dissipate, and to run into blocking signals, especially as the target cells are so closely related to the normal constituency of the body. There is every prospect that neoplastic variants, under selective pressure for survival against host defenses, will find loopholes and escape routes from host attack, by adaptation or by the selection of resistant clones.

These defeating impediments could be circumvented only if it were possible to recruit and concentrate at will those immunological reactants which will selectively carry out desired functions. It is very difficult to conceive of such accomplishment in the intact organisms. It may be reasonable to set this goal, however, for sensitization *in vitro*. There, negative and inhibiting elements can be excluded or minimized, and conditions set empirically for elicitation of specified end results of antigenic excitation. Cellular (and humoral) effectors produced *in vitro* could then be utilized for passive/adoptive immunotherapy.

Large attention has been given to this approach in our laboratories during the past several years. ELI KEDAR and his group have established the optimal conditions for specific *in vitro* sensitization of splenic and other lymphoid cells against four mouse lymphomas and leukemias of both syngeneic and allogeneic origin [52, 53]. The sensitized effector cells obtained by this modified one-directional lymphoid cell - tumor cell culture method display strong cytotoxic activity in *in vitro* ^{51}Cr liberation tests, and have powerful tumor neutralizing potency in Winn assays [53, 54]. Animals surviving Winn assays in which the protecting lymphoid cells (apparently, T lymphocytes) were of either syngeneic or allogeneic source acquire solid resistance to massive second challenge: this acquisition appears to involve a recruitment of host immunocytes by the passively administered effector cells. Administration of the *in vitro* educated effectors to mice already bearing leukemic and lymphomatous tumors has revealed the immunotherapeutic efficacy of the cells. Under circumstances where all animals succumb to the neoplastic challenge, and chemotherapy alone aids only a small proportion, combination treatment with chemotherapy and *in vitro* sensitized effectors cures 80 to 100% of the subjects [54, 55].

Recently, the methodology of *in vitro* sensitization has been applied to human peripheral blood lymphoid cells (PBL) and human leukemic target cells. With certain technical modifications, it has proven feasible to generate appreciable anti-leukemia cell cytotoxicity in PBL populations, as assayed *in vitro* [56].

MER in microgram amounts magnifies significantly the *in vitro* generation of specifically cytotoxic effector cells, and also provokes a degree of nonspecific cytotoxic activity [3, 57]. Moreover, the agent prevents the development of suppressor cell activity in lymphoid tissue cultures, even in amounts much above the levels at which maximum potentiation of cytotoxic reactivity occurs (KEDAR E., observations to be published). With the help of MER, cytotoxic effector cells are generated *in vitro* against poorly immunogenic neoplastic cells, even in circumstances where no sensitization takes place in the absence of the agent. It has also been shown that tumor cells can be made more powerful stimulators of the sensitization process by haptenization and enzymatic treatment [58].

Experiments now in progress suggest that conditions can be defined for synergistic magnification of *in vitro* education to anti-tumor cytotoxicity, by simultaneous resort to both MER immunomodulation and modification of the neoplastic stimulator cells in cultures consisting of defined immunocyte subpopulations.

Tumor cells can be preserved at low temperatures without loss of stimulator capacity, and lymphoid cells withstand cryopreservation without reduction in ability to undergo sensitization after thawing, or in effector activity where education preceded freeze-preservation.

These findings thus support the practicability of creating *in vitro* immunological microcosms in which specific sensitization and nonspecific cytotoxic excitation of effector cells can be achieved to a greater magnitude, with more precision, and much more rapidly (within 4 to 6 days) than is possible in the whole organism. Neither patient nor any normal donor is exposed to tumor cells or their modifying agents as vaccine, or to immunomodulators. The lymphoid cells retain the ability to be sensitized or to serve as effectors for many months in liquid nitrogen or air, and perhaps indefinitely, and at least in several animal leukemia models they are highly efficacious therapeutically. *In vitro* sensitization and passive/adoptive immunotherapy with the effectors thereby produced offers a challenging new treatment modality.

That large problems must be overcome in translating the success of this approach from the laboratory animal to the patient is obvious [54]. It is not certain whether sensitized effector cells retain, especially after cryopreservation, the full viability and functionality required to establish themselves in the patient for sufficiently long to seek out and destroy their neoplastic targets, or to effect an adequate recruitment, by whatever means, of host immunocytes to anti-tumor reactivity; time relationships in the clinical situation are very different from those in the usual animal models where death of tumor-challenged controls is a matter of weeks, and the protective activities of passively administered effectors are probably played out within several days. The numbers of "residual" tumor cells remaining in patients in whom tumor burden has first been reduced by conventional means may still be very large. The numbers of effector cells required to destroy or inhibit these may not be tolerated by the patient, and they may be difficult to obtain. Patients in remission may not be able to supply adequate quantities of white blood cells for sensitization, and use of presensitized allogeneic effector cells derived from normal donors or long-term survivors of similar malignant disease is accompanied by the dilemma of graft-versus-host (GvH) reactivity on the one hand, and of rapid rejection of the therapeutic implant on the other.

These problems may not be beyond solution, however. Where autochthonous neoplastic cells are available as stimulators, close HL-A matching between patient and effector cell donor would lower the dangers of GvH disease and of premature graft rejection. Techniques have been developed [59] for selective immunoadsorption of clones reactive to normal cell antigens (such clones could be generated *in vitro* even within autochthonous lymphoid populations [60]). Induction *in vitro* of partial tolerance to histocompatibility antigens of the stimulating or target tumor cells may not be entirely out of the question [61], especially with the definition of HL-A structure [62].

There are other possibilities. For instance, if we can assume TATA cross-reactivity between related neoplasms, it may be possible to sensitize allogeneic donor PBL against neoplastic cells derived from one patient, and to use the effector cells produced in another. Effector and stimulator cells should then, perhaps, be as close as possible in histocompatibility make-up, so as to reduce the generation of cytotoxicity against normal cell components; in contradistinction, the HL-A types of the stimulator cells and of the patient to be treated should be as distant as possible, to lessen GvH initiation due to whatever sensitization did occur against common normal self markers. However, multiple effector cell donors may have to be sought to obtain an adequate effector cell supply. It may be necessary, in that event, to use successively effector cells from donors far-removed from each other in HL-A characteristics, so as to reduce accelerated immune rejection of the effector inoculums. Even then, the operative principle should be retained: the greatest possible restriction in overlap of normal cell antigens between the tumor stimulators *in vitro* and the tumor targets to be attacked in the patient, and the closest possible proximity between stimulator and effector cells This could be attained by seeking for each new sensitization episode stimulator-effector combinations closely related in histocompatibility characteristics, while preserving the distance of each combination from the others and from the particular patient.

A large impediment to such attempts at cross-sensitization may lie with the restrictions imposed by major histocompatibility antigens on sensitization-reaction responses to other, weaker antigens [63]. It might be possible to overcome this difficulty, however, for instance by resort to sequential exposure of macrophages and T-cells to the TATA and the ensuing helper-mediated generation of cytostatic effectors [64].

Even with solution of the formidable problem of histocompatibility relationships, the efficacy of passive/adoptive immunotherapy alone is likely to be limited. Combined treatment with *in vitro* sensitized cells and active immunostimulation of the host, together with conventional therapy, would appear to hold greater promise [55, 65].

To assure ingress of the largest possible numbers of cytotoxic effector cells to foci of solid tumors, efforts to facilitate the movement of cells across blood vessels supplying neoplastic tissue may be fruitful; the elicitation of Shwartzman-like reactions at tumor sites, or resort to small quantities of tumor necrotizing factor (TNF) come to mind. Direct introduction of effector cells into vessels afferent to large tumor deposits could also be taken into account in some cases.

Separation of purified populations of cytotoxically reactive clones from the lymphoid cell preparations sensitized *in vitro* could allow marked reduction in the numbers of cells that must be administered. It is also conceivable that anti-tumor effects short of the destruction of all residual neoplastic cells — killing of a portion of the targets, injury of some, and cytostatic action on still others (*) — may have significant therapeutic benefits in affording patients the chance of coping with fewer malignant cells, impaired in growth capacity.

(*) Observations suggesting that cytostasis may be a functional property of certain lymphoid cells distinct from cytotoxicity have been reported from our laboratories [66], as well as by other workers.

Ultimately, the attempt may be warranted to isolate soluble transforming factors from sensitized effector cells, for recruitment of host immunocytes to specific anti-tumor activity. There are other eventualities of immunological engineering on the horizon, based on availability of a large complement of effector cells brought to potent anti-tumor reactivity *in vitro* by specific education and nonspecific immunomodulation.

Summary

The purpose of this presentation has been to bring into focus the variegated possibilities of potentiation of resistance to neoplastic disease by nonspecific immunomodulators of microbial derivation. The attempt to group the potentialities of such substances according to likely mechanism and orientation of action is seen necessary, to bring into clearer light the scope of the therapeutic and prophylactic goals that might be achieved, and to direct further work towards their realization.

The MER mycobacterial fraction has been taken in this discussion as the main model of microbial immunomodulators able to elevate resistance to progressive neoplasia. Recent findings on the magnification by MER of the *in vitro* generation of anti-tumor cytotoxic effector cells for employment in passive/adoptive immunotherapy of cancer have been reviewed.

It appears that judicious resort to nonspecific immunomodulators, directly in the tumor host and as an adjunct to specific activation *in vitro* of immunocytes reactive against neoplastic target cells, may come to have an important role in the overall strategy of cancer treatment and prevention.

REFERENCES

[1] WEISS D. W., KUPERMAN O., FATHALLAH N. and KEDAR E., *Mode of action of mycobacterial fractions in anti-tumor immunity: Preliminary evidence for a direct nonspecific stimulatory effect of MER on immunologically reactive cells.* « Ann. N. Y. Acad. Sci. », *276*, 536-549 (1976).

[2] BEN-EFRAIM S. and DIAMANTSTEIN T., *Mitogenic and adjuvant activity of a methanol extraction residue (MER) of tubercle bacilli on mouse lymphoid cells "in vitro".* « Immunol. Communic. », *4*, 565-577 (1975).

[3] KEDAR E., NAHAS F., UNGER E. and WEISS D. W., *"In vitro" induction of cell-mediated immunity to murine leukemia cells. III. Effect of the methanol extraction residue (MER) fraction of tubercle bacilli on the generation of antileukemia cytotoxic lymphocytes.* « J. Natl. Cancer Instit. », in press.

[4] GALLILY R., STAIN E. and WEISS D. W., *Potentiation of macrophage activities by the MER fraction "in vitro".* « J. Reticuloendothel. Soc. », in press.

[5] BEN-EFRAIM S., ULMER A., SCHMIDT M. and DIAMANTSTEIN T., *Differences between lymphoid cell populations of guinea pigs and mice as determined by the response to mitogens "in vitro".* « Int. Archs. Allergy Appl. Immun. », *51*, 117-130 (1976).

[6] BEN-EFRAIM S. and WEISS D. W., *Effects of MER on lymphoid cell division and antibody synthetis "in vitro".* « Cellul. Immunol. », submitted for publication (1978).

[7] *Immunopotentiation*, Ciba Foundation Symposium 18 (New series), Elsevier - North Holland, Amsterdam (1973).

[8] YAGEL S., GALLILY R. and WEISS D. W., *Effect of treatment with the MER fraction of tubercle bacilli on hydrolytic lysozomal enzyme activity of mouse peritoneal macrophages.* « Cell. Immunol. », *19*, 381-386 (1975).

[9] GERY I., BAER A., STUPP Y. and WEISS D. W., *Further studies on the effects of the Methanol Extraction Residue fraction of tubercle bacilli on lymphoid cells and macrophages.* In: « Immnological parameters of Host-Tumor relationships », Weiss D. W., ed., Academic Press, Vol. III, N. Y., pp. 170-177 (1974).

[10] WHITE R. G., *Antigens and adjuvants.* « Proc. Royal Soc. Med. », *61*, 1-5 (1968).

[11] GERY I. and WAKSMAN B. H., *Potentiation of the T-lymphocyte response to mitogens. II. The cellular source of the potentiating mediator(s).* « J. Exp. Med. », *136*, 143-155 (1972).

[12] EVANS R. and ALEXANDER P., *Mechanisms of immunologically specific killing of tumor cells by macrophages.* « Nature », *236*, 168-170 (1972).

[13] FIDLER I. J., *Recognition and destruction of target cells by tumoricidal macro phages.* In: « Immunological parameters of Host-Tumor relationships », Weiss D. W., ed., Academic Press, Vol. V, 1978, N. Y., in press.

[14] WEISS D. W., *Neoplastic diseases and tumor immunology from the perspective of host-parasite relationships.* « Nat. Cancer Instit. Monog. », *44*, 115-122 (1976).

[15] SCHLAGER S. I. and DRAY S., *Complete regression of a guinea pig hepato-carcinoma by immunotherapy with "tumor-immune" RNA or antibody to fibrin fragment E.* « Israel J. Med. Sci. », *12*, 344-359 (1976).

[16] RADOV L. A., HASKILL J. S. and KORN J. H., *Host immune potentiation of drug responses to a murine mammary adenocarcinoma.* « Int. J. Cancer », *17*, 773-779 (1976).

[17] MANTOVANI A., *Rationalized approaches to cancer chemoimmunotherapy.* In: « Tumor-associated antigens and their specific immune response ». Proceedings of the Milano Conference, June 1977, Spreafico F., ed., Academic Press, N. Y., in press.

[18] WEISS D. W., *Perspectives in tumor immunotherapy.* « Adv. Cancer Res. », submitted for publication.

[19] YRON I., COHEN D., ROBINSON E., HABER M. and WEISS D. W., *Effects of methanol extraction residue and therapeutic irradiation against established isografts and simulated local recurrence of mammary carcinomas.* « Cancer Res. », *35*, 1779-1790 (1975).

[20] SHARMA B., TUBERGEN D. G., MINDEN P. and BRUNDA M. J., *"In vitro" immunisation against human tumour cells with bacterial extracts.* « Nature », *267*, 845-847 (1977).

[21] MINDEN P., McCLATCHY J. K., WAINBERG M. and WEISS D. W., *Shared antigens between "Mycobacterium bovis (BCG)" and neoplastic cells.* « J. Natl. Cancer Instit. », *53*, 1325-1331 (1974).

[22] HENNEY C. S., TRACEY D. E. and WOLFE S. A., *BCG induced natural killer cells: Immunotherapeutic implications.* In: « Immunological parameters of host-tumor relationships », Weiss D. W., ed., Academic Press, Vol. V, N. Y., 1978, in press.

[23] SHUSTIK C., COHEN I. R., SCHWARTZ R. S., LATHAM-GRIFFIN E. and WAKSAL S. D., *T lymphocytes with promiscuous cytotoxicity.* « Nature », *263*, 699-701 (1976).

[24] BEVAN M. J., LANGMAN R. E. and COHN M., *H-2 antigen-specific cytotoxic T cells induced by concanavalin A: estimation of their relative frequency.* « Eur. J. Immunol. », *6*, 150-156 (1976).

[25] GALLILY R., STAIN E. and WEISS D. W., *Potentiation of macrophage activities following incubation with factor(s) released from lymphocytes treated "in vitro" with MER.* « J. Reticuloendothel. Soc. », *22*, 64a (1977).

[26] GALLILY R., DUCHAN Z. and WEISS D. W., *Potentiation of mouse peritoneal macrophage antibacterial functions by treatment of the donors with the methanol extraction residue (MER) fraction of tubercle bacilli.* « Inf. and Imm. », 1977, in press.

[27] SACHS L., *Contour of immune receptors and the development of leukemia.* In: « Tumor-associated antigens and their specific immune response ». Proceedings of the Milano Conference, June 1977, Spreafico F., ed., Academic Press, N. Y., in press.

[28] IZAK G., STUPP Y., MANNY N., ZAJICEK G. and WEISS D. W., *The immune response in acute myelocytic leukemia. Effect of the methanol extraction residue fraction of tubercle bacilli (MER) on T and B cell functions and their relation to the course of the disease.* « Israel J. Med. Sci. », *13*, 677-693 (1977).

[29] WEISS D. W., *Animal models of cancer immunotherapy.* In: « Immunotherapy of human cancer », Hersh E. M. and Sinkovics J. G., eds., Raven Press, N. Y., in press.

[30] TERRY Wm. and WINDHORST D., « Immunotherapy of cancer », Raven Press, N. Y., in press.

[31] WEISS D. W., *Discussion.* In: « Immunotherapy of cancer », Terry Wm. and Windhorst D., eds., Raven Press, N. Y., in press.

[32] BEKESI J. G. and HOLLAND J. F., *Active immunotherapy in leukemia with neuraminidase-modified leukemic cells.* In: « Recent results in cancer research », Vol. 62, Mathé G., ed., Springer-Verlag, N. Y., 1977, pp. 78-89.

[33] WEISS D. W., *The questionable immunogenicity of certain neoplasms: What then the prospects for immunological intervention in malignant disease?* « Cancer Immunol. Immunotherapy », *2*, 11-19 (1977).

[34] RIBI E., *Immunotherapy with compounds derived from microorganisms and with synthetic analogs of some of these.* In: « Immunotherapy of human cancer », Hersh E. M. and Sinkovics J. G., eds., Raven Press, N. Y., in press.

[35] FIDLER I. J. and BUCANA C., *Mechanism of tumor cell resistance to lysis by syngeneic lymphocytes.* « Cancer Res. », *37*, 3945-3956 (1977).

[36] FIDLER I. J., GERSTEN D. M. and RIGGS Ch. W., *Relationship of host immune status to tumor cell arrest, distribution, and survival in experimental metastasis.* « Cancer », *40*, 46-55 (1977).

[37] HOLLAND J. F., BEKESI J. G. and CUTTNER J., *Chemoimmunotherapy of acute myelocytic leukemia.* In: « Immunotherapy of human cancer », Hersh E. M. and Sinkovics J. G., eds., Raven Press, N. Y., in press.

[38] TREVES A. J., COHEN I. R., FELDMAN M. and WEISS D. W., *Effect of treatment with the methanol extraction residue fraction of killed tubercle bacilli (MER) on the development of spontaneous pulmonary metastases from syngeneic implants of tumor 3LL in C57Bl mice.* In: « Immunological parameters of host-tumor relationships », Vol. IV, Weiss D. W., ed., Academic Press, N. Y., 1976, pp. 384-387.

[39] WEISS D. W., *MER and other mycobacterial fractions in the immunotherapy of cancer.* « Med. Clin. N. America », *60*, 473-497 (1976).

[40] BEN-EFRAIM S., *Methanol extraction residue: Effects and mechanisms of action.* « Pharmac. Ther. A. », *1*, 383-410 (1977).

[41] WEISS D. W., *Nonspecific stimulation and modulation of the immune response and of states of resistance by the MER fraction of tubercle bacilli.* « Natl. Cancer Instit. Monog. », *35*, 157-171 (1972).

[42] Weiss D. W. and Yashphe D. J., *Nonspecific stimulation of antimicrobial and antitumor resistance and of immunological responsiveness by the MER fraction of tubercle bacilli*. In: « Dynamic aspects of host-parasite relationships », Zuckerman A. and Weiss D. W., eds., Academic Press, N. Y., 1973, pp. 163-223.

[43] Hart I. R., Fidler I. J., Hanna M. G. Jr., Cardy R. H., Gutterman J. U. and Hersh E. M., *The effects of intravenous administration of methanol extraction residue (MER) of tubercle bacilli in the dog*. « Cancer Immunol. Immunotherapy », in press.

[44] Vogl S. E., Lumb G., Bekesi J. G. and Holland J. F., *Preclinical study of IV administration of the methanol extraction residue of Bacillus Calmette-Guérin*. « Cancer Treat. Rpts. », *61*, 901-903 (1977).

[45] Moertel C. G., Ritts R. E., Schutt A. J. and Hahn R. G., *Clinical studies of methanol extraction residue fraction of Bacillus Calmette-Guérin as an immunostimulant in patients with advanced cancer*. « Cancer Res. », *35*, 3075-3083 (1975).

[46] Cuttner J., Glidewell O. J. and Holland J. F., *A controlled trial of chemo-immunotherapy in acute myelocytic leukemia (AML)*. « Proc. Amer. Soc. Clin. Oncol. », 1978, in press.

[47] Wainberg M. A., Deutsch V. and Weiss D. W., *Stimulation of anti-tumour immunity in guinea-pigs by methanol extraction residue of BCG*. « Brit. J. Cancer », *34*, 500-508 (1976).

[48] Cohen D., Yron I., Haber M., Robinson E. and Weiss D. W., *Effect of treatment with the MER tubercle bacilli fraction on the survival of mice carrying mammary tumor isografts: Injection of MER at the tumour site or at a distal location*. « Brit. J. Cancer », *32*, 483-489 (1975).

[49] Wainberg M. A., Margolese R. G. and Weiss D. W., *Differential responsiveness of various substrains of inbred Strain 2 guinea pigs to immunotherapy with the methanol extraction residue (MER) of BCG*. « Cancer Immunol. Immunotherapy », *2*, 101-108 (1977).

[50] Wainberg M. A., Margolese R. G. and Weiss D. W., *Tumor immunoprophylaxis and immunotherapy in guinea pigs treated with the methanol extraction residue (MER) of BCG*. In: « BCG in cancer immunotherapy », Lamoreux G., Turcotte R. and Portelance V. eds., Grune and Stratton, N. Y., 1976, pp. 39-50.

[51] Markson Y., Doljansky F. and Weiss D. W., *Effects of prophylactic treatment with the MER tubercle bacillus fraction on the development of Rous sarcomas of chickens following challenge with the Rous sarcoma virus*. In: « Immunological parameters of host-tumor relationships », Vol. V, Weiss D. W. ed., Academic Press, N. Y., 1978, in press.

[52] Kedar E., Unger E. and Schwartzbach M., *"In vitro" induction of cell-mediated immunity to murine leukemia cells. I. Optimization of tissue culture conditions for the generation of cytotoxic lymphocytes*. « J. Immunol. Methods », *13*, 1-19 (1976).

[53] Kedar E., Schwartzbach M., Raanan Z. and Hefetz S., *"In vitro" induction of cell-mediated immunity to murine leukemia cells. II. Cytotoxic activity "in vitro" and tumor-neutralizing capacity "in vivo" of anti-leukemia cytotoxic lymphocytes generated in macrocultures*. « J. Immunol. Methods », *16*, 39-58 (1977).

[54] KEDAR E., NAHAS F., SCHWARTZBACH M., UNGER E., RAANAN Z., HEFETZ S. and WEISS D. W., *Generation "in vitro" of cytotoxic effector cells against syngeneic and allogeneic mouse leukemias and lymphomas*. In: « Tumor-associated antigens and their specific immune response », Spreafico F., ed., Academic Press, N. Y., in press.

[55] KEDAR E., RAANAN Z. and SCHWARTZBACH M., *"In vitro" induction of cell-mediated immunity to murine leukemia cells. VI. Adoptive chemoimmunotherapy of leukemia in mice using lymphocytes sensitized "in vitro" to leukemia cells*. « Cancer Immunol. Immunotherapy », 1978, in press.

[56] RAANAN Z., WEISS D. W., BEKESI G., HOLLAND J. F., SCHWARTZBACH M. and KEDAR E., *"In vitro" induction of cell-mediated immunity to human tumor cells. I. Sensitization of normal donor peripheral white blood cells to human leukemia cells*. « Cancer Immunol. Immunotherapy », 1978, submitted for publication.

[57] WEISS D. W., *Host mechanisms for control of tumor growth which can be modulated by nonspecific immunotherapy*. In: « Immunotherapy of human cancer », Hersh E. M. and Sinkovics J. G., eds., Raven Press, N. Y., in press.

[58] KEDAR E. and LUPU T., *"In vitro" induction of cell-mediated immunity to murine leukemia cells. IV. Amplification of the generation of cytotoxic lymphocytes by enzymatically and chemically modified stimulator leukemia cells*. « Cancer Immunol. Immunotherapy », 1978, in press.

[59] BONAVIDA B. and KEDAR E., *Transplantation of allogeneic lymphoid cells specifically depleted of graft-versus-host reactive cells*. « Nature », 249, 658-659 (1974).

[60] COHEN I. R., WEKERLE H. and FELDMAN M., *The regulation of self-tolerance. Implications for immune surveillance against tumor cells*. « Israel J. Med. Sci. », 10, 1024-1032 (1974).

[61] STOLLAR B. D. and BOREL Y., *Nucleoside specificity in the carrier IgG-dependent induction of tolerance*. « J. Immunol. », 117, 1308-1313 (1976).

[62] FUKS A., KAUFMAN J. F., ORR H. T., PARHAM P., ROBB R. R., TERHORST C. and STROMINGER J. L., *Structural aspects of the products of the human major-histocompatibility complex*. « Transp. Proc. », 9, 1685-1689 (1977).

[63] ZINKERNAGEL R. M. and DOHERTY P. C., *H-2 compatibility requirement for T-cell-mediated lysis of target cells infected with lymphocytic choriomeningitis virus. Different cytotoxic T-cell specificities are associated with structures coded for in H-2K or H-2D*. « J. Exp. Med. », 141, 1427-1436 (1975).

[64] TREVES A. J., FELDMAN M. and KAPLAN S. H., *Macrophage-mediated "in vitro" sensitization of T-lymphocytes. I. Detection of murine leukemia virus-associated antigens*. « J. Natl. Cancer Instit. », 58, 1527-1530 (1977).

[65] KEDAR E., SCHWARTZBACH M., RAANAN Z. and HEFETZ S., *"In vitro" induction of cell-mediated immunity to murine leukemia cells. V. Adoptive immunotherapy of leukemia in mice with lymphocytes sensitized "in vitro" to leukemia cells*. « Cancer Immunol. Immunotherapy », 1978, in press.

[66] STEINITZ M., FEIGIS M. and WEISS D. W., *Studies on the physiological manifestations of cell mediated cytotoxicity. II. Inhibition of ^{3}H-thymidine incorporation by plasmacytoma cells exposed "in vitro" to sensitized splenocytes*. « Cell. Immunol. », 17, 181-191 (1975).

DISCUSSION

NOSSAL

I would like to address a comment to the alleged non-specific action of MER acting to produce lytic capacity against the various tumor lines. I wonder whether you would accept an alternative explanation based on the work of my former colleague John Marbrook who cultures T-lymphocytes at limit dilution to produce single clones of cells, each of which has a specific and restricted capacity for lysis of one sort of allogeneic or tumor target or on occasion even one sort of autologous cells. Is it not possible that the MER is acting as a polyclonal T-cell stimulator, allowing each particular T cell to express its innate genetic pre-programmed reactivity so that the end result is a mixture of specificities coming up, which, if you put the cells into limit dilution culture, would disappear and would allow each clone to express itself?

WEISS

It has been shown by Dr. Shlomo Ben-Efraim of Tel Aviv University that MER is indeed a potent polyclonal mitogen for B cells; and it may have such activity for some T cell populations as well. It should be noted, however, that MER potentiates the production of specific antibodies and the generation of specifically reactive cytotoxic lymphocytes in amounts orders of magnitude below the threshold of polyclonal mitogenicity. Information has recently developed in our and in Dr. Ben-Efraim's laboratories pointing to a helper function by MER, i.e., the providing of necessary second signal(s) for the production of antibodies and the generation of cytotoxic effector cells. Whatever the mechanisms may be, MER appears to stimulate the functionality and the proliferation of immunocytes reacting to specific antigenic stimuli, as well as to effect polyclonal cell expansion. It might also be noted that even a very limited degree of cross-reactivity between determinants on mycobacterial moieties and the membrane of a variety of tumor cells — shown quite convincingly by Dr. Percy Minden of Denver, and by other workers — might aid in the *selective* stimulation of multiplication of clones programmed for these antigens.

ROSENBERG

The tumors you have used have been around for many years, probably fifteen years or more. Have you repeated any of these experiments with recently developed tumors in the first few generations or spontaneous human tumors?

WEISS

I have been arguing for many years, viz., Weiss D. W., Immunology of spontaneous tumors, *In*: Proceedings of the Fifth Berkeley Symposium on Mathematical Statistics and Probability, Lecam, L. and Neyman, J., eds., University of California Press, Berkeley, 1967, (pp. 657-706) that work in tumor immunology, if not in all areas of tumor biology, must be conducted with spontaneous tumors, preferably in the autochthonous host or at least in animals of proven isogenicity and in the first or second tumor transplant generation, if the experiments are to have true relevance to neoplasia in nature. And yet, for nefarious considerations of cost and convenience, I and my colleagues too have made large resort to hoary "tumors" whose resemblance to freshly arisen neoplastic growths is most dubious.

I might point out, nonetheless, that we have remained true to our convictions at least on occasion, attempting to conduct representative experiments with spontaneously appearing neoplasms of very recent origin in animals of established isogenicity — although even then, the caveat holds that many of our "spontaneous" tumors of inbred mice are probably still a far distance removed from naturally occurring tumors in outbred animal populations.

In this instance, we have conducted sample experiments, with similar results, employing lymphomas arising in C57B1 mice following whole body irradiation or infection with newly isolated Radiation Leukemia Virus — the model worked out so elegantly by Dr. Nechamah Haran-Ghera of the Weizmann Institute. We have then turned our attention to human leukemic cells — AML blasts and "hairy cell" leukemia cells freshly obtained by plasmapharesis from the patient, frozen, and then used — for our *in vitro* sensitization experiments; the effector cells in these studies have been fresh normal donor peripheral blood leukocytes, or separated lymphocytes. With the reservation that the cytotoxic capacity of the human effector cells, as measured by an *in vitro* ^{51}Cr short-term assay, is lower than that of mouse splenocytes in allogeneic systems, the results in these human models are in every respect very similar to those obtained in mouse allogeneic and syngeneic systems; this is true for the kinetics and limits of specificity of the reactions, and for the ability to potentiate them with MER and by various modifications of the tumor stimulator cells. It must be added, however, that the optimum conditions for *in vitro* sensitization vary appreciably for different test models, and must be determined empirically.

The difficult question now before us is how to test the cytotoxic abilities of human effector cells against human tumors *in vivo*. It is questionable whether experiments in animals severely compromised immunologically — for instance, nude mice, or animals exposed to near-lethal irradiation of chemical immunosuppression — would have categorically greater biological significance than the *in vitro* tests for CMI. Are such highly artifactual animal experiments nonetheless a necessary step before one may attempt to intervene clinically with *in vitro* sensitized effector cells? This problem is now under active discussion in the department of Dr. James Holland of Mt. Sinai Hospital in New York, where I am currently on sabbatical leave.

OETTGEN

Can you use the chromium release assay with adherent human tumor cells, or does this type of cell require a longer period of incubation? When we use that type of assay with chemically-induced tumors of the mouse, we find a very high degree of nonspecific reactivity with *in vitro* sensitization as opposed to *in vivo* sensitization.

WEISS

I agree that the nude mouse cannot be viewed as immunologically sterile; T cells are certainly not the only arm of defensive immunological responsiveness. And I must reiterate: the nude mouse bearing a human tumor xenograft is an exceedingly artifactual test system. Specifically with regard to your question: the possibility that human neoplastic cells growing in a nude mouse will not express certain antigens is a very real one. With regard to your first point, all I can say is that we have utilized the short-term labeled chromium release assay so far, in the studies with murine and human leukemia cells. We are only now beginning to turn our attention to *in vitro* sensitization against several solid tumors of experimental animals, and for this work we shall employ both the chromium release assay and several other tests that are feasible with adherent target cells — the *terminal* chromium labeling assay developed by Dr. More in our laboratories (this is a modification of the Klein-Takasugi technique), the immunoadherence test described by Dr. Mark Wainberg during his time with us in Jerusalem, and several others. I do not yet have results to report on sensitization to solid neoplasms or on the employment of the other assay methods.

RAPP

I like your chicken system very much. You are at least dealing with a primary tumor and these are allogeneic animals. This might be a good system to study *in vitro* education and sensitization.

WEISS

The tumors in chicken are sarcomas arising in the autochthonous test animal after infection with Rous Sarcoma Virus (RSV). The chickens are outbred birds of the White Leghorn ond of other breeds. Yes, we have begun *in vitro* sensitization studies with effector cells from the autochthonous and from allogeneic donors in this system, work done in collaboration with Dr. Fanny Doljanski and Mr. Yossi Markson, but we have no data as yet.

RAPP

Do you think antiviral immunity has anything to do with the success that you had in that system?

[9] *Weiss* · p. 38

WEISS

I am not certain. Remember that these sarcomas grew progressively for a time in every bird, and that the effect of prophylactic MER treatment was expressed by a subsequent regression. If we were dealing here simply with antiviral immunity, I might have anticipated inhibition of any initial tumor development in at least some instances. This was not seen. On the other hand, I cannot rule out the possibility that continued viral replication and infection of target cells is not requisite for progressive tumor development; in that event, antiviral immunity as well as cytotoxic reactivity to the transformed cells themselves could play a role in the regression of growing tumors.

SELA

I would like to make one comment if I may. During the last three hours we heard so much about MER and I almost forgot that it has something to do with BCG, at least it is isolated from it. I would like to hear from you a short comment as to where it is similar and where it differs. I know that BCG is still a complete organism, I know that BCG causes lesions and so forth.

WEISS

The situation is the other way round, Dr. Sela! MER is indeed a derivative of BCG, but a nonliving entity. Many other investigators have found MER to induce at least the same degree of heightened resistance to tumor cells — I believe I can cite some of Dr. Baldwin's work here — and the same degree of immunopotentiation as living BCG. That alone constitutes an excellent reason for favoring MER over BCG. If there are levels of impurity in the "Dreckapotheke", then living BCG is certainly at the lowest level. MER is a preparation free of a portion of the complex lipids of the whole bacterium; it is nonviable; and it is highly stable, less toxic than the intact organism, and subject to standardization even though its active components are still not known.

When MER is given to human subjects at a standardized amount and frequency, as was done in the original clinical trials, severe ulcerating skin lesions develop after a time in some patients, and treatment must be terminated. What is now being done, however, is to titrate the amount of MER at first administration over several orders of magnitude, in the skin of each recipient. Treatment is then given with a quantity that induces, in that patient, only a moderate and well tolerated local skin reaction; as the patient becomes more strongly reactive with continued use — it must be remembered that MER itself is immunogenic, and evokes delayed hypersensitivity reactions to itself and to PPD (although of a lower order than does living BCG or intact killed BCG organisms) — the amount is again reduced. There is no evidence that very severe local reactions are a condition for the systemic efficacy of this agent.

It is clear from what we have heard at this conference that the biological activities of living BCG vary markedly from strain to strain, and also with uncontrolled variables that accompany employment of this living agent, even when the same strain and the same parameters of administration are utilized. This is not at all surprising. The amount of material introduced at administration is very small, and there is reliance, accordingly, on the further multiplication of the bacteria in the recipient. The replicatory abilities of living BCG are a very unstable property, however, varying from strain to strain, and differing as a function of the preparation of the inoculum, its handling, and the immune status of the treated subject. Little has been done in the way of objective comparisons of different living BCG preparations, tested simultaneously under rigidly controlled conditions, and even less for objective comparisons of "BCG" with the standardized MER agent. What I can say is that whenever we have essayed such comparisons, we have found MER to be more likely to bestow heightened protection against tumor cells and against pathogenic microorganisms than living BCG, and have found the latter to tend not infrequently to elicit changes in immunological reactivity manifested by *enhanced* tumor growth. With MER, in contrast, enhancement is almost never seen; this is true especially when the moiety is administered in treatment schedules which include therapeutic irradiation of tumor masses or chemotherapy. Regarding T and B cell functions and macrophage activities, we have also found MER to be a consistently more effective potentiating agent. I should point out in fairness, however, that I speak here of comparisons in our hands — and we are far more familiar with the proclivities of MER than we are with the vagaries of living BCG. I do not know, therefore, whether MER is inherently a superior immunomodulator and resistance-inducing substance than living

[9] *Weiss* - p. 40

BCG, or whether the maximum and equal capacities of the latter have eluded us because the preparations are so unstable and fickle. We tend to believe quite strongly that MER is indeed a more effective, and otherwise a more desirable agent. Certainly, it is not inferior to living BCG by any criterion of comparison — and the question must be posed therefore: why continue using the much more difficult and problematic and potentially hazardous living organisms when a material like MER is at hand?

CHEDID

Chemically or physicochemically, MER is a composite material which even contains ghosts of whole bacterial cells and in which certain mycobacterial components such as tuberculin can be demonstrated by biological testing. This preparation contains also cord factor and probably phospholipids which could explain why such a material is easily suspended in water. This represents a major advantage and there is good evidence in the literature that MER is extremely potent in several infectious and tumoral experimental models. I completely agree that using an inert material rather than a viable proliferating microorganism represents a definite advantage.

RAPP

There is one slight correction: these dead materials were developed by Edgar Ribi originally. But speaking in terms of the desire to have this meeting be relevant to the handling of clinical cancer, I have to take exception to some of the things Dr. Weiss has been saying. I think if we are going to compare MER and BCG, we have to talk about therapy models in which established tumors as well as metastasis are eliminated. The guinea pig hepatoma model so far has yielded results in general agreement with clinical results. When we directly compared MER and BCG for their activity against the line 10 hepatoma in the same foundation colony of animals in which the tumor was originally induced, MER did not work very well at all, whereas living BCG worked very well.

OETTGEN

In one human tumor situation — malignant melanoma — the local effects of intralesionally injected BCG and MER are quite comparable.

WEISS

I should like to stress once again, at the risk of repeating myself, that I have no emotional attachment to MER. The development of this model agent of immunomodulation was not the result of great insight, ingenuity, or inductive experimentation. Rather, I came across MER by chance: Dr. René Dubos asked me in the early 1950's to repeat, at the Rockefeller Institute, the earlier work of Negrè and Boquet which demonstrated the specific immunizing capacities of a methanol *soluble* fraction of tubercle bacilli; it materialized that the soluble preparations afforded protection against experimental tuberculosis only when they were contaminated with the extraction residue, MER; and it the turned out that mice and guinea pigs treated with MER exhibited nonspecifically heightened resistance as well, against a variety of challenges. MER has the definite advantages of standardizability, stability, nonviability, and, often, superiority of performance — but the latter not always. Dr. Rapp is perfectly right: In the guinea pig hepatoma model, MER at best cures somewhat over 50% of animals treated under optimum circumstances, whereas living BCG effects cures in up to 90% of the hosts. In many other tumor test models, however, MER is as effective as living BCG, or more so. As I have said repeatedly on this and on other occasions, there is no one ideal test model of human neoplasia, and it may be that different adjuvants will have different degrees of therapeutic efficacy in human neoplasia; there is no one human model of human malignant disease, either. At this time, it can be said that MER is a felicitous model of immunotherapeutic agents, with proven and repeatedly demonstrable efficacy in a broad spectrum of animal tumors, and apparently with efficacy as well in at least some human cancers.

SELA

Thank you; I think it is obvious that it is better to have two possibilities rather than one, and I think that we would like to have Dr. Chedid tell us about twenty more possibilities which will increase the chances for a positive solution.

THERAPEUTIC POTENTIAL
OF IMMUNOREGULATING
SYNTHETIC GLYCOPEPTIDES

LOUIS CHEDID

C.N.R.S., Institut Pasteur
75015 Paris, France

Cancer immunotherapy is based on ample evidence that the immune response to unrelated antigens and resistance to tumors can be enhanced by a variety of microbial agents. The ever-growing list of such agents includes viruses, bacteria, fungi, plants and their products [1-11]. Indeed it is not exaggerated to state that micro-organisms are the strongest and most persistent exogenous regulators of the immune system.

In recent years, thanks to the pioneering work of Mathé, several clinical investigators have been very active in this field [12]. Most if not all of their studies have been done either with whole micro-organisms [13, 14, 15], or complex fractions such as cell walls or MER [16, 17].

Since investigations with BCG or *C. parvum* will be reviewed elsewhere the aim of the present paper is to attract attention on Freund's complete adjuvant (FCA) and more particularly on small glycopeptides which have been recently synthesized.

Current attempts at isolating chemically well-defined substances are justified and timely, as they may lead to preparations that retain the therapeutic effects which are required yet cause less toxicity. Indeed although BCG and *C. parvum* have been shown to be dra-matically effective in certain experimental models, investigators are well aware of the fact that they contain a great variety of heterogenous antigens, some of which could cross-react to host tissues [18, 19, 20] and also that they are endowed with undesirable pharmacological side effects. Moreover, following dose and mode of administration, immune modulation can be unruly (for instance tumor enhancement instead of rejection) [20 *bis*].

Since Freund's original observation on the effect of paraffin oil and mycobacteria on antibody formation and sensitization, these adjuvants have been considered as the most potent enhancing agents of the immune response [21, 22]. The utilization of the remarkable activity of FCA, other than in experimental procedures, has been restricted by the toxic reactivity of mycobacteria which can induce various side effects. Such side effects (increased susceptibility to endotoxin, granuloma formation and lymphoid hyperplasia, adjuvant arthritis, sensitization to tuberculin, etc.) are related to their content in cord factor or PPD and probably also to yet non-identified components. Last but not least clinical applications have been greatly limited by the presence of non-metabolizable oil in FCA.

In his early studies, Freund suggested the existence of a rather widely dispersed common adjuvant unit when he wrote: "It would be of great interest to identify the fraction or fractions which exert the adjuvant effect of mycobacteria and to know whether the effect could be produced without sensitizing to tuberculin" [23].

The difficult problem of determining the chemistry of fractions of mycobacteria with adjuvant activity has been pursued for many years but only recently have important relevant structures been identified. Early investigations revealed that the whole organisms could be replaced by purified cell walls [24] or by wax D which was extracted and solubilized in lipid solvents [25, 26]. More recently an important advance has been made in the identification of water soluble fractions [27, 28, 29, 30, 31].

Thus a preparation containing arabinogalactan linked to peptidoglycan was obtained after lysozyme treatment of *M. smegmatis* by Adam *et al.* [27-29] and found capable of substituting for whole mycobacterial cells in FCA. In contrast to whole cells or crude cell walls, this fraction termed Water Soluble Adjuvant (WSA) did not induce side effects [32] and was not arthritogenic although it could induce delayed hypersensitivity and under the same circumstances auto-immune diseases [33, 34]. *In vitro* experiments have shown that WSA amplified the immune response to other T-independent antigens and that this activity might be exerted at the level of macrophage [35]. However these adjuvants may have multiple effects and WSA has been shown to be active in the mixed lymphocyte reaction and to be capable of restoring the immune response in mice depleted of rosette-forming cells [36]. In these instances mediation may occur through the thymus-derived cells.

The chemical breakdown of WSA revealed that the minimal cell wall unit capable of replacing whole mycobacterial cells in FCA was a monosaccharide tripeptide [37], part of which, N-acetyl muramyl-L-alanyl-D-isoglutamine (hereafter referred to as MDP for muramyl dipeptide), was subsequently synthesized and shown to be the minimal unit with immunoregulatory properties [37, 38, 39]. The formula for WSA and MDP are shown in Figure 1 which also shows their relationship to the mycobacterial cell wall skeleton and wax C structures, as stipulated by E. LEDERER [40, 41].

Like WSA, MDP was devoid of several of the side effects elicited by the administration of whole mycobacterial cells. Thus it did not render mice susceptible to endotoxins, did not induce granuloma formation or lymphoid hyperplasia, was not arthritogenic and did not sensitize guinea pigs to tuberculin [42]. Moreover, even when administered in FCA, MDP does not sensitize guinea pigs to itself. This small molecule which is not immunogenic, can be coupled however to a carrier and thus persuaded to induce anti-MDP antibodies (C. REICHERT et al., unpublished results). Moreover, no detectable toxicity was observed in normal or even adrenalectomized mice [43]. KOTANI et al. demonstrated however that administration of MDP to rabbits elicited a febrile response [44]. This observation has been recently confirmed by DINARELLO et al. [45] who also demonstrated that MDP could release endogenous pyrogens from rabbit granulocytes or macrophages in vitro. A similar although weaker release was observed using human blood cells. However two analogs having the same degree of adjuvant activity were markedly less pyrogenic and all three molecules were negative in the limulus test.

In contrast to other adjuvant fractions, MDP was found to be very active when injected in an aqueous medium [42]. More-

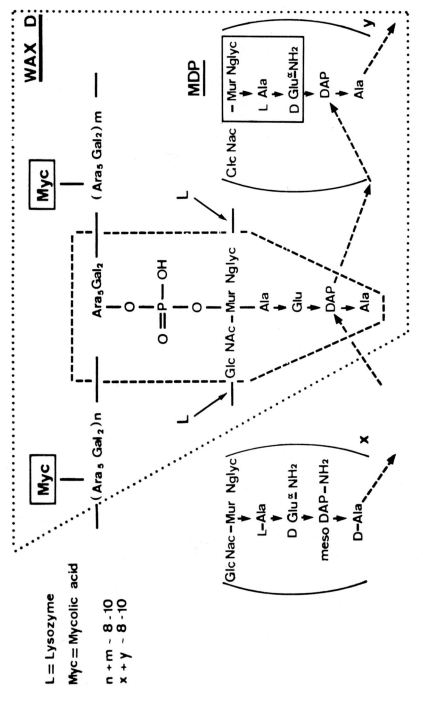

FIG. 1 — Simplified scheme of the mycobacterial cell wall and its adjuvant-active derivatives wax D, water-soluble adjuvant (WSA), and N-acetylmuramyl-L-alanyl-D-isoglutamine (MDP). Myc = mycolic acid. L = lysozyme. The WSA unit shown here has a molecular weight of about 2,000.

over, its activity was demonstrable by various routes including oral administration [46].

The data summarized in Figure 2 make it evident that it is not necessary to administer the antigen and MDP by the same route to observe an increase of the humoral antibody response and that MDP was active even after oral administration.

D-isoglutamine which is essential for the activity of MDP is not hydrolyzable by enzymes of mammalian hosts and thus cannot be degraded. Substitution of the L isomer at this point results

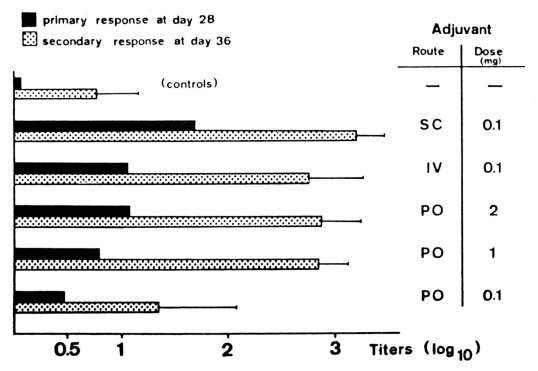

Fig. 2 — Adjuvant activity of MDP administered by various routes including the oral route.
Mice (10 per group) received subcutaneously 500 µg of BSA with or without adjuvant administered in PBS and 30 days later a recall of 100 µg of antigen alone. Antibody titers are estimated by passive hemagglutination of BSA-sensitized sheep red blood cells. In the four first experimental groups titers are highly significantly elevated (P < 0.01) as compared with the controls by Student's t test.

in an inactive product. One might speculate then that the former non-degradable form may be a distinct asset compared to natural mediators which probably have short biological half-lives. In this respect it is interesting to note that recently synthetic pentapeptides related to Met-enkephalin were shown to have prolonged parenteral and oral analgesic activity. In these molecules D-alanine had been substituted to the glycine residue in position 2 [47].

The various aspects of biological activity of MDP and its analogs have been reviewed recently [48, 49] and mechanisms of action studied in various systems [50, 51, 52, 53, 54, 55, 56]. Multiple analogs of MDP have now been synthesized with minor modifications and correlations between biological activity and chemical structure are beginning to be made [57, 58]. To illustrate, certain derivatives such as an MDP stereoisomer where D-alanyl was substituted for the L form, were capable of inhibiting the immune response, suggesting their possible use as immunosuppressants [46]. It is also of importance that certain of these synthetic adjuvants were shown to stimulate phagocytosis as measured by carbon clearance [59] and to increase non-specific resistance to infection [43]. MDP and 4 other synthetic adjuvants enhance non-specific immunity of mice infected by *K. pneumoniae*. These compounds were active by various routes including oral administration (Figure 3). They were also effective when administered after challenge. Of the 17 analogs tested none was able to increase resistance to infection although 7 of these molecules were adjuvant active in saline. It must be recalled that in contrast to lipopolysaccharides these synthetic adjuvants are devoid of immunogenicity and toxicity in normal or adrenalectomized mice (Figure 3).

Although most of the data obtained when this synthetic adjuvant was administered in saline concern systems involving humoral antibody production, it must be recalled that when administered in Freund's incomplete adjuvant (FIA), MDP can induce delayed hypersensitivity [37, 39, 60, 61, 62] and even auto-immune disease [47, 48]. In this last very recent report auto-immune disease was induced by administering a synthetic encephalitogen antigen either with FCA or with FIA containing very small amounts of MDP. In all previous studies which were made with FCA in guinea pigs, this synthetic auto-antigen (a tryptophan nona-

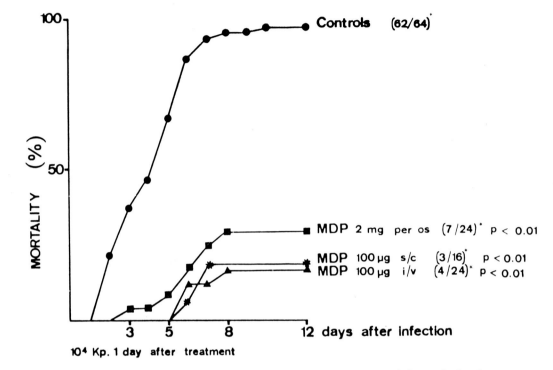

FIG. 3 — Protective effect of MDP injected by different routes before infection by intramuscular route (10^4 K.pneumoniae 1 day after treatment).
* Number of dead/total number of mice per group at day + 12.

peptide) had been shown to be the shortest active encephalitogen peptide. However auto-immune encephalomyelitis was also induced by a tri-heptapeptide administered with MDP in FIA, but not with FCA. In contrast, administration with either adjuvant of even shorter peptides (containing 6 or less aminoacids) had no effect, showing how critical is the presence of a single amino-acid in this system.

These experiments are remarkable, not only because they show a maximal amplification of the immune response under the influence of a synthetic antigen and of a synthetic adjuvant but also because they provide a most interesting model for cell-mediated

[10] *Chedid* - p. 7

auto-immune reactions since such haptenic synthetic peptides did not induce antibody production.

It has also been reported that the enhancement of the antibody response to Sheep red blood cells administered with MDP *in an aqueous medium* was produced via the T cells [51].

Recently YAMAMURA has shown that allogenic cell-mediated cytotoxicity was enhanced by MDP *in vitro* but not *in vivo* whereas a mycoloyl derivative of MDP was active *in vivo* [52]. Adminis-tered *in vivo* to C57B1/6 J mice, 6-0-mycoloyl MDP was found to be as effective as BCG cell walls for the generation of cell-mediated cytotoxic effector cells against P815-X$_2$ mastocytoma. However it was less active as adjuvant than BCG cell walls or MDP in enhanc-ing circulating antibodies to a T-independent antigen (DNP-Ficoll) and on the generation of helper function of carrier-primed T cells. It was also inactive as a mitogen on murine spleen cells.

It must also be remembered that MDP administered in saline activated macrophages, enabling them to inhibit the growth of tumor target cells [50]. Oppenheim and Mizel have observed that MDP induces mitogenic activity to appear in the supernatant of mouse peritoneal exudate cells and human peripheral mononuclear cells. This activity is made by the cell population which is enriched for adherent cells. It is therefore likely to be similar to lymphocyte-activating factor (LAF), however the adherent cells contain some lymphocytes and they may be making a mitogenic factor (MF) (unpublished results).

In all these studies the synthetic molecules were administered in an aqueous medium.

More investigation should be made to see whether aqueous MDP or perhaps some other analogs can stimulate cell-mediated immunity as powerfully as FCA so that this type of synthetic adjuvant can be used in conjunction with future vaccines against tumors.

However in view of the findings reported here, several ap-proaches concerning the use of these synthetic molecules in cancer immunotherapy should be considered. They can be summarized as follows: *a*) potentiation of immunization by a neo-antigen; *b*) enhancement of non-specific tumor immunity; *c*) utilization of immunosuppressive analogs; *d*) enhancement of non-specific immunity against infections.

It is indeed generally recognized that intercurrent infections with often a fatal outcome constitute one of the greatest hazards for cancer patients.

For a long time there have been conceptual differences between chemotherapy and immunotherapy, sometimes to the point of the two being in opposition. Yet it must be recalled that cancer chemotherapy has rendered available since decades several synthetic cytostatic but also immunosuppressive molecules. The availability of synthetic compounds representing analogs of natural structures existing in prokaryotes and capable of regulating the immune response may also bridge the gap existing between these two approaches to tumor therapy. Various conjugations of synthetic adjuvants to synthetic antigens such as certain modified peptides which are now available may also be a promising field for future immunological manipulations. To summarize, the experimental evidences already accumulated in a short period of time with immunoregulating synthetic molecules augur favorably of their potential therapeutic value.

REFERENCES

[1] OLD L.J., CLARKE D.A. and BENACERRAF B., *Effect of Bacillus Calmette-Guérin infection on transplanted tumours in the mouse.* « Nature », *184*, 291-292 (1959).

[2] MATHÉ G., *Active immunotherapy.* « Advan. Cancer Res. », *14*, 1-36 (1971).

[3] WEISS D.W., BONHAG R.S. and DE OME K.B., *Protective activity of fractions of tubercle bacilli against isologous tumours in mice.* « Nature », *190*, 889-891 (1961).

[4] ZBAR B., BERNSTEIN I., TANAKA T. and RAPP H.J., *Tumor immunity produced by the intradermal inoculation of living tumor cells and living* Mycobacterium bovis (strain BCG). « Science », *170*, 1217-1218 (1970).

[5] LAUCIUS J.F., BODURTHA A.J., MASTRANGELO M.J. and CREECH R.H., *Bacillus Calmette-Guérin in the treatment of neoplastic disease.* « J. Reticuloendothel. Soc. », *16*, 347-373 (1974).

[6] CHEDID L., LAMENSANS A., PARANT F., PARANT M., ADAM A., PETIT J.F. and LEDERER E., *Protective effect of delipidated mycobacterial cells and purified cell walls against Ehrlich carcinoma and a syngeneic lymphoid leukemia in mice.* « Cancer Res. », *33*, 2187-2195 (1973).

[7] LAMENSANS A., CHEDID L., LEDERER E., ROSSELET J.P., LUDWIG B., BERGER F.M., GUSTAFSON R.H. and SPENCER H J., *Enhancement of immunity against murine syngeneic tumors by a fraction extracted from non-pathogenic mycobacteria.* « Proc. Natl. Acad. Sci. USA », *72*, 3656-3660 (1975).

[8] LECLERC C., LAMENSANS A., CHEDID L., DRAPIER J.C., PETIT J.F., WIETZERBIN J. and LEDERER E., *Nonspecific immunoprevention of L1210 leukemia by cord factor (6-6' dimycolate of thehalose) administered in a metabolizable oil.* « Cancer Immunol. Immunother. », *1*, 227-232 (1976).

[9] BAST R.C. and SIMPSON-BAST B., *Critical review of previously reported animal studies of tumor immunotherapy with non-specific immunostimulants.* Int. Conf. on Immunotherapy of Cancer, C.M. Southam and H. Friedman eds, « The New York Academy of Sciences », *277*, 60-93 (1976).

[10] ZBAR B., RAPP H.J. and RIBI E., *Tumor suppression by cell walls of Mycobacterium bovis attached to oil droplets.* « J. Nat. Cancer Inst. », *48*, 831-835 (1972).

[11] GRAY G.R., RIBI E., GRANGER D.L., PAEKER R., AZUMA I. and YAMAMOTO K., *Immunotherapy of cancer: tumor suppression by cell walls of Mycobacterium phlei attached to oil droplets.* « J. Nat. Cancer Inst. », *55*, 727-729 (1975).

[10] *Chedid* · p. 10

[12] MASTRANGELO M.J., BERD D. and BELLET R.E., *Critical review of previously reported clinical trials of cancer immunotherapy with non-specific immunostimulants*. Int. Conf. on Immunotherapy of Cancer, C.M. Southam and H. Friedman eds, « The New York Academy of Sciences », *277*, 94-123 (1976).

[13] HERSCH E.M., GUTTERMAN J.U., MAVIGLIT G.M., ROOED R.C. and RICHMAN S.P., *BCG vaccine and its derivatives: potential, practical considerations and precautions in human cancer immunotherapy*. « J. Amer. Med. Ass. », *235*, 646-650 (1976).

[14] POUILLART P., MATHÉ G., PALANGIÉ T., SCHWARZENBERG L., HUQUENIN P., MORIN P., GAUTIER M. and PARROT R., *Trial of BCG immunotherapy in the treatment of resectable squamous cell carcinoma of the bronchus* (stages I and II). « Cancer Immunol. Immunoth. », *1*, 271-276 (1976).

[15] ISRAEL L., *Immunochemotherapy with* Corynebacterium parvum *in disseminated cancer*. Int Conf. on Immunotherapy of Cancer, C.M. Southam and H. Friedman eds, « The New York Academy of Sciences », *277*, 209-227 (1976).

[16] YAMAMURA Y., AZUMA I., TANIYAMA T., SUGIMURA K., HIRAO F., TOKUZEN R., OKABE M., NAKAHARA W., YASUMOTO K. and OHTA M., *Immunotherapy of cancer with cell wall skeleton of* Mycobacterium bovis-*Bacillus Calmette-Guérin: experimental and clinical results*. Int. Conf. on Immunotherapy of Cancer, C.M. Southam and H. Friedman eds, « The New York Academy of Sciences », *277*, 209-227 (1976).

[17] PERLOFF M., HOLLAND J.F., LUMB G.J. and BEKESI J.G., *Effect of methanol extraction residues of* Bacillus Calmette-Guérin *in Humans*. « Cancer Res. », *37*, 1191-1196 (1977).

[18] BUCANA C. and HANNA M.G. Jr., *Immunoelectron microscopic analysis of surface antigens common to* Mycobacterium bovis (BCG) *and tumor cells*. « J. Nat. Cancer Inst. », *53*, 1313-1323 (1974).

[19] BORSOS T. and RAPP H.J., *Antigenic relationship between* Mycobacterium bovis (BCG) *and a guinea pig hepatoma*. « J. Nat. Cancer Inst. », *51*, 1085-1102 (1973).

[20] VANDENBARD A.A., BURGER D.R. and VETTO R.M., *Cell-mediated immunity in experimental allergic encephalomyelitis. Cross reactivity between myelin basic protein and mycobacteria antigens*. « Proc. Soc. Exp. Biol. Med. », *148*, 1233-1236 (1975).

[20bis] WERNER G.H., MARAL R., FLOC'H F. and JOUANNE M., *Toxicological aspects of immunopotentiation by adjuvants and immunostimulating substances*. « Bull. Inst. Pasteur », *75*, 5-84 (1977).

[21] FREUND J., *The mode of action of immunologic adjuvants*. « Adv. Tub. Res., S. Karger Basel/N. Y. », *7*, 130-148 (1956).

[22] WHITE R.G., *The adjuvant effect of microbial products on the immune response*. « Ann. Rev. Microb. », *30*, 579-600 (1976).

[23] FREUND J., *Some aspects of active immunization*. « Ann. Rev. Microb. », *1*, 291-308 (1947).

[24] AZUMA I., KISHIMOTO S., YAMAMURA Y. and PETIT J.F., *Adjuvanticity of mycobacterial cell walls*. « Japan. J. Microbiol. », *15*, 193-197 (1971).

[25] RAFFEL S., *The components of the tubercle bacillus responsible for the delayed type of infectious allergy.* « J. Infect. Dis. », *82*, 267-293 (1948).

[26] WHITE R.C., JOLLÈS P., SAMOUR D. and LEDERER E., *Correlation of adjuvant activity and chemical structure of wax D fractions of mycobacteria.* « Immunology », *7*, 185-171 (1964).

[27] ADAM A., CIORBARU R., PETIT J.F. and LEDERER E., *Isolation and properties of a macromolecular, water soluble, immunoadjuvant fraction from the cell wall of* Mycobacterium smegmatis. « Proc. Natl. Acad. Sci. USA », *69*, 851-854 (1972).

[28] MIGLIORE-SAMOUR D. and JOLLÈS P., *A hydrosoluble adjuvant active mycobacterial polysaccharide-peptidoglycan. Preparation by a single extraction technique of the bacterial cells* (strain peurois). « FEBS Lett. », *25*, 301-304 (1972).

[29] ADAM A., CIORBARU R., PETIT J.F., LEDERER E., CHEDID L., LAMENSANS A., PARANT F., PARANT M., ROSSELET J.P. and BERGER F.M., *Preparation and biological properties of water soluble adjuvant fraction from delipidated cells of* Mycobacterium smegmatis *and* Nocardia opaca. « Infect. Immun. », *7*, 855-861 (1973).

[30] HIU I.J., *Water soluble and lipid-free fraction from BCG with adjuvant antitumor activity.* « Nature (London) New Biol. », *238*, 241-242 (1972).

[31] STEWART-TULL D.E.S., SHIMONO T., KOTANI S., KATO M., OGAWA Y., YAMAMURA Y., KOGA T. and PEARSON C.M., *Adjuvant activity of a non-toxic, water soluble glycopeptide present in large quantities in the culture filtrate of* Mycobacterium tuberculosis *strain OT.* « Immunology », *29*, 1-15 (1975).

[32] CHEDID L., PARANT M., PARANT F., GUSTAFSON R.H. and BERGER F.M., *Biological study of non-toxic, water soluble immunoadjuvant from mycobacterial cell walls.* « Proc. Natl. Acad. Sci. USA », *69*, 855-858 (1972).

[33] TOULLET F., AUDIBERT F., CHEDID L. and VOISIN G.A., *Production d'une orchiépididymite aspermatogénétique auto-immune (OAAI) chez le cobaye à l'aide d'un adjuvant hydrosoluble extrait de* Mycobacterium smegmatis. « Ann. Immunol. (Inst. Pasteur) », *125C*, 901-910 (1974).

[34] LEBAR R. and VOISIN G.A., *Production d'une encéphalomyélite allergique expérimentale auto-immune (EAE) chez le cobaye à l'aide d'un adjuvant hydrosoluble extrait de* Mycobacterium smegmatis. « Ann. Immunol. (Inst. Pasteur) », *125C*, 911-916 (1974).

[35] MODOLELL M., LUCKENBACH G.A., PARANT M. and MUNDER P.G., *The adjuvant activity of a mycobacterial water soluble adjuvant (WSA) in vitro. I. The requirement for macrophages.* « J. Immunol. », *113*, 395-403 (1974).

[36] BONA C., HEUCLIN C. and CHEDID L., *Enhancement of human mixed lymphocyte cultures by a water soluble adjuvant.* « Recent Results Cancer Res. », *47*, 197-200 (1974).

[37] ELLOUZ F., ADAM A., CIORBARU R. and LEDERER E., *Minimal structural requirements for adjuvant activity of bacterial peptidoglycan derivatives.* « Biochem. Biophys. Res. Commun. », *59*, 1317-1325 (1974).

[38] ADAM A., ELLOUZ F., CIORBARU R., PETIT J.F. and LEDERER E., *Peptidoglycan adjuvants: minimal structure required for activity.* « Z. Immunitätsforsch.», *149S*, 341-348 (1975).

[39] MERSER C., SINAY P. and ADAM A., *Total synthesis and adjuvant activity of bacterial peptidoglycan derivatives.* « Biochem. Biophys. Res. Commun.», *66*, 1316-1322 (1975).

[40] LEDERER E., *Natural and synthetic immunostimulants related to the mycobacterial cell wall.* Proceedings of the 5th International Symposium on Medicinal Chemistry, 1977, Elsevier Scientific, Amsterdam.

[41] LEDERER E., ADAM A., CIORBARU R., PETIT J.F. and WIETZERBIN J., *Cell walls of mycobacteria and related organisms: chemistry and immunostimulant properties.* « Molec. Cell. Biochem.», *7*, 87-104 (1975).

[42] AUDIBERT F., CHEDID L., LEFRANCIER P. and CHOAY J., *Distinctive adjuvanticity of synthetic analogs of mycobacterial water soluble components.* « Cell. Immunol.», *21*, 243-249 (1976).

[43] CHEDID L., PARANT M., PARANT F., LEFRANCIER P., CHOAY J. and LEDERER E., *Enhancement of non-specific immunity to* Klebsiella pneumoniae *infection by a synthetic immunoadjuvant (N-acetylmuramyl-L-alanyl-D-isoglutamine) and several analogs.* « Proc. Natl. Acad. Sci. USA », *74*, 2089-2093 (1977).

[44] KOTANI S., WATANABE Y., SHIMONO T., HARUDA K., SHIBA T., KUSUMOTO S., YOKOGAWA K. and TANIGUCHI M., *Correlation between immunoadjuvant activities and pyrogenicities of synthetic N-acetyl muramyl-peptides or -aminoacids.* « Biken J.», *19*, 9-13 (1976).

[45] DINARELLO C.A., ELIN R.J., CHEDID L. and WOLFF S.M., *The pyrogenicity of synthetic adjuvants.* Submitted to publication.

[46] CHEDID L., AUDIBERT F., LEFRANCIER P., CHOAY J. and LEDERER E., *Modulation of the immune response by a synthetic adjuvant and analogs.* « Proc. Natl. Acad. Sci. USA », *73*, 2472-2475 (1976).

[47] ROEMER D., BUESCHER H.H., HILL R.C., PLESS J., BAUER W., CARDINAUX F., CLOSSE A., HAUSER D. and HUGUENIN R., *A synthetic enkephalin analogue with prolonged parenteral and oral analgesic activity.* « Nature », *268*, 547-549 (1977).

[48] CHEDID L. and AUDIBERT F., *Recent advances in the use of the synthetic immunoadjuvant muramyl dipeptide and analogues.* In « Microbiology-1977 », pp. 388-394, D. Schlessinger ed., American Soc. for Microbiol., Washington, 1977.

[49] The Lancet, Editorial: *Immunological adjuvantes: less alchemy and more science?* July 30, vol. II for 1977, 230-231.

[50] JUY D. and CHEDID L., *Comparison between macrophage activation and enhancement of nonspecific resistance to tumors by mycobacterial immunoadjuvants.* « Proc. Natl. Acad. Sci. USA », *72*, 4105-4109 (1975).

[51] LÖWY I., BONA C. and CHEDID L., *Target cells for the activity of a synthetic adjuvant: muramyl dipeptide.* « Cell. Immunol.», *29*, 195-199 (1977).

[52] YAMAMURA Y., AZUMA I., SUGIMURA K., YAMAWAKI M., UEMIYA M., KUSUMOTO S., OKADA S. and SHIBA T., *Adjuvant activity of 6-O-mycoloyl-N-acetyl-muramyl-L-alanyl-D-isoglutamine.* « Gann », *67*, 867-877 (1976).

[53] TOULLET F., AUDIBERT F., VOISIN G.A. and CHEDID L., *Production d'orchiépididymite aspermatogénique autoimmune chez le cobaye, à l'aide de différents adjuvants hydrosolubles*. « Ann. Immunol. (Inst. Pasteur) », *128C*, 267-269 (1977).

[54] NAGAI Y., *Modulation of the immunologic response of myelin basic protein by extrinsic and intrisic factors*. « Neurology », *26*, 45-46 (1976).

[55] DAMAIS C., PARANT M. and CHEDID L., *Nonspecific activation of murine spleen cells* in vitro *by a synthetic immunoadjuvant (N-acetylmuramyl-L-alanyl-D-isoglutamine)*. « Cell. Immunol. », *33*, in press (1977).

[56] SPECTER S., FRIEDMAN H. and CHEDID L., *Dissociation between the adjuvant vs mitogenic activity of a synthetic muramyl dipeptide for murine splenocytes*. « Proc. Soc. Ex. Biol. Med. », *155*, 349-352 (1977).

[57] DAMAIS C., PARANT M. and CHEDID L., In vitro *spleen cell responsiveness to various analogs of MDP (N-acetylmuramyl-L-alanyl-D-isoglutamine), a synthetic immunoadjuvant, in MDP high-responder mice*. « Cell. Immunol. », in press.

[58] AUDIBERT F., CHEDID L., LEFRANCIER P., CHOAY J. and LEDERER E., *Relationship between chemical structure and adjuvant activity of some synthetic analogs of N-acetylmuramyl-L-alanyl-D-isoglutamine (MDP)*. « Ann. Immunol. (Inst. Pasteur) », *128C*, 643-661 (1977).

[59] TANAKA A., NAGAO S., SAITO R., KOTANI S., KUSUMOTO S. and SHIBA T., *Correlation of stereochemically specific structure in muramyl dipeptide between macrophage activation and adjuvant activity*. « Biochem. Biophys. Res. Commun. », *77*, 621-627 (1977).

[60] KOTANI S., WATANABE Y., KINOSHITA F., SHIMONO T., MORISAKI I., SHIBA T., KUSUMOTO S., TARUMY Y. and IKENAKA K., *Immunoadjuvant activities of synthetic N-acetyl muramyl-peptides or -aminoacids*. « Biken J. », *18*, 105-111 (1975).

[61] AZUWA I., SUGIWURA K., TANIYAWA T., YAMAWAKI M., YAMAMURA Y., KUSUMOTO S., OKADA S. and SHIBA T., *Adjuvant activity of mycobacterial fractions. Adjuvant activity of synthetic N-acetylmuramyl-dipeptide and the related compounds*. « Infect. Immun. », *14*, 18-27 (1976).

[62] TANAKA A., SAITO R., SUGIYAMA K., MORISAKI I., KOTANI S., KUSUMOTO S. and SHIBA T., *Adjuvant activity of synthetic N-acetylmuramyl peptides in rats*. « Infect. Immun. », *15*, 332-334 (1977).

DISCUSSION

WEISS

I should like to congratulate Dr. Chedid on his elegant work and its presentation, and to ask him one specific question: what is known so far about the ability of these analogues in tumor immunoprophylaxis and immunotherapy? You alluded to this aspect of their activities only briefly; is there much data available so far?

CHEDID

To my knowledge there is no data available concerning *in vivo* tumor systems; results have been obtained, however, with *in vitro* systems such as enhancement of allogenic cytotoxicity. Moreover, I would like to remind you that these molecules administered in an aqueous medium are only effective for the enhancement of the humoral antibody response. However, since they are cleared so rapidly and since we have many indications of some T cell affinity, we should not rule out a possible role in cell mediated immunity before repeating experiments with conjugated or polymerized molecules. Such synthetic preparations will be phagocytized, channeled in different cellular compartments, and retained in the host for longer periods.

WESTPHAL

I wonder whether you tried repeated injections of these materials? Would tolerance be induced?

CHEDID

No.

WESTPHAL

So, in principle, if these substances would be infused, they should produce a continuous fever.

G. KLEIN

I was intrigued by the difference between the three mouse strains you demonstrated, particularly since C57B1 is a high responder in many other systems. Have you studied the genetics? What happens with F_1 crosses? Is anything known about backcrosses?

CHEDID

Evidence obtained in Dr. Benacerraf's laboratory showed that certain inbred strains can respond very strongly to BSA (agglutination titers of 100,000 were obtained versus 10 for the controls). Since we were using different strains in our *in vitro* experiments, we tested these sublines and found the results which have just been shown to you. There is a great probability that different immunogenetic patterns will be found by using different adjuvants. Some immunogenetic studies have been performed with Dr. Edna Mozes and Dr. Sela. These experiments were undertaken using the native peptidoglycan molecule which is a water soluble adjuvant and which we call WSA. They showed that bad responders to the (T,G)-A—L antigen administered in Freund's complete adjuvant became good responders when WSA was added. Similar experiments are being repeated with MDP.

SELA

I would like to add to this that synthetic antigens built on multichain polyproline are under genetic control, and we found that polyadenylic acid-polyuridylic acid double strand corrected the genetic defect of DBA/1 mice in mounting an immune response to (T,G)-Pro—L (based on multichain polyproline) but not to (T,G)-A—L (based on multichain poly-DL-alanine). On the other hand, we found now that the water-soluble adjuvant of Dr. Chedid does not affect the immune response to (T,G)-Pro—L but corrects the poor response to (T,G)-A—L in C3H/HeJ and SJL/J mice.

[10] *Chedid* - p. 16

I would also like to mention that when we recently attached a peptidoglycan, obtained from Dr. Nauciel in Strasbourg, to a synthetic branched polypeptide containing the P2 peptide, a fragment of the coat protein of bacteriophage MS2, the resulting conjugate provoked efficient formation of antiviral antibodies in incomplete Freund's adjuvant, in contrast to the synthetic antigen without the peptidoglycan attached, which led to an immune response only in the presence of complete Freund's adjuvant (Langbeheim, Arnon and Sela, Proc. Natl. Acad. Sci. U.S. 73, 4636 (1976).

CHEDID

I may add 2 comments to what Dr. Sela has just said. The first is to mention that in his laboratory glycopeptide was conjugated to their P2 synthetic viral antigen and that this conjugate administered in Freund's incomplete adjuvant had a greater activity. Similar experiments are being repeated, conjugating MDP and synthetic antigens such as (T,G)-A—L or P2, on polylysine-alanine chains. My second remark is related to the activity of MDP by oral route. We believe that the ability of MDP to be active orally is related to the terminal D-isoglutamine which is resistant to degradation by mammalian enzymes. This result comforted us because endotoxin is only active if administered parenterally and since in all experiments a contamination by endotoxin is always possible.

BARCINSKI

I want to ask if in the reversion of the (T,G)-A—L system it is already known in which cell water soluble adjuvant acts: in the macrophage or in the lymphocyte?

SELA

The genetic defect may be mainly in the T cell or mainly in the B cell, depending on the antigen and on the strain. Macrophages seem also to be definitely involved.

TERRY

We have some new information that partially answers Dr. Barcinski's questions. Some recent work has been done by Dr. Singer and Dr. Hodes in our laboratory. Using a primary *in vitro* immunization system to soluble antigens, including the synthetic polypeptides, it has been shown that an adherent cell, apparently neither a T cell nor a B cell is responsible for determining responsiveness and nonresponsiveness. The regulator cell may be a macrophage, but that has not been proved vigorously. This would be an ideal *in vitro* system for examining the cell stimulated by Dr. Chedid's materials.

RAPP

Do BCG cell wall skeletons in oil have adjuvant activity?

CHEDID

Yes.

RAPP

So does that mean that there are different fractions in the BCG which contribute to adjuvant activity, and are they independent or do they work together — what is your opinion?

CHEDID

The MDP structure is a constituent of the cell wall of most bacteria not only acid fast but also gram-negative and gram-positive. This structure has even been found in blue-green algae.

RAPP

And there is no quantitative difference in adjuvanticity between the living BCG and the cell wall skeleton?

CHEDID

You may indeed have differences. Thus, a well purified cell wall skeleton does not sensitize to tuberculin, does not increase the mouse's

[10] *Chedid* - p. 18

susceptibility to endotoxin and in certain cases is not arthritogenic. This requires that a very well purified preparation has been obtained and contains no longer detectable amounts of tuberculin or cord factor.

OETTGEN

In your long list of analogues that were tested for pyrogenicity and adjuvanticity, the absence of pyrogenicity usually also meant loss of adjuvanticity. There were two exceptions. Are these two compounds, in terms of their adjuvant activity, quite up to the potency of the pyrogenic analogue?

CHEDID

Since we do endpoints in our experiments I can answer you very positively that adjuvant activity can be separated from pyrogenicity. However, we have not succeeded yet in separating adjuvant from antibacterial activity: whereas all the anti-bacterial products are also adjuvant, all the adjuvants do not necessarily enhance resistance to bacterial challenge.

ROSENBERG

If this MDP is so ubiquitous, what is it about the BCG or the mycrobacteria that makes it such a good adjuvant in oil when other bacteria containing MDP are not good adjuvants?

CHEDID

I believe that the answer is that in certain bacterial species, the peptidoglycan structure is not well presented or can even be antagonized by other bacterial products. Thus, for instance, in gram-negative organisms, lipopolysaccharides not only conceal the peptidoglycan but also can commit the immune response towards humoral antibody formation.

NOSSAL

It is a pity that our friend Christian De Duve is not yet here, so

I will ask you a question that he would have asked you, had he been here. If the purpose of nonspecific cancer immunotherapy is to activate the macrophage to become angry and kill tumor cells, might it be interesting to hook muramyl dipeptide on to coacervates of DNA, constituting a lysosomotropic agent? If so, would you expect superb tumor regression to follow?

CHEDID

I quite agree and we are probably going to have a second and a third generation of such synthetic molecules. The second generation will consist in modifications of the structure, whereas the third will be obtained by coupling these molecules to carriers or by hooking them to antigens. Furthermore, and since we are in this realm of thinking and as these ideas are rather germane to the concept of "guided missiles", one could very well envision conjugation of synthetic immunoregulators to DNA.

THE INTERPLAY OF VIRAL TRANSFORMATION, ENVIRONMENTAL FACTORS AND CHROMOSOMAL CHANGES IN THE CAUSATION OF BURKITT'S LYMPHOMA

GEORGE KLEIN

Department of Tumor Biology Karolinska Institutet
S 104 01 Stockholm 60 - Sweden

This paper will deal with the causation of Burkitt's lymphoma. It is the first human tumor where the role of a known virus has been defined. Moreover, it represents an intriguing interplay of viral transformation, the environmental promotion and cytogenetic changes, all involved in the development of frank neoplasia.

EPSTEIN-BARR virus (EBV) is a lymphotropic herpesvirus in man [1]. Its main target is the human B lymphocyte [2]. Only B lymphocytes and most if not all B lymphocytes have specific EBV receptors [3]. It has been recently shown that the complement receptor of the B lymphocyte serves as the receptor for EBV [4, 5, 6, 7]. However, the complement receptors of other cell types, e.g. T-cells, macrophages, granulocytes, erythrocytes, do not serve as EBV-receptors.

It is interesting that the virus should have "chosen" a pre-existent receptor of the B-lymphocyte as its receptor during its evolution. On the one hand, this explains the exclusive infectivity of EBV for the B-lymphocyte, among all potential target cells so far tested. On the other hand, it may also give some functional clues. At least some immunologists believe that the complement receptor of the B-lymphocyte plays a role in triggering cellular DNA synthesis and opening the way towards blastogenesis, following the attachment of appropriate antigen-antibody-complement complexes. EBV acts as a B-cell mitogen by itself. It induces DNA synthesis in the infected B lymphocyte [8, 9] and activates B-lymphocytes to polyclonal IgM production [10]. Induction of cellular DNA synthesis appears to be a prerequisite for EBV induced immortalization. A variant strain of the virus, derived from the P3HR-1 line, fails to induce DNA synthesis and also fails to immortalize [9, 11]. Prevention of DNA synthesis by cytosine arabinoside completely prevents the induction of EBV-determined nuclear antigen (EBNA) in normal lymphocytes by transforming strains of the virus. EBNA induction is the first step on the way towards immortalization [12]. The variant B3HR-1 virus prevents the DNA synthesis induced by the transforming virus and thereby prevents transformation, if added before, simultaneously with or shortly after the transforming virus [13]. Due to its release of a growth inhibitory, cytopathic virus, this line has lost EBV and complement receptors, as a result of internal selection [14]. Non-producer sublines can regain both receptors after long periods (years) of continuous culture.

EBV induced immortalization of normal lymphocytes that have an otherwise limited life span in vitro, leads to permanently growing cell lines [15, 16, 17, 18, 19, 20]. Such "immortalized" lines have a diploid or near-diploid karyotype [21, 22] carry multiple copies of the viral genome per cell [23, 24, 25, 26] and express EBV-specific nuclear antigen (EBNA) [27]. A smaller part of the viral genomes (perhaps only one or a few copies) are present in a covalently integrated form with the host cell genome, whereas the major part is present as covalently closed circles, probably propagated as free plasmids [28]. The exact relationship between the integrated and the free genomes is not known in detail.

EBNA is a virally determined or virally altered chromosomal protein, the only known viral product expressed in all EBV-DNA carrying cells, independent of virus production. It has been recently purified to homogeneity [29]. We have recently found that the amount of EBNA per nucleus is directly proportional to the number of EBV-genome copies per cell [30]. Moreover, EBNA seems to be an autonomous function of the viral genome. It is fully expressed in e.g. human/mouse hybrids that are otherwise completely non-permissive and non-inducible with regard to all other EBV determined functions [31, 32, 33, 34, 35]. Also, EBNA is a DNA binding protein, a fact that was widely utilized for concentration and purification [36, 37, 38] and also for the definite demonstration that EBNA was identical with the previously known, EBV-associated complement fixing soluble antigen. Following concentration and purification, the CF antigen was added to acid fixed nuclei of various EBNA-negative cells. Brilliant EBNA specific staining was obtained, both with metaphase chromosomes and interphase nuclei [39].

The autonomous expression of EBNA, together with its DNA binding properties, raise the question whether it might be a virally determined regulatory protein. The most interesting possibility is that it may play a role in preventing the multiple EBV genomes from entering the viral cycle, a process that inevitably leads to cell death. Repression of the viral cycle is an obvious prerequisite for prolonged viral latency in vivo and for the multiplication of established EBV-carrying cell lines in vitro.

EBV-DNA and EBNA carrying lymphoblastoid cell lines can be regularly established from the peripheral blood or lymph nodes of EBV-seropositive donors, but not from seronegatives [40, 41]. EBV can also transform the B lymphocytes of certain simian hosts [42, 43]. Some of the derived lines can grow progressively after reimplantation and kill the original, autochthonous host [44, 45]. In marmosets [45, 46, 47] and owl monkeys [48], the virus also has a direct oncogenic activity. The induced lymphomas carry the viral genome and contain EBNA.

EBV infects the majority of all adult human populations in all countries [49, 50]. Its seroepidemiology resembles other horizontally transmitted viruses, with the regular presence of passively transmitted antibody in the newborn, its subsequent decline and the reappearance of actively induced antibody after infection. The timing and extent of seroconversion are strongly related to socioeconomic status. In low socioeconomic groups, infection occurs during early childhood, as a rule. It is not accompanied by any recognized disease, and the route of transmission is unknown. Only a minority of young children become infected in high socio-

[11] *G. Klein* - p. 3

economic groups where a later (teen-age) infection predominates. Although at least half the teen-age infections appear without recognized symptoms, primary infection is accompanied by heterophile-positive infectious mononucleosis in the other half [51, 52, 53, 54].

Despite the unclear pathogenesis of the infectious mononucleosis syndrome, infectious (transforming) EBV can be regularly recovered from throat washings of patients with the disease [55, 56, 57, 58]. During the acute phase, these patients' peripheral blood contains specific killer T-lymphocytes that can lyse EBV-genome positive but not EBV-negative target cells [59, 60]. In parallel, large blast cells appear in the B-cell fraction, containing the EBV-determined nuclear antigen, EBNA [61]. Part of the infectious mononucleosis syndrome may reflect an acute rejection reaction against virally converted lymphocytes. Recently, we have examined the lymphoid tissues of a three-year old girl who died of acute IM. Her thymus, tonsils and spleen contained up to 19% EBNA positive cells. Her T-cells showed only a weak activity against EBV carrying lines in cytotoxic tests [62]. All this supports the concept that, under normal conditions, a T-cell mediated rejection reaction stops what could otherwise develop into a lethal proliferation of virus carrying B-cells.

Two human neoplasias, nasopharyngeal carcinoma and African Burkitt's lymphoma, show a remarkably consistent association with EBV both by serology [63, 64] and by EBV-genome tests [65, 66, 67]. African Burkitt's lymphoma can be regarded as the neoplastic proliferation of an EBV-genome carrying clone [68] in 97% of the cases [69]. The very rare cases of Burkitt's lymphoma occurring outside the high endemic regions of Africa do not show a similar association with EBV either by serology [70] or EBV-genome tests [71], as a rule. Recently, however, five EBV-genome carrying European and American Burkitt lymphomas have been identified, comprising approximately 15-20% of all similarly examined cases [for reference see 72]. Since the histopathological diagnosis of Burkitt's lymphoma is not based on unequivocal criteria, it remains to be seen whether the EBV-carrying and the EBV negative Burkitt lymphomas represent the same disease. This can only be decided by correlated and, eventually, prospective EBV-related, histopathological and clinical studies.

Like the EBV-carrying established lines, biopsies of African Burkitt's lymphoma carry multiple copies of the viral genome per cell [65, 66, 67]. Part of these genomes exist in a covalently closed, free circular form [73], whereas another part is integrated with the cell genome. The biopsies contain the same type of circles as established lines [73, 74].

EBV carrying Burkitt's lymphoma cells grow into established in vitro lines more readily than explants from infectious mononucleosis or normal seropositive donors. In the majority of the cases studied, the clonal characteristics of established lymphoma-derived lines correspond to the in vivo clone [75], but contaminating EBV-positive B cells can occasionally overgrow the lymphoma cells [76]. Representative lymphoma lines differ from "lymphoblastoid lines", i.e. in vitro EBV-transformed cells and lines derived from non-lymphomatous sources, with regard to a number of morphologic, functional and growth characteristics [21]. Lymphoma lines are relatively uniform, but lymphoblastoid lines show great heterogeneity. EBV-carrying African Burkitt's lymphomas are already uniclonal in vivo [68], however, whereas lines derived from normal donors are polyclonal [77]. This diversity may explain some of the differences. Alternatively, lymphoma development may involve the appearance of a special neoplastic cell type, not present in EBV-transformed normal lymphocyte populations. The latter possibility is supported by the recent observation [22, 78, 79] that a highly specific chromosome 8 to 14-translocation can be found in biopsies of Burkitt's lymphoma and derived lines but is not observed in EBV-carrying lymphoblastoid lines of non-lymphoma origin. A similar 14q+ marker has also been found in a number of other B-cell derived neoplasias [80]. The implications of these findings are discussed in more detail below.

Some EBV-genome-negative B-type lymphomas have been established as continuous lines [31, 32, 33, 34], but only with considerable difficulty. The easy overgrowth of EBV-carrying normal cells is one of the main problems. EBV-negative lymphoid lines have never been established from normal tissues, however. Human lymphocytes can probably only grow as established lines if they are derived from a lymphoma or if they carry the EBV-genome or both. African Burkitt's lymphoma is the only known condition in which lymphoma derivation and EBV-positive status coincide.

This unique position of Burkitt's lymphoma as the only known EBV-carrying lymphoproliferative neoplasia in man, together with the known transforming and oncogenic properties of the virus, keep EBV as an important etiologic candidate for oncogenesis. Before accepting that a causative association may exist, alternatives must be considered, however. Numerous early commentators have favored the "passenger hypothesis". This idea implies that lymphoma cells, arising in EBV-carrying persons for EBV-unrelated reasons, pick up the virus as a passenger, just like normal lymphocytes, carry it along as they proliferate and thereby increase the antigenic load and induce antibody production. But, the very fact that non-Burkitt lymphomas that arise in EBV-seropositive patients do not pick up the virus is in itself a strong argument against this idea. It may be argued that such lymphoma cells are insensitive to EBV infection. However, some of the EBV-genome negative lymphoma lines, derived from EBV-negative Burkitt-like lymphomas that have arisen in seropositive patients could be infected with EBV in vitro [31, 32, 33, 34], followed by permanent conversion into EBV-DNA and EBNA-carrying lines [31, 32, 33, 34, 61, 81]. This finding confirms that EBV-sensitive lymphoma cells that arise in seropositive patients do not necessarily become infected by horizontal virus spread in vivo, presumably owing to the regular presence of neutralizing antibodies. It also suggests that EBV-genome-positive Burkitt's lymphomas originate from a genome-carrying cell. If this speculation is accepted, we are left with essentially two interpretations that are usually referred to as the immunologic and the co-factor hypotheses.

Arguments can be found for both interpretations. Lines derived from in vitro EBV transformed normal lymphocytes can have a neoplastic potential, although we have recently found that EBV-transformed diploid lines of recent origin do not kill nude mice, whereas long established, aneuploid lines do [82]. Earlier, NILSSON and PONTÉN [21] showed that EBV-carrying lymphoblastoid lines derived from normal donors or from benign conditions, including infectious mononucleosis, differed from EBV-carry-

[11] G. Klein - p. 6

ing, Burkitt's lymphoma-derived lines with regard to a whole series of morphologic, functional and growth characteristics.

Perhaps the most important difference lies in the cytogenetic constitution of the BL lines, as contrasted to EBV-carrying lines of non-neoplastic origin. It was originally discovered by MANOLOV and MANOLOVA [79] and recently confirmed and extended by JARVIS et al. [78] and by ZECH et al. [22], that definite chromosome differences exist between normal and lymphoma-derived lines. Normal diploid lines were only found among EBV-carrying lymphoblastoid lines derived from non-Burkitt's lymphoma donors. In contrast, all lymphoma lines so far examined were characterized by various chromosomal anomalies. The majority contained the characteristic chromosome-14 marker, recently identified as an 8-14 translocation [22]. Thus, EBV is fully capable of "immortalizing" B lymphocytes with a normal diploid karyotype in vitro, but EBV-carrying lymphomas in vivo have genetic changes in addition, probably of a rather specific kind. Such an interaction of viral transformation and cytogenetic changes is not as unique as it may appear at first sight. There are many experimental examples showing that known oncogenic viruses do not transform all or even the majority of appropriate target cells. Transformability is dependent on an obscure but probably specific "state of competence". Competence may be determined by the differentiation state or the genetic constitution of the cell (or both). The importance of the genetic constitution is emphasized by increasing evidence [83, 84, 85, 86, 87, 88] that both chemically and virally induced tumors may display highly specific chromosomal changes, different for tumors induced by different agents.

Some forms of viral oncogenesis may require specific genetic changes as a prerequisite for full development of cancer in vivo. Cells with a normal diploid karyotype possess regulatory mechanisms that could counteract the neoplastic change, even in cells that contain integrated genomes of a potentially oncogenic virus. Basilico's temperature-sensitive transformants [89] exemplify a situation in which a cellular function can influence the phenotype of virally transformed cells. Somatic cell hybridization experiments [90,

91, 92] have shown that the highly malignant behavior of established, polyomainduced or other tumors could be suppressed by fusion with normal diploid cells.

The importance of cellular genetics for virus-induced neoplastic transformation is also illustrated by the wholly unexpected finding [93, 94, 95, 96, 97, 98, 99, 100] that SV40 transforms with a higher efficiency if the target cells are derived from hosts with a known tendency for increased chromosomal variation or mitotic anomalies (e.g. Fanconi or Klinefelter syndromes, ataxia teleangiectasia, or xeroderma pigmentosum). The increased SV40 transformability of normal diploid human fibroblasts with ageing and accumulating chromosomal aberrations may be a further example.

ZECH et al. [22] have recently found that the Burkitt's lymphoma-associated chromosome-14 translocation was also present in some-EBV-negative Burkitt's and non-Burkitt's lymphomas, but never in EBV-transformed cells derived from normal donors or from patients with infectious mononucleosis. This cytogenetic change may somehow promote transformation to a malignant lymphoma. A relation between abnormal lymphocyte growth and structural rearrangement of the long arm of chromosome 14 is also suggested by recent studies of cells from patients with ataxia-teleangiectasia [101, 102]. Since a minority of African EBV-carrying Burkitt lymphomas lack the chromosome 14 translocation [22, 78, 79] (although they have other chromosomal anomalies), the visible manifestation of this particular translocation is not an absolute requirement for the development of full-fledged lymphomas. A similar situation may exist in chronic myelogenous leukemia where the Ph$_1$ chromosome (another translocation) is present in the majority but not all the cases.

Studies on the genetics of experimental carcinogenesis provide ample evidence [103, 104] that genetic factors may influence the probability of neoplastic transformation at the level of the target cell itself. Thus, a given genetic change — here expressed by the chromosome 14 translocation — may influence the probability of lymphoma induction by EBV and also by other, as yet unknown agents. This idea does not preclude the possibility that EBV and

[11] G. Klein - p. 8

other agents may occasionally induce lymphomas in the absence of this particular genetic aberration.

A discussion about the possible role of EBV in human neoplasia would not be complete without considering the relation between EBV and nasopharyngeal carcinoma (NPC). In contrast to Burkitt's lymphoma, there appears to be no major geographic variation in the EBV-carrying status of NPC [66, 105, 106] but there is a striking histologic restriction. Only poorly differentiated or anaplastic tumors have been found to carry the viral genome so far [107]. In contrast to earlier interpretations it is now clear [31, 32, 33, 34, 108, 109] that the viral genomes are not carried by the tumor-infiltrating lymphocytes (largely T cells [110]) but by the carcinoma cells themselves. They also express the EBNA antigen [31, 32, 33, 34, 108, 111]. Recent preliminary evidence suggests that the NPC associated genome may be slightly different from the Burkitt's lymphoma-associated genome. PAGANO et al. [24, 71] found that certain sequences were missing from the EBV-DNA of a Tunisian NPC as compared with a Burkitt's lymphoma-derived viral probe. In two nude mouse carriers of NPC, purified from infiltrating human lymphocytes by heterologous passage, KASCHKA-DIERICH et al. [74] found covalently closed EBV circles. It remains to be established whether these circles have the same characteristics as the Burkitt's lymphoma-associated circles. If they are different, this may be due to a variation in the virus strains associated with the different individual donors, in analogy with the molecular variations between different herpes simplex isolates [112], or may have a disease-associated importance.

At this stage, the NPC-EBV relation raises many interesting questions. The exclusive and regular presence of the viral genome in one histologically distinct tumor type, independently of geographic location and high or low endemicity, strongly suggests that the association must have some etiologic relevance, but it is impossible to state a preference for a causative versus a promoting relation. Genetic factors are known to play an important role in some high endemic ethnic groups, Chinese in particular [113]. In addition to the possible existence of an NPC-associated viral subtype, it would be important to obtain some information about the EBV susceptibility of the normal progenitor cells in the naso-pharyngeal epithelium. It would not be surprising if a co-operative interaction of viral transformation and host-cell genetics eventually emerged in this case as well. If so, the picture may resemble the situation postulated above for Burkitt's lymphoma — at least in principle, although the details may be quite different.

[11] G. *Klein* - p. 10

REFERENCES

[1] EPSTEIN M.A., ACHONG B.G. and BARR Y.M., « Lancet », *1*, 702 (1964).

[2] JONDAL M. and KLEIN G., « J. Exp. Med. », *138*, 1365 (1973).

[3] GREAVES F.M., BROWN G. and RICKINSON A.B., « Clin. Immunol. Immuno pathol. », *3*, 514 (1975).

[4] JONDAL M., KLEIN G., OLDSTONE M.B.A., BOKISH V. and YEFENOF E., « Scand. J. Immunol. », *5*, 401 (1976).

[5] YEFENOF E. and KLEIN G., « Int. J. Cancer », *20*, 347 (1977).

[6] YEFENOF E., KLEIN G., JONDAL M. and OLDSTONE M.B.A., « Int. J. Cancer », *17*, 693 (1976).

[7] YEFENOF E., KLEIN G. and KVARNUNG K., « Cell. Immunol. », *31*, 225 (1977).

[8] GERBER P. and HOYER B., « Nature », *267*, 52 (1977).

[9] MILLER G., ROBINSON J., HESTON L. and LIPMAN M., « Proc. Nat. Acad. Sci USA », *71*, 4006 (1974).

[10] ROSÉN A., BRITTON S., GERGELY P., JONDAL M. and KLEIN G., « Nature », *267*, 52 (1977).

[11] MENEZES J., LEIBOLD W. and KLEIN G., « Exp. Cell. Res. », *92*, 478 (1975).

[12] EINHORN L. and ERNBERG I., « Int. J. Cancer », *21*, 157 (1978).

[13] STEINITZ M., BAKACS T. and KLEIN G., « Int. J. Cancer », *22*, 251 (1978).

[14] KLEIN G., YEFENOF E., FALK K. and WESTMAN A., « Int. J. Cancer », (1978).

[15] CHANG R.S. and GOLDEN D.H., « Nature », *234*, 259 (1971).

[16] GERBER P., WHANG-PENG J. and MONROE J.H., « Proc. Nat. Acad. Sci. USA », *63*, 740 (1969).

[17] HENLE W., DIEHL V., KOHN G., ZUR HAUSEN H. and HENLE G., « Science », *157*, 1064 (1967).

[18] MILLER G., « Yale J. Biol. Med. », *43*, 358 (1971).

[19] MILLER G., LISCO H., KOHN H.I. and STITT D., « Proc. Soc. Exp. Biol. Med. », *137*, 1459 (1971).

[20] POPE J.H., HORNE M.K. and SCOTT W., « Int. J. Cancer », *4*, 225 (1969).

[21] NILSSON K. and PONTÉN J., « Int. J. Cancer », *15*, 321 (1975).

[22] ZECH L., HAGLUND U., NILSSON K. and KLEIN G., « Int. J. Cancer », *17*, 47 (1976).

[23] NONOYAMA M. and PAGANO J.S., « Nature (New Biol.) », *233*, 103 (1971).

[24] PAGANO J.S., « Cold Spring Harbor Symp. Quant. Biol. », *39*, 797 (1975).

[25] ZUR HAUSEN H. and SCHULTE-HOLTHAUSEN H., « Nature », 227, 245 (1970).

[26] ZUR HAUSEN H., DIEHL V., WOLF H., SCHULTEPHOLTHAUSEN H. and SCHNEIDER U., « Nature (New Biol.) », 237, 189 (1972).

[27] REEDMAN B.M. and KLEIN G., « Int. J. Cancer », 11, 499 (1973).

[28] LINDAHL T., ADAMS A., BJURSELL G., BORNKAMM G.W., KASCHKA-DIERICH C. and JEHN U., « J. Mol. Biol. », 102, 511 (1976).

[29] LUKA J., LINDAHL T. and KLEIN G., « J. Virol. », 27, 604 (1978).

[30] ERNBERG I., ANDERSSON M., KLEIN G., LUNDIN L. and KILLANDER D., « Nature », 266, 269 (1977).

[31] KLEIN G., WIENER F., ZECH L., ZUR HAUSEN H. and REEDMAN B., « Int. J. Cancer », 14, 54 (1974).

[32] KLEIN G., LINDAHL T., JONDAL M., LEIBOLD W., MENEZES J., NILSSON K. and SUNDSTRÖM CH., « Proc. Nat. Acad. Sci. USA », 71, 3283 (1974).

[33] KLEIN G., SUGDEN B., LEIBOLD W. and MENEZES J., « Intervirology », 3, 232 (1974).

[34] KLEIN G., GIOVANELLA B.C., LINDAHL T., FIALKOW P.J., SINGH S. and STEHLIN J.S., « Proc. Nat. Acad. Sci. USA », 71, 4737 (1974).

[35] STEPLEWSKI Z., KOPROWSKI H., ANDERSON-ANUROT M. and KLEIN G., « J. Cell. Physiol. », 97, 1 (1978).

[36] BARON D.W., BEZ W.C., CARMICHAEL G., YOCUM R.R. and STROMINGER J.L., « IARC technical report », 75, 003 (1975).

[37] LENOIR G., BERHELON M.C., FAVRE M.C. and DE THÉ G., « J. Virol. », 17, 672 (1976).

[38] LUKA J., SIEGERT W. and KLEIN G., « J. Virol. », 22, 1 (1977).

[39] OHNO S., LUKA J., LINDAHL T. and KLEIN G., « Proc. Nat. Acad. Sci. USA », 74, 1605 (1977).

[40] DIEHL V., HENLE G., HENLE W. and KOHN G., « J. Virol. », 2, 663 (1968).

[41] NILSSON K., KLEIN G., HENLE W. and HENLE G., « Int. J. Cancer », 8, 443 (1971).

[42] FALK L., WOLFE K., DEINHARDT F., PACIGA J., DOMBOS L., KLEIN G., HENLE W. and HENLE G., « Int. J. Cancer », 13, 363 (1974).

[43] MILLER G., SHOPE T., LISCO H., STITT D. and LIPMAN M., « Proc. Nat. Acad. Sci. USA », 69, 383 (1972).

[44] LEIBOLD W., HULDT G., FLANAGAN T.D., ANDERSSON M., DALENS M., WRIGHT D.H., VOLLER A. and KLEIN G., « Int. J. Cancer », 17, 533 (1976).

[45] SHOPE T., DECHARRO D. and MILLER G., « Proc. Nat. Acad. Sci. USA », 70, 2487 (1973).

[46] MILLER G., « J. Infect. Dis. », 130, 187 (1974).

[47] WERNER J., WOLF H., APODACA J. and ZUR HAUSEN H., « Int. J. Cancer », 15, 1000 (1975).

[48] EPSTEIN M.A., HUNT R.D. and RABIN H., « Int. J. Cancer », 12, 309 (1973).

[49] HENLE G. and HENLE W., « J. Infect. Dis. », 121, 303 (1970).

[50] NIEDERMAN J.C., EVANS A.S., SUBRAHMANYAN L. and McCOLLUM R.W., « N. Engl. J. Med. », *282*, 361 (1970).

[51] EVANS A.S., NIEDERMAN J.C. and McCOLLUM R.W., « N. Engl. J. Med. », *279*, 1121 (1968).

[52] HENLE W. and HENLE G., « N. Engl. J. Med. », *288*, 263 (1973).

[53] HENLE G., HENLE W. and DIEHL V., « Proc. Nat. Acad. Sci. USA », *59*, 94 (1968).

[54] NIEDERMAN J.C., McCOLLUM R.W., HENLE G. and HENLE W., « J. Amer. Med. Ass. », *203*, 205 (1968).

[55] GERBER P., NONOYAMA M., LUCAS S., NONOYAMA M., PERLIN E. and GOLD- STEIN L.I., « Lancet », *2*, 988 (1972).

[56] GOLDEN H.D., CHANG R.S., LOU J.J. and COOPER T.Y., « J. Infect. Dis. », *124*, 422 (1971).

[57] MILLER G., NIEDERMAN J.C. and ANDREWS L.L., « N. Engl. J. Med. », *288*, 229 (1973).

[58] PEREIRA M.S., FIELD A.M., BLAKE J.M., RODGERS F.G., BAILEY L.A. and DAVIES J.R., « Lancet », 710 (1972).

[59] BAKACS T., SVEDMYR E., KLEIN E. and ROMBO L., « Cancer Letters », *4*, 185 (1978).

[60] SVEDMYR E. and JONDAL M., « Proc. Nat. Acad. Sci. USA », *72*, 1622 (1975).

[61] KLEIN G., SVEDMYR E., JONDAL M. and PERSSON P.O., « Int. J. Cancer », *17*, 21 (1976).

[62] BRITTON S., ANDERSSON M., GERGELY P., HENLE W., JONDAL M., KLEIN G., SANDSTEDT B. and SVEDMYR E., « N. Engl. J. Med. », *298*, 89 (1978).

[63] HENLE G., HENLE W., CLIFFORD P., DIEHL V., KAFUKO G.W., KIRYA B.B., KLEIN G., MORROW R.H., MUNUBE G.M.R., PIKE P., TUKEI P.M. and ZIEGLER J.L., « J. Nat. Cancer Inst. », *43*, 1147 (1969).

[64] HENLE G., HENLE W., KLEIN G., GUNVÉN P., CLIFFORD P., MORROW R.H. and ZIEGLER J.L., « J. Nat. Cancer Inst. », *46*, 861 (1971).

[65] LINDAHL T., KLEIN G., REEDMAN B.M., JOHANSSON B. and SINGH S., « Int. J. Cancer », *13*, 764 (1974).

[66] NONOYAMA M., HUANG C.H., PAGANO J.S., KLEIN G. and SINGH S., « Proc. Nat. Acad. Sci. USA », *70*, 3265 (1973).

[67] ZUR HAUSEN H., SCHULTE-HOLTHAUSEN H., KLEIN G., HENLE W., HENLE G., CLIFFORD P. and SANTESSON L., « Nature (London) », *228*, 1056 (1970).

[68] FIALKOW P.J., KLEIN G., GARTLER S.M. and CLIFFORD P., « Lancet », *1*, 384 (1970).

[69] KLEIN G., « Cold Spring Harbor Symp. Quant. Biol. », *39*, 783 (1975).

[70] LEVINE P.H., In: *Oncogenesis and Herpesviruses.* (P.M. Biggs, G. de Thé, L. N. Payne, eds.). Lyon, IARC Scientific Publications, pp. 384-389 (1972).

[71] PAGANO J.S., Proc. Second Internat. Symposium on Oncogenesis and Herpes- viruses, Nuremberg. (H. zur Hausen, G. de Thé, M.A. Epstein, eds.). Lyon, IARC Scientific Publications, in press (1974).

[72] ZIEGLER J.L., ANDERSSON M., KLEIN G. and HENLE W., « Int. J. Cancer », *17*, 701 (1976).

[73] ADAMS A. and LINDAHL T., « Proc. Nat. Acad. Sci. USA », *72*, 1477 (1975).

[74] KASCHKA-DIERICH G., ADAMS A., LINDAHL T., BORNKAMM G., BJURSELL G., KLEIN G., GIOVANELLA B.C. and SINGH S., « Nature », *260*, 302 (1976).

[75] KLEIN E., VAN FURTH R., JOHANSSON B., ERNBERG I. and CLIFFORD P., In: *Oncogenesis and Herpesviruses*. (P.M. Biggs, G. de Thé, L.N. Payne, eds.). Lyon, IARC Scientific Publications, pp. 253-257 (1972).

[76] FIALKOW P.J., KLEIN G., GIBLETT E.R., GOTHOSKAR B. and CLIFFORD P., « Lancet », *1*, 883 (1971).

[77] BECHET J.M., FIALKOW P.J., NILSSON K., KLEIN G. and SINGH S., « Exp. Cell. Res. », *89*, 275 (1974).

[78] JARVIS J.E., BALL G., RICKINSON A.B. and EPSTEIN M.A., « Int. J. Cancer », *14*, 716 (1974).

[79] MANOLOV G. and MANOLOVA Y., « Nature », *237*, 33 (1972.

[80] MARK J., « Adv. Cancer Res. », *24*, 165 (1977).

[81] CLEMENTS G.B., KLEIN G. and POVEY S., « Int. J. Cancer », *16*, 125 (1975).

[82] NILSSON K., GIOVANELLA B.C., STEHLIN J.S. and KLEIN G., « Int. J. Cancer », *19*, 337 (1977).

[83] KURITA Y., SUGIYAMA T. and NISHIZUKA Y., « Cancer Res. », *28*, 1738 (1968).

[84] LEVAN G., « Hereditas », *78*, 273 (1974).

[85] MITELMAN F., « Hereditas », *70*, 1 (1972).

[86] NOWELL P.C. and HUNGERFORD D.A., « Science », *132*, 1497 (1960).

[87] SINGER H. and ZANG K.D., « Humangenetik », *9*, 172 (1970).

[88] YAMAMOTO T., HAYASHI M., RABINOWITZ Z. and SACHS L., « Int. J. Cancer », *11*, 555 (1973).

[89] RENGER H.C. and BASILICO C., « Proc. Nat. Acad. Sci. USA », *69*, 109 (1972).

[90] HARRIS H., MILLER O.J., KLEIN G., WORST P. and TACHIBANA T., « Nature », *22*, 363 (1969).

[91] KLEIN G., BREGULA U., WIENER F. and HARRIS H., « J. Cell. Sci. », *8*, 639 (1971).

[92] WIENER F., KLEIN G. and HARRIS H., « J. Cell. Sci. », *8*, 681 (1971).

[93] JENSEN F., KOPROWSKI H. and PONTÉN J.A., « Proc. Nat. Acad. Sci. USA », *50*, 343 (1963).

[94] KERSEY J.H., GATTI R.A., GOOD R.A., AARONSON S.A. and TODARO G.J., « Proc. Nat. Acad. Sci. USA », *69*, 980 (1972).

[95] MUKERJEE D., BOWEN J. and ANDERSON D.E., « Cancer Res. », *30*, 1769 (1970).

[96] PITOT H.C., « J. Nat. Cancer Inst. », *53*, 905 (1974).

[97] POTTER C.W., POTTER A.M. and OXFORD J.S., « J. Virol. », *5*, 293 (1970).

[98] SANDBERG A.A. and SAKURAI M., *Cancer Chromosomes. The Molecular Biology of Cancer* (H. Busch, ed.). Academic Press, New York, pp. 81-106 (1973).

[99] TODARO G.J., « Proc. Soc. Exp. Biol. Med. », *124*, 1232 (1967).

[100] Todaro G.J., Wolman S.R. and Green H., « J. Cell. Comp. Physiol. », *62*, 257 (1963).

[101] McCaw B.K., Hecht F., Harnden D.G. and Teplitz R.L., « Proc. Nat. Acad. Sci. USA », *72*, 2071 (1975).

[102] Cohen M., Personal communication.

[103] Heston W.E. and Vlahakis G., 20th Annual Symposium on Fundamental Cancer Research. (R.W. Cumley, Williams and Wilkins Co., Baltimore) (1966).

[104] Prehn R.T., « J. Nat. Cancer Inst. », *13*, 859 (1953).

[105] Desgranges C., Wolf H., de Thé G., Shanmugaratnam K., Cammoun N., Ellouz R., Klein G., Lennert K., Munoz N. and zur Hausen H., « Int. J. Cancer », *16*, 7 (1975).

[106] de Schryver A., Friberg S. Jr., Klein G., Henle W., Henle G., de Thé G., Clifford P. and Ho H.C., « Clin. Exp. Immunol. », *5*, 443 (1969).

[107] Andersson-Anvret M., Forsby N., Klein G. and Henle W., « Int. J. Cancer », *20*, 486 (1977).

[108] Wolf H., zur Hausen H. and Becker V., « Nature (New Biol.) », *244*, 245 (1973).

[109] Wolf H., zur Hausen H., Klein G., Becker V., Henle G. and Henle W., « Med. Microbiol. Immunol. », *161*, 15 (1975).

[110] Jondal M. and Klein G., « Biomedicine », *23*, 163 (1975).

[111] Huang D.P., Ho J.H.C., Henle W. and Henle G., « Int. J. Cancer », *14*, 580 (1974).

[112] Roizman B., Proc. Second Internat. Symposium on Oncogenesis and Herpes-viruses, Nuremberg. (H. zur Hausen, G. de Thé, M. A. Epstein, eds.). Lyon, IARC Scientific Publications, pp. 3-38.

[113] Ho J.H.C., « Adv. Cancer Res. », *15*, 57 (1972).

DISCUSSION

RAPP

The paradox that you told us about relating to DNA synthesis interested me because of some current studies in our laboratory. Drs. Schlager, Ohanian and Borsos have been studying the mechanisms of the killing of line 10 tumor cells *in vitro* by specific antibody and complement. Tumor cells are difficult to kill *in vitro* using antibodies and complement, even though the mechanism seems to be about the same as it is for the immune lysis of red blood cells, which are easy to kill. By treating these tumor cells with metabolic inhibitors, they found that the cells became sensitive to killing *in vitro*. For example, actinomycin, puromycin and certain chemotherapeutic agents were active but increased susceptibility to immune cytotoxicity could not be related to DNA synthesis. It turns out that what is important here is lipid synthesis. Since you are dealing with complement receptors, it may be that your paradox is due to the fact that lipid synthesis rather than DNA synthesis is important in the phenomenon you described.

ROSENBERG

You mentioned that infectious mononucleosis was polyclonal and Burkitt's lymphoma monoclonal — now what was the evidence for that?

G. KLEIN

The monoclonality of Burkitt's lymphoma was shown by the G6PD method (FIALKOW *et al.*, 1970). The polyclonality of infectious mononucleosis was shown by polyclonal immunoglobulin markers. This is in line with the polyclonality of in vitro EBV-induced transformation (ROSÉN *et al.*, 1977).

TERRY

You did not have the opportunity to discuss nasopharyngeal carcinoma (NPC) but let me ask you a question about that disease. There have been reports of tumors that very much resemble nasopharyngeal carcinoma in Chinese pigs. Pigs with those tumors are found only in areas where the disease occurs in high frequency in man. Are you aware of any serologic studies in such pigs?

G. KLEIN

I am afraid I do not know about the pig NPC, although it would be very interesting to study them. About human NPC, one can state that the tumor has been found 100% positive so far, provided it has the right histology (low differentiated or anaplastic carcinoma) and the biopsy pieces examined were histologically shown to contain viable tumor tissue. This means that this type of tumor is an EBV-carrying epithelial neoplasia, no matter whether it occurs in the high frequency Chinese population, the lower or medium frequency African population, or in the very low frequency Western populations. This is a stricter EBV-correlation than in Burkitt's lymphoma but of course it is easier to make the histological diagnosis.

MATHÉ

We consider that only 20% of the non-African so-called Burkitt's lymphomas are acceptable as Burkitt's lymphomas according to W.H.O. Reference Center. This fits very well with your 20% EBNA positive proportion.

G. KLEIN

It would be very important indeed to do the histology and the EBV DNA and EBNA tests on the same material, as on the NPC system.

WEISS

Infectious mononucleosis as "civil war" between transformed and

[11] *G. Klein* - p. 18

potentially malignant B cells, and cytotoxic T cells — please let me understand this more clearly! You said that such T cells can be demonstrated in the peripheral blood only with difficulty; that they disappear with convalescence, and are not found in chronic cases. Are you then invoking other arms of the immune response as responsible for maintaining the necessary balance between the transformed B cells and the host, so that progressive neoplastic disease does not occur?

G. KLEIN

The data that we have indicate the killer T-cell reaction is important during the acute phase. In the chronically infected person, the controls may be partly immunological and partly non-immunological. We know that the EBV-transformed diploid B-lymphocyte is not yet capable of growing in immunosuppressed animals, or in nude mice. This means that it may still obey some of the normal regulatory mechanisms. If immunological controls are also involved, antibodies and antibody dependent lymphocytotoxicity would be good candidates, since infection is always followed by life-long maintenance of several EBV-induced antibodies, including the one that reacts with the membrane of the virus-carrying cells.

CLERICI

There is a point of your beautiful lecture that I did not understand. You said that the EB virus has a special affinity for the complement receptors of B-lymphocytes. And then you mentioned the C3b receptor. However, is it likely that C3d, rather than C3b, is the receptor for the EB virus, because only B-lymphocytes have the C3d receptor, while the C3b receptor is found also on the membranes of macrophages and granulocytes which, as far as I know, are not affected by the EB virus. Suppose that you prepare an EAC3d indicator by treating EAC3b with the C3b inactivating enzyme and then you add EAC3d and EB virus to a B-lymphocyte suspension. Probably there will be a competition for the C3d receptor on B-lymphocytes, between the indicator and the virus and, maybe, the B-lymphocytes will not be infected by the EB virus. In other words, can you specify if the EB virus reacts with the C3d rather than C3b receptor on B-lymphocytes?

[11] G. Klein - p. 19

G. KLEIN

We have tried to block the C3d and C3b receptor separately, but had great difficulties in doing these experiments in a clean way. We could block viral adsorption to the cells with C3 and anti C3. Conversely, we could block EAC rosetting with viral concentrates (JONDAL et al., 1976). One reason to believe that C3d receptors can function as EBV receptors relates to the fact that the Daudi cell lacks C3b but has C3d receptors, and it has also a high EBV-receptor concentration. The same can be said about BJAB.

CHAGAS

First of all, I would like to tell this meeting that we have tried to bring Dr. Olweny here but without any success. I would ask: is there any serological or biological evidence that malaria is a promoting element in Burkitt's lymphoma?

G. KLEIN

I am indeed sorry that Dr. Olweny could not come. As to the relationship with malaria, Burkitt's suggestion is that chronic holoendemic malaria (not just malaria) serves as a promoting factor. There is fairly good concordance between the occurrence of a heavy parasite load and the occurrence of Burkitt's lymphoma (BURKITT, « J. Nat. Cancer Inst. », 42, 19, 1969).

NOSSAL

The International Agency for Research on Cancer is conducting a large-scale malaria eradication trial in northwestern Tanzania, which is designed to ask the question of whether getting rid of malaria gets rid of Burkitt's lymphoma. So we will have an answer to this question within five years.

CHAGAS

The malaria eradication essays in Latin America have been very unsuccessful.

[11] *G. Klein* - p. 20

OETTGEN

I have two questions. First, patients who acquire infectious mononucleosis are VCA-antibody negative prior to that time. Are they also
negative with respect to antibodies to all other EBV-associated antigens?

G. KLEIN

Yes.

OETTGEN

Second, EBV being almost as ubiquitous as endotoxin, do you think
it plays a physiological role in maintaining expansions of the differentiated
B cell system?

G. KLEIN

All EBV-negative (pre-IM) persons were negative for all EBV-related
antibodies. During primary infection, IgM-anti VCA appears first,
followed by anti-EA. Anti-EBNA antibodies appear with a long delay
of several months. Presumably, a number of EBNA carrying cells must
be destroyed by the immune response before EBNA antibodies are induced.
Whether the successful symbiotic relationship between EBV and human
B lymphocytes is due to some advantage for the host, e.g. in maintaining
the volume of the B-cell system, is a very interesting question that is very
hard to answer.

SELA

What do the killer cells recognize? I understand that the EB virus
receptor cannot be the site because the main producers do not possess
the virus.

G. KLEIN

The T-killer cells that appear during acute IM recognize a membrane
change present in all viral genome carrying cells. We cannot detect it

serologically and we therefore called it LYDMA (lymphocyte detected membrane antigen). Superficially at least, it reminds one of the polyoma-associated TSTA. In that case, the membrane antigen was shown to be a modified form of the intranuclear T-antigen. This raised the interesting question whether LYDMA could be some modified form of EBNA, but we have no information on this.

[11] *G. Klein* · p. 22

MACROPHAGE ACTIVATION AS A COMPONENT OF THE ANTI-TUMOR RESPONSE

ROBERT J. NORTH

The Trudeau Institute

Saranac Lake, N.Y. 12983

There has been a significant resurgence of interest in recent years in the role of macrophages in defense against tissue colonization by neoplastic cells. The earlier observations [1] that animals with macrophage systems activated by microbial infection display an acquired capacity for inhibiting the growth of tumor cell implants, have been recently confirmed [2, 3, 4], and subjected to *in vitro* analysis. This has resulted in the generation of a large body of evidence from numerous laboratories [5, 6, 7, 8, 9, 10, 11] which supports the proposition that activated macrophages display a potent capacity for destroying or inhibiting the growth of tumor cells *in vitro*. Needless to say, however, this information would be relatively meaningless, if it were not for the additional though limited number of observations that activated macrophages are not cytotoxic for normal cells in culture.

Even so, it is well to realize that some of this *in vitro* evidence is open to criticism. In some cases, for example, the purity of macrophage populations employed was neither investigated nor documented; a serious problem in view of accumulating evidence [12, 13] to show that experimental manipulations that result in macrophage activation in vivo may also result in an accompanying increase in the number of natural killer cells. Again, the popular technique of measuring macrophage-mediated inhibition of tumor cell replication by inhibition of ^{3}H-thymidine into tumor cell DNA has been thrown into doubt by the revelation that activated macrophages secrete thymidine [14]. It has also been shown [15] that activated macrophages are capable of rapidly depleting the culture medium of arginine, an essential amino acid for cell growth *in vitro*. On top of these problems is the relative scarcity of publications which compare macrophage cytotoxicity for tumor cells with cytotoxicity for normal cells. In spite of these criticisms, however, the *in vitro* evidence appears so reproducible at face value that it is difficult to avoid hypothesizing that activated macrophages are responsible for the acquired non-specific antitumor activity displayed by animals infected with BCG or other microbial agents, and that activated macrophages possess a potential for participating in the host's antitumor response. The important point to realize about this evidence, however, is that it is practically all based on results obtained, not from tumor-bearing animals, but from animals either infected with microbial parasites, or treated with a variety of agents known to cause non-specific systemic macrophage activation. Therefore, most published experiments do not represent a legitimate analysis of antitumor defense mechanism as such, since this would require a knowledge about macrophage activation in the tumor-bearing host.

There is evidence to show that macrophages do indeed undergo adaptive changes in response to progressive neoplastic colonization of host tissues. For instance, tumor-bearing humans [16], as well as tumor-bearing animals [17, 18, 19] have been shown to acquire a systemically activated macrophage system as measured by a greatly increased capacity for clearing intravenously infused colloids. That this increased phagocytic potential of the fixed macrophage system may be linked to an augmentation of macrophage numbers is indicated by additional finding [20] that subcutaneous growth of murine sarcomas can result in a significant increase in the rate of replication of macrophages in the peritoneal cavity. This fits with the evidence [21] that tumor-bearing animals can possess increased numbers of cells in bone marrow capable of forming macrophage colonies *in vitro*: a possible indicator of an increased production of precursors of blood monocytes.

An antitumor response by macrophages is also evidenced by the so called stromal reaction that surrounds solid tumors. The fact that the stromal tissue can contain significant numbers of lymphocytes and macrophages and that this can be used as a prognostic indicator has been discussed for some time. It seems highly likely, moreover, that it is the macrophage content of the stromal reaction and not the tumor proper which is responsible for the surprisingly large proportion of macrophages seen in single cell suspensions of enzyme-dissociated tumors. This procedure has shown that some murine tumors can be made up of more than 60% macrophages [22]. In fact, it has been suggested [23], on the basis of a comparative study of the macrophage content of a variety of murine tumors, that the macrophage content of a tumor is inversely related to its capacity for disseminating systemically. There is also recent evidence [24, 25, 26] to show that macrophages isolated from solid tumors can display tumoricidal activity *in vitro*. In spite of the presence of all of these macrophages, however, the simple fact remains that malignant tumors continue to grow to kill their hosts.

Macrophage activation as a component of concomitant antitumor immunity. Recent experimental results from this laboratory give credence to the proposition that systemic macrophage activation is a component of the host's antitumor response, in that it is a consequence of the generation of T cell-mediated concomitant antitumor immunity. Concomitant immunity refers to the paradoxical state of progressive tumor growth in the face of a state of systemic antitumor immunity capable of suppressing the growth of cells of the same tumor implanted at a distant site. This form of antitumor immunity has been described for autochthonous as well as syngeneic tumors [27], and there is limited evidence to suggest [28] that it may also be generated by tumor-bearing humans.

Concomitant immunity generated against the transplantable SA1 sarcoma in syngeneic A/J mice was shown to have the following properties [29]:

a) The generation of immunity depends on progressive growth of the tumor, and is independent of the latency period before tumor growth becomes manifest.

b) Immunity is not generated in mice made T cell-deficient by thymectomy and lethal X-irradiation, and restored with bone marrow cells.

c) Immunity is associated with the presence of Thy-1-positive T cells in the node draining the primary tumor which are capable of passively transferring immunity to normal recipients.

The most important finding relative to this discussion, however, is that the generation of concomitant immunity is associated with the generation by the host of a strikingly enhanced capacity for rapidly inactivating a lethal intravenous challenge inoculum with the bacterial parasite, *Listeria monocytogenes*. Since there is overwhelming evidence [30] that immunity to this organism is expressed by activated macrophages, there is little doubt that the immune response to the tumor also resulted in the generation of a highly activated macrophage system. This finding serves to show, therefore, the reciprocal of the much repeated finding of an acquired antitumor mechanism in animals infected with microbial parasites. It is apparent that macrophage activation in response to either agent serves to protect the host against the other. Thus, there is striking similarity between cell-mediated concomitant antitumor immunity and cell-mediated antibacterial immunity, in that the T cell response to both agents, in the presence of adequate antigen, results in the systemic generation of activated macrophages. If activated macrophages do, in fact, possess the capacity to destroy tumor cells *in vivo*, then their presence in a tumor-bearing host makes the state of concomitant immunity appear even more paradoxical than ever.

The possibility that tumors possess mechanisms that subvert macrophage function. Recent experiments published from this laboratory [31, 32] indicate one possible reason why malignant tumors continue to grow in spite of the presence of an activated macrophage system. They point to the distinct possibility that tumors are naturally selected, at least in part, on the basis of their ability to subvert macrophage function. It was shown, for instance, that subcutaneous implantation of cells of any one of five unselected, syngeneic murine tumors rapidly resulted in 24 hours in a severe suppression of the capacity of mice to resist sublethal infection with the bacterial parasite, *Listeria monocytogenes*. It is well established that immunity to this parasite is mediated by specifically sensitized T cells and is expressed by activated macrophages. It was further shown that the state of supressed anti-*Listeria* resistance resulted from a severe reduction in the capacity of preexisting fixed phagocytes in the liver and spleen to destroy, during the first 12 hours of infection, the bacterial load taken up by these organs. Again, tumor cell implantation also greatly suppressed the increased *in vivo* listericidal activity of a macrophage system activated by BCG infection, although an above normal level of activation persisted. Serum transfer experiments showed, in addition, that suppression of macrophage function was mediated by a factor in circulation which was small enough to pass through a dialysis membrane, and had a functional half-life of about 24 hours in normal recipients. The tumor-induced state of suppressed macrophage function was short-lived, however, in that the emergence and growth of the tumor implant was associated with conversion from a suppressed to a greatly enhanced state of antimicrobial resistance. This conversion was concordant with the generation of concomitant antitumor immunity. However, in spite of the conversion to a state of systemically enhanced antimicrobial resistance, tumor-bearing mice continued to show the presence of enough suppressor factor in their serum to suppress antimicrobial resistance in normal recipients. It was apparent, therefore, that macrophages had become activated enough to overcome the effects of the factor systemically. The possibility remained, however, that macrophage function was nevertheless suppressed in the tumor itself, because of the predicted presence of much higher concentrations of the suppressor factor at this site. It was predicted on the basis of this reasoning that in spite of enhanced systemic anti-*Listeria* resistance, the host should be incapable of destroying a *Listeria* inoculum injected directly into its tumor.

This prediction proved to be true, as shown by the results of experiments which compared the fate of *Listeria* inoculated subcutaneously into a normal footpad with its growth in a footpad bearing a progressive SA1 sarcoma. It was found [33] that whereas the organism grew for 24 hours and was then efficiently eliminated from the normal footpad, it was not eliminated from the tumor-bearing footpad. Instead, it either continued to multiply, or its growth plateaued at high level. The host, however, did not die from progressive bacterial infection. In fact, the suppressed expression of anti-microbial resistance in the tumor was associated with a contrasting state of greatly enhanced systemic anti-microbial resistance that occurred as a consequence of the generation both of T cell-mediated concomitant antitumor immunity and T cell-mediated antibacterial resistance. Indeed, this acquired greatly enhanced systemic anti-microbial resistance was not only capable of protecting the mice against those bacteria that were constantly seeded from the tumor into the circulation, but also protected them against a lethal intravenous challenge infection. It is important to realize, moreover, that all of these findings also apply to tumors growing in the ascites form intraperitoneally [33], where there was no necrotic core, no mechanical barriers to the movement of host cells, and where inoculated bacteria were shown to be rapidly ingested by available macrophages.

The foregoing results show, then, that there are parallels between concomitant antitumor immunity and cell-mediated antimicrobial immunity, in that while both types of immunity can be expressed systemically, neither type can be fully expressed within an established progressive tumor. It is apparent, therefore, that conditions within a progressive tumor are antagonistic not only to the expression of antitumor immunity, but also to the expression of host defenses in general. Thus, the function of cells is either suppressed inside the tumor, or these cells are prevented from entering the tumor.

In support of the second alternative, there is now a number of publications which show that tumor cells can secrete factors that suppress the emigration of leukocytes across small blood vessels into sites of inflammation. Apart from the earlier observations [34] that the cellular response to inflammatory stimuli within tumor tissue is much lower than in normal tissues, there are additional publications which show that tumor-bearing humans [36, 37, 38] as well as animals [39, 40, 41, 42] display a reduced cellular response to inflammatory stimuli in general. This evidence is supported in turn by the direct demonstrations [43, 44] that extracts of murine tumors contain small molecular weight factors that suppress leukocyte emigration into inflammation and inhibit the chemotaxis of mononuclear phagocytes *in vitro*.

SUMMARY

The purpose of this presentation was to draw attention to evidence which shows that systemic macrophage activation can be a component of the host response to progressive tumor growth, and that this happens by way of the generation of T cell-mediated concomitant antitumor immunity. The fact that progressive tumor growth occurs in spite of the possession of activated macrophages serves to further underscore the paradox of concomitant antitumor immunity, and suggests the hypothesis that conditions within an established tumor are locally antagonistic to the functioning of macrophages as well as cytotoxic T cells. Evidence consistent with this hypothesis was supplied by the results of experiments which tested whether systemically acquired, macrophage-mediated antibacterial resistance could be expressed within a progressive tumor. It was found that although intralesional inoculation of the bacterial parasite, *Listeria monocytogenes* resulted in the generation and expression of very high levels of antibacterial immunity systemically, this immunity was not expressed in an established solid or ascites tumor. It is apparent, therefore, that malignant neoplastic cells are naturally selected, at least partly, on the basis of their capacity for subverting macrophage function. This possibility must surely be considered by those who are interested in causing the regression of tumors by immunotherapy.

REFERENCES

[1] OLD L.J., CLARK D.A., BENACERRAF B. and GOLDSMITH M., « Ann. N.Y. Acad. Sci. », *88*, 264-280 (1960).

[2] HIBBS J.B., LAMBERT L.H. and REMINGTON J.S., « J. Infect. Dis. », *124*, 587-592 (1971).

[3] HIBBS J.B., LAMBERT L.H. and REMINGTON J.S., « Science », *177*, 998-1000 (1972).

[4] HIBBS J.B., LAMBERT L.H. and REMINGTON J.S., « Proc. Soc. Exp. Biol. Med. », *139*, 1053-1056 (1972).

[5] HIBBS J.B., LAMBERT L.H. and REMINGTON J.S., « Proc. Soc. Exp. Biol. Med. », *139*, 1049 (1972).

[6] HIBBS J.B. Jr., « Transplantation. », *19* (1), 77 (1975).

[7] CLEVELAND R.P., MELTZER M.S. and ABAR B., « J. Natl. Cancer Inst. », *52*, 1887-1895 (1974).

[8] KELLER R., « J. Exp. Med. », *138*, 625-644 (1973).

[9] KRAKENBUHL J.L. and LAMBERT L.H., « J. Natl. Cancer Inst. », *54*, 1433-1437 (1975).

[10] GERMAIN R.N., WILLIAMS R.M. and BENACERRAF B., « J. Natl. Cancer Inst. », *54*, 709-720 (1975).

[11] NORBURY K.C. and FIDLER I.J., « J. Immunological Methods », *7*, 109-121 (1975).

[12] TRACEY D.E., WOLFE S.A., DURDIK J.M. and HENNEY C.S., « J. Immunol. », *119*, 1145 (1977).

[13] WOLFE S.A., TRACEY D.E. and HENNEY C.S., « J. Immunol. », *119*, 1152 (1977).

[14] OPITZ H.G., NEITHAMMER D., JACKSON R.C., LEMKE H., HUGET R. and FLAD H.D., « Cell Immunol. », *18*, 70-75 (1975).

[15] KUNG J.T., BROOKS S.B., JAKWAY J.P., LEONARD L.L. and TALMAGE D.W., « J. Exp. Med. », *146*, 665 (1977).

[16] MAGAREY C.J. and BAUM M., « Brit. J. Surg. », *57*, 748-752 (1970).

[17] KAMPSCHIDT R.F. and UPCHURCH H.F., « J. Reticuloendothel Soc. », *5*, 510-519 (1968).

[18] BLAMEY R.W., CROSBY D.L. and BAKER J.M., « Cancer Res. », *29*, 335-337 (1969).

[19] KAMPSCHIDT R.F. and PULLIAM L.A., « J. Reticuloendothel. Soc. », *11*, 1-10 (1972).

[12] *North* - p. 8

[20] NELSON D.S. and KEARNEY R., « Brit. J. Cancer. », *34*, 221-226 (1976).

[21] BAUM M. and FISHER B., « Cancer Res. », *32*, 2813-2817 (1972).

[22] EVANS R., « Transplant. », *14*, 468-473 (1972).

[23] ECCLES S.A. and ALEXANDER P., « Nature », *250*, 667-669 (1974).

[24] HASKILL J.S., PROCTOR J.W. and YAMAMURA Y., « J. Nat. Cancer Inst. », *54*, 387-393 (1975).

[25] VANLOVEREN H. and DEN OTTER W., « J. Natl. Cancer Soc. », *53*, 1057 (1974).

[26] RUSSEL S.W., DOE W.F. and McINTOSH A.T., «« J. Exp. Med. », *146*, 1511 (1977).

[27] VAAGE J., « Cancer Res. », *31*, 1655-1662 (1971).

[28] SOUTHAM C.M. and BRUNSCHWIG A., « Cancer », *14*, 971-978 (1961).

[29] NORTH R.J. and KIRSTEIN D.P., « J. Exp. Med. », *145*, 275-292 (1977).

[30] NORTH R.J., *Cell-mediated immunity and the response to infection*. In: Mechanisms of Cell-Mediated Immunity. R.T. McCluskey and S. Cohen, eds. John Wiley and Sons, Inc., New York and London, pp. 185-220 (1974).

[31] NORTH R.J., KIRSTEIN D.P. and TUTTLE R.L., « J. Exp. Med. », *143*, 559-573 (1976).

[32] NORTH R.J., KIRSTEIN D.P. and TUTTLE R.L., « J. Exp. Med. », *143*, 574-584 (1976).

[33] SPITALNY G.L. and NORTH R.J., « J. Exp. Med. », *145*, 1264 (1977).

[34] MAHONEY M.J. and LEIGHTON J., « Cancer Res. », *22*, 334-339 (1962).

[35] DIZON Q.S. and SOUTHAM C.M., « Cancer », *14*, 1288-1292 (1963).

[36] JOHNSON M.W., MAIBACH H.I. and SALMON S.E., « N. Engl. J. Med. », *284*, 1255-1257 (1971).

[37] JOHNSON M.W., MAIBACH H.I. and SALMON S.E., « N. Engl. J. Med. », *286*, 1162-1165 (1972).

[38] JOHNSON M.W., MAIBACH H.I. and SALMON S.E., « J. Natl. Cancer Inst. », *51*, 1075-1076 (1973).

[39] BERNSTEIN I.D., ZBAR B. and RAPP H.J., « J. Natl. Cancer Inst. », *49*, 1641-1647 (1972).

[40] FAUVE R.M., HEVIN B., JACOB H., GAILLARD J.A. and JACOB F., « Proc. Natl. Acad. Sci. USA », *71*, 4052-4056 (1974).

[41] SNYDERMAN R., PIKE M.C., BLAYLOCK B.L. and WEINSTEIN P., « J. Immunol. », *116*, 585-589 (1976).

[42] MELTZER M.S. and STEVENSON M.M., « J. Immunol. », *118*, 2176 (1977).

[43] PIKE M.C. and SNYDERMAN R., « J. Immunol. », *117*, 1243-1249 (1976).

[44] SCHECHTER M. and MOROSON H., « Cell Immunol. », *34*, 57 (1977).

DISCUSSION

NOSSAL

Thank you very much, Dr. North, for your most interesting and conservatively presented report, and I wonder whether I could start by asking you just to stick your neck out a tiny little bit and give us some advance clues to your thinking as to what the nature of these local resistance mechanisms may be.

NORTH

Well, there are a lot of people now describing soluble subversive factors. Snyderman at Duke University, for instance, is describing anti-inflammatory factors produced by tumors. Meltzer at NCI has recently confirmed the observations of Snyderman; similar factors are being described which prevent the chemotaxis of monocytes *in vitro*. These factors are anti-inflammatory, in that if you inject them into an animal they will prevent leukocyte immigration into inflammatory exudates. So that is one possibility. Another possibility is that a tumor creates an anti-inflammatory environment that prevents host effector cells from entering it. In our case that does not seem to be so, because when we put *Listeria* into a peritoneal tumor there is a massive influx of macrophages and lymphocytes, which is associated with a little bit of tumor cell killing. However, this does not last for very long. So, we would think that everything is O.K. until these effector cells reach the environment of the tumor. As far as knowing what is really happening, I do not know. Presumably the listericidal activity of the macrophages is turned off.

G. KLEIN

Did you find the local anti-inflammatory environment only in solid tumors or did you also find it in ascites tumors and in leukemias?

NORTH

Yes, we found it with ascites tumors.

G. KLEIN

And in generalized leukemias?

NORTH

We have not looked.

CHEDID

Dr. North, I have a technical question to ask you. How do you evaluate the presence of *Listeria* in the tumor? Is it histologically? It seems difficult to discriminate between the presence or absence of growth on one side because of local problems of clearance and of hemodynamic disturbances due to inflammation *in situ.*

NORTH

We do not really know the answer to that question, but that is why we irradiate the animal.

CHEDID

Could it not be non-removal rather than proliferation that you are measuring? I also would like you to explain, since you have only one tumor-bearing parabiont, why his partner is not invaded by the neoplastic cells. As you know, there is continuous blood filtration between 2 parabionts since their blood vessels communicate freely by anastomosis and that erythrocytes circulate from one to the other.

NORTH

Well, we only inject one peritoneal cavity with tumor cells.

[12] *North* - p. 12

CHEDID

Could you please comment about problems of local immunity such as those which have recently been studied by Fauve and Jacob in relation to absence of inflammation in the tumor environment.

NORTH

Yes, well, that paper showed that tumor cells secrete anti-inflammatory factors. It was one of the first. There is old literature which shows that tumors have anti-inflammatory properties. Such factors could be operating in our system. Certainly in the case of an ascites tumor growing in the peritoneal cavity we can induce a very massive influx of host cells. Indeed, if you count the cells already in the peritoneal cavity, there are a lot of macrophages, about four times normal. So macrophages are coming in, but they do not seem to be operating. When you inject *Listeria* I.P. and look to see where these Listeria are, they are always in macrophages, and a few in polymorphs. So it would appear that the macrophages in the vicinity of tumor cells are somehow turned off.

OETTGEN

Dr. North, you said that regression does not occur in T cell deficient animals. Could you qualify that statement by distinguishing between the initial necrotic response and the subsequent regressions? With LPS, we can induce acute necrosis of tumor grafts in lethally irradiated mice and also in mice treated with antilymphocytic serum.

NOSSAL

I wonder whether I can ask you, Dr. Oettgen, just to remind us about tumor necrosis factor in these mice. It would seem to be the ideal tool for answering this question of T-cells involvement.

OETTGEN

We have not yet tested whether we can induce necrosis in nude mice. What we do know is that we cannot induce the production of

tumor necrosis factor in the nude mouse, which of course lacks mature
T cells. But this does not mean that the tumor-necrotizing effect of the
factor depends on T cells. It only indicates that T cells are apparently
needed in whatever interaction leads to the production of tumor necrosis
factor.

ROSENBERG

Do you have any reason to believe that the micro environment which
allows the Listeria to grow is in any way related to the reason that the
tumor grows? Could not this be a function of the fact that the blood
supply, for example, of the tumor might be altered in such a way as to
affect the Listeria to grow but is really unrelated to the reason all
activated macrophages or sensitized lymphocytes will not destroy the
tumor. Obviously in these experiments you can show a correlation, but
to prove that there is any cause and effect, or at what level the correlation
exists, is very difficult. Could you, for example, take a solid tumor that is
in the process of regressing, something like the Moloney sarcoma virus-
induced tumor, and show that in that tumor, for which there is an
efficient rejection mechanism in progress, Listeria in that setting would
also not grow?

NORTH

Well, we have done it with allogeneic tumors, and what happens
in an allograft is that you get the same result until the allograft begins
to be rejected; at that stage Listeria is killed. What we do know is that
with ascites tumors Listeria goes into macrophages: it is not extracellular,
and there are a lot of macrophages there. So if we could just show that
there is a suppression of macrophage antitumor function, it would be
very satisfactory. But I am not sure that I completely understand your
question. Is there a subtleness in your question that I am missing?
It seems to me that what we are showing here is that maybe macrophages
are turned off at the site of a tumor, but nowhere else.

ROSENBERG

Is there any way, for example, to inject a new tumor inoculum into

[12] *North* - p. 14

an already established tumor to see if that concomitant immunity exists within the tumor as well as at a different site?

NORTH

Well, I would not like to have to do that experiment — but if you lethally irradiate the animal, there is very little difference in the growth rate of the tumor. In other words, if there was concomitant immunity, one would expect some sort of difference in growth rate after irradiation. One thing you should remember is that if concomitant immunity does not develop in these animals the tumor growth rate does not increase, but metastases come up earlier and they grow much more quickly. It does not stop metastases, but it appears to be holding them back. This has been recorded by others.

WEISS

Could your observations be related to the findings of Dr. Isaac Witz of Tel Aviv University that tumor cells are sometimes able to produce enzymes which degrade immunoglobulin molecules, and may actually produce Ig fragments capable of protecting the neoplastic cells from other immunological attack by blocking antigenic determinants? Tumor cells also appear able to produce other substances that cause alterations on the surface of T cells and macrophages, and may compromise their effector capacities. Dr. Lucien Israel has recently reviewed these defensive, or escape mechanisms of neoplastic cells. It is possible that the concentration of such neutralizing and blocking factors is very low, and that they may not be detectable systemically although playing an important role in the host-tumor interaction *in situ*.

NORTH

Yes, we have also reported on a small molecule weight factor which suppresses macrophage function in terms of antibacterial resistance.

NOSSAL

We have got to keep a little bit of order in this meeting. Now we

will hear from Dr. Terry briefly and then we will go through the sequence
that I have down here: Baldwin, Rapp, etc.

TERRY

Built in to this whole discussion is the assumption that macrophage
function is indeed important in terms of destroying local tumor, and that
is something about which no data have been presented here or discussed.
The importance of macrophages is being accepted as an article of faith,
but I am not sure that it is one that we should accept so easily.

NORTH

Yes, I agree with you.

BALDWIN

I could confirm that we can isolate this small peptide from tumors
that will inhibit macrophage function and it is particularly relevant.
As I showed you yesterday, we have several tumors that, as they grow,
have a different level of infiltration of macrophages. The tumors that
have low level of macrophage infiltration, you can isolate from them the
peptide — and the tumors that do not have this infiltration, you do not
isolate the material. So I think this positive effect of the tumor is
stopping infiltration. But I think perhaps more important: have you
looked at macrophages from tumors to show that they are cytotoxic to
tumor cells *in vitro*? It seems to me that in your system where you
have intraperitoneal tumors you have a much better opportunity getting
peritoneal macrophages. Have you looked to see whether those peritoneal
macrophages are switched off?

NORTH

That is going on now, we are doing exactly that.

RAPP

You mentioned that you looked at other tumors, in early transplant generations. Did you find with some of them that if you left the tumor in place concomitant immunity did not develop?

NORTH

Oh yes, sure.

RAPP

We found with line 10 that if you take the tumors out at the right time — not too early — the animals do develop transplantation resistance.

NORTH

Right. Sure, I think there is probably some suppressor mechanism operating. Suppressive T-cells are probably going to explain a lot of things in the future. This may be one small part of a very complex mechanism.

RAPP

Just one comment, about macrophages: Dr. Bernstein in our lab years ago showed that autologous macrophages could prevent the growth of tumors in animals that were never immunized, by placing the macrophages and tumor cells together in the skin of the animal.

OETTGEN

Dr. North, with respect to the phenomenon of concomitant immunity, have you found it expressed as well in experiments with tumors that metastasize fairly early? In other words, is there any correlation between the expression of concomitant immunity as you have tested it, and the ability of a tumor to metastasize?

NORTH

Yes, if you use a T-cell-deficient animal, you see micrometastases at the same time you see them in normal mice when you look at the draining lymph nodes, but the growth is greatly increased and the T-cell deficient animal dies much earlier. This has been reported by others also. So, if concomitant immunity does not occur, metastatic spread and growth is increased. This is what the experiments tell us. But the immunity is not absolute.

CLERICI

I have only a comment. During our experiments in Milano on the mechanism of the immunodepression in cancer-bearing mice, we observed that these animals become quickly unable to react not only against their own tumoral antigens, but also against heterologous antigens, like SRBC. While trying to find out what is the mechanism of such immunodepression, we realized that tumor-bearing mice have a significantly increased number of macrophages in peripheral lymphoid tissues and a decreased number of T-lymphocytes, while that of B-lymphocytes remained unvaried, as compared to controls. This behavior may explain the mechanism of protection against *Listeria monocytogenes*, which is an intracellular parasite which is killed by activated macrophages. Since Koprowski has found that an increased number of macrophages decreases the antibody synthesis, I would suggest that your tumor-bearing animals may have more macrophages than controls, so that they can express a non-specific immunity against *Listeria monocytogenes* infections, but they cannot specifically react against their own tumoral antigens (or heterologous antigens). Did you check the number of macrophages in your tumor-bearing animals?

NORTH

No, we did not do that.

NOSSAL

I think it is fair to comment that in our work to date we really have not spent enough time thinking about immuno-resistance and the possible reasons therefor, and I think it is a very good thing that George Klein reminded us today that induction of tumor development is distinctly a multistage process — there is absolutely no reason to believe that those

[12] *North* - p. 18

metastasizing cells that are lodging in the lungs are absolutely identical to the cells which would have been put into the footpad and have caused concomitant immunity. Is that a straight comment?

NORTH

Yes, it would be worth looking at.

NATURAL KILLER CELLS

EVA KLEIN

Department of Tumor Biology
Karolinska Institutet
S-104 01 Stockholm 60, Sweden

Cell mediated cytotoxic tests in tumor immunology

Immune response against experimental tumors, both chemically and virally induced, was discovered in transplantation studies two decades ago. Immunization of inbred animals with syngeneic transplanted tumors or the autochtonous hosts with their primary tumors has been shown to elicit various degrees of protection against subsequent challenge with viable cells of the same tumor [1].

Cellular immunity was first shown by adoptive transfer in neutralization experiments in which lymphoid cells derived from immune donors admixed to tumor grafts inhibited their outgrowth [2, 3].

Following the demonstration that cell mediated reactions were probably more important for tumor rejection than serum antibodies, much emphasis was put on the *in vitro* lymphocytotoxicity tests. Many investigators assumed that these tests would reflect the *in vivo* events. However, it became evident that these assumptions are largely wrong. One of the important inconsistencies often mentioned, is the *in vitro* cross reactivity of chemically induced tumors, also with embryo cells, and their individual antigenicity in rejection tests [4, 5].

Initially, the cell mediated cytotoxicitic studies, performed in experimental systems and with patients with different tumor types were almost invariably interpreted to show tumor specific selective reactivities [6].

The base lines taken for calculation of the tumor related effects were either the survival of target without or after the addition of lymphocytes derived from appropriate controls. Effects by the control cells were ascribed to the conditions in the culture system or were not noticed if controls without lymphocytes were not included. Taking these control cultures into consideration later, it was revealed that cells with the capacity to attack certain tumor cell lines are present in the blood of healthy persons [7, 8, 9, 10].

Similarly, in mice, using lymphomas as targets, it was discovered that certain cultured lymphoma lines are affected by spleen cells from young unmanipulated animals [11, 12]. Apart from spleen cells, blood lymphocytes were found to be highly active [13]. Lymph node and bone marrow cells were somewhat less and thymus cells inactive. In man, the effect was first shown with blood lymphocytes, lymph node cells and tumor infiltrating lymphocytes were found to be active only occasionally [14].

Natural killer cells

This discovery initiated intensive studies motivated mainly for two reasons: 1) Characterization of a new cytotoxic phenomenon and 2) In order to achieve a test condition which could be used for tumor immunity studies, revealing disease related effects, it is necessary to characterize and remove the subpopulation responsible for this effect.

In mice, the reactivity varied widely among different strains. A pronounced age influence was also found with peak activity around 2 months. Spleen cells from newborn as well as from old mice invariably showed lower, if any activity. Thymus-less, nude mice with a variety of genetic backgrounds were active [11, 12]. The effect designated as NK — natural killer effect — was found to represent a hitherto unknown cell mediated cytotoxicity inasmuch as it is not performed by T cells and is different from the antibody dependent lymphocyte cytotoxicity. Only cultured lines were highly sensitive, cells harvested from animals were insensitive or weakly affected. The sensitivity of various mouse and rat cell lines was found to

[13] E. *Klein* · p. 2

vary. It was suggested that the target on the cell's surface is determined by C-type viruses [12]. However, when a number of cell lines were tested, there was no correlation between sensitivity for the mouse NK effect and the expression of the known viral antigens on the cell surface [15]. Mouse cells were found to kill human cell lines and *vice versa*, though the homologous reactivities were stronger [16, 17].

There is considerable interest presently in the NK effect of the animal systems since one of the important questions is the *in vivo* relevance of the phenomenon. Transplantation tests with a lymphoma line showed indeed that the rejection of small inocula by semisyngeneic mice paralleled the *in vitro* reactivity of the strain [18].

When an *in vitro* carried sensitive lymphoma line YAC-1 was retransplanted and propagated in mice its sensitivity declined [19]. These experiments and the rule that only cultured lines are highly sensitive would indicate that this type of host response is extremely efficient and only such cells can be established for longer time in the host which lack the sensitivity to this mechanism. Consequently, the NK system may represent a potent surveillence mechanism. Sensitivity is not an obligatory feature of tumor cells. However, it may be assumed that if during oncogenesis malignant cells with sensitivity to the NK cell arise, these must be eliminated.

On the other hand, there is no indication yet for the role of NK effect in oncogenesis, though the spleen NK activity was found to be relatively decreased in tumor bearing animals (both induced and transplanted) [12, 13] and tumor patients [14, 20]. Arguments against this role: 1) There is no correlation between the NK efficiency and sensitivity to Moloney virus induced leukemogenesis when different strains are compared. Admittedly, leukemogenesis is the outcome of several factors, some unrelated to immune response. 2) MSV induced sarcomas regress in A mice as regularly as in other strains but in this strain in contrast to CBA or CBA × C57B1 F_1 mice no cytotoxic activity was seen when spleens or tumor infiltrating lymphocytes were tested against the YAC-1 cells — one of the most sensitive NK targets [13]. 3) Mice infected neonatally with Moloney leukemia virus (a measure which leads to leukemia development) did not differ in spleen cell exerted cytotoxic activity (anti YAC-1) when tested in parallel with uninfected age matched controls [21]. 4) Mice which carry methylcholanthrene pellets and thus will develop sarcomas were shown not to have any change in spleen NK efficiency when compared with age matched controls [22]. Such mice were reported to have decreased numbers of antibody producing cells in the spleen [23].

However, indicative for the role of NK cells in immune surveillance is the low incidence of naturally occurring tumors in nude mice [24], expected to be unprotected since they lack T cell mediated and T cell dependent mechanisms considered to be crucial in graft rejection. As mentioned above nude mice have NK effector cells.

The nature of surface structure recognized by the effector cells is not known. Since cells from long term cultures are usually sensitive, incorporation of calf serum component in the cell membrane was proposed as at least one of the factors [25]. However, this possibility was not confirmed [26]), cell lines cultured with medium substituted with human serum were found as sensitive to the effect of human lymphocytes as the ones carried in parallel in fetal calf serum.

Selectivity is not apparent but seems to depend on the general sensitivity of the cell line. However, in studies with a panel of human cell lines and several blood donors, selectivity was indicated [27].

Similarly to the mouse, also in man, the active lymphocytes are not the well characterizable T or B cells and the effect is not histocompatibility restricted.

Several authors have attempted to define the effectors in the human NK system. Separation of subsets with monitoring of surface markers parallel with functional studies revealed that the so-called "null" fraction, *i.e.* the population non-adherent to nylon wool and depleted of SRBC rosette forming lymphocytes, is the most active [28, 29]. This population is rich in FC receptor positive cells [30]. Most authors agree, based on results with various targets, that the active cells do not carry SIg and are Fc receptor positive [30, 31]. Inconsistencies in the opinions about the other markers may partly be due to variation in the methodology of fractionation and surface marker detection. There is also a difference in the way the results are viewed. A cell subset can be highly active — like the "null"

[13] *E. Klein* - p. 4

— but its representation in the lymphocyte population may be relatively low. Other subsets may be low in activity when calculated on a per cell basis, but they may be more representative for the total population, like the E rosetting T subset.

The results of at least two studies agree that part of the active cells can be rosetted with SRBC depending on the condition of the rosetting [30, 32]. According to our results these T cells carry FC receptors [30]. The highly active "null" subset was shown to have high proportion of C_3 receptor carrying cells [33]. Mature T cells with high avidity SRBC receptors and devoid of FC receptors are not active. Thus Fc and low avidity E and C_3 receptors have been demonstrated on the human NK cells. Real "null" cells *i.e.* without markers were also shown to be active [29].

It is conceivable that more than one cell type contributes with different functions. PETER *et al.* supposed that one subset produces a soluble factor upon contact with target cells and another exerts the killing [34]. Similarly, TAKASUGI *et al.* [35] and PERLMANN *et al.* [36] assume that the effect is essentially ADCC, the effector cells either carrying cytophylic antibodies on their surface and/or a small number of admixed antibody producing cells contribute during the *in vitro* incubation. The subsets active in NK thus far were shown to be efficient in ADCC also. Even the organ distribution of the two types of effect overlaps.

In an attempt to differentiate these two functions in man we studied the cation requirements and kinetics of killing in NK, ADCC, and MLC generated killer cells using the same target cells. We found no difference [37]. Inhibition of ADCC but not NK by addition of protein A, inhibition of NK but not ADCC by trypsin treatment led HERBERMAN *et al.* to suppose that the mechanism of the two effects may be different.

In lack of knowledge about its initiation, the effect is designated with the attribute "natural" though it is not excluded that it might be generated by classical immunization.

By *in vitro* cultivation with allogeneic cells or syngeneic tumor cells cytotoxic T cells can be generated [38]. When spleen cells of mice or blood lymphocytes of man are cultured alone, NK activity declines [12, 39].

In mice, cocultivation with syngeneic NK sensitive target cells generate cytotoxic activity with NK characteristics *i.e.* the effector cells do not regularly kill the subline known to be insensitive to the NK effect when tested with fresh spleen cells [40]. This was shown also with the A mouse strain which is low reactive when tested directly, without cocultivation. Thus, killer cells may be present in the A spleen in low proportion and are selected out by cocultivation with the target.

Such experiments in man are more complex since a similar set-up requires autologous combination, otherwise histocompatibility differences generate cytotoxic cells. The K562 lymphoblastoid line, widely used as target for the NK effect lacks HLA and Ia determinants [41]. Theoretically this would eliminate the possibility for generation of cytotoxic T cells. Using K562 as sensitizer cell *in vitro*, we found that the cytotoxicity of the cultured lymphocytes is strongly increased [39]. The cultivation was carried out in the presence of serum from the lymphocyte donor. When the culture was fractionated into subsets, the activity was bound to the presence of blast transformed lymphocytes and Fc receptor carrying cells. Characteristics of the cytotoxicity was found to be similar to those in the fresh blood, in that cells with SIg and those which sediment with SRBC on Ficoll, were not active. Distinctive for the cultured population compared to fresh cells was the higher proportion of cells which adhered to nylon wool, among them also E receptor carrying ones.

Disease related cytotoxicity

Since specific cellular recognition is considered to reside in the T cell population and mature T cells have no NK effect — either in man or mice and rats, detection of disease related cytotoxicity on cell lines is expected to be possible by using subsets enriched in these cells.

The T cell mediated effects can be investigated *in vitro* directly or after *in vitro* sensitization by culturing the effector population cells in the presence of antigen carrying cells [38].

A new aspect of the T effector system directed against virally or chemically altered cells has recently evoked considerable general interest when it was discovered that effector and target cells have to share histocompatibility antigens [42, 43]. The present view is that the restriction is not absolute and can be overridden to some extent especially in long term cytotoxic assays [44].

In view of this restriction it is questionable whether established cell lines can be used as prototype targets in the human studies. It is possible that experiments have to be restricted to autologous systems. However, at least in one human disease — infectious mononucleosis — T cell mediated cytotoxicity was demonstrated in short term assay on allogeneic target cells.

This study is interesting from several aspects. One important point is that it was possible to show the disease related effects either after elimination of NK active cells from the blood lymphocyte population [45] or testing the isolated mature T subset [46]. The targets used were lymphoblastoid cell lines and only those which carried the EBV genetic information, and thus probably express an EBV related cell surface antigen, were damaged. This study illustrates also the relative ease for designing experiments for demonstrating specific effects if target cell characteristics with regard to the disease studied are known. This condition is not easily met in the human tumor systems except in Burkitt's lymphoma and nasopharyngeal carcinoma. In a few of such patients, selective EBV related cytotoxicity was demonstrated with lymph node derived lymphocytes and those infiltrating the tumors [47].

We have tested 10 patients with breast tumor for cytotoxicity on cell lines established from breast cancer. There was no indication for specific effect exerted by the purified T cell fraction [48]. The negative outcome may be ascribed to histoincompatibility of effector and target cells.

In an effort to eliminate at least some of the factors which hamper interpretation of results with cell lines, two tests, measuring cell-mediated antitumor recognition in man have been designed in our laboratory. In both tests, tumor cells separated from biopsy specimens were allowed to react with autologous lymphocytes.

The advantage of using biopsy cells is that the antigen source is not subjected to the modification and selective conditions of tissue culture. Its main disadvantages are the variability of the quality, the quantitative limitation and the laboriosity of tumor cell separation.

The autologous tumor stimulation (ATS)-test, [49], detects DNA synthesis of lymphocytes following cocultivation with mitomycin-treated tumor cells. At least part of the responding cells belong to the T subset since the lymphocytes attached to the tumor cells during the early period of cocultivation and the blast transformed cells at the end of the 6 day cocultivation formed rosettes with SRBC. Also, when prefractionated populations were used, the T-enriched fraction reacted while the T-depleted fractions did not.

ATS was obtained in 30% of 197 tumors tested. Cells derived from non-malignant tissue did not stimulate.

The autologous lymphocytotoxicity (ALC) test was worked out recently using a short term ^{51}Cr-release microtest [50]. In 30 of 90 cases killing of biopsy cells by autologous blood derived lymphocytes was obtained. In 8 tests allogeneic combinations could be used simultaneously, allowing also criss-cross combination. Only one showed cross reaction. Biopsy cells are only rarely sensitive to the killing effect of blood lymphocytes of healthy donors, thus the NK effect does not disturb in this assay.

In a further step, generation of secondary cytotoxic cells was attempted by cocultivating for 6 days the lymphocytes with autologous tumor biopsy cells — a procedure which has been shown to operate in some experimental tumor systems. In 8/15 cases (2 also showed primary ALC) secondary ALC was obtained.

Cytotoxic effects aimed to demonstrate disease related selective cellular recognition in experimental systems and in man are now performed with the awareness that at least three known effector mechanisms exist in which lymphocytes participate. Targets can be damaged by cells equipped with specific antigen recognizing receptors — probably T —, cells recognizing targets which have already been selected out by the recognition of antibodies — ADCC effect — and cells exerting the destructive effect on seemingly indiscriminative basis by unknown mechanism.

The work upon which this publication is based was performed pursuant to Contract NO1-CB-64023 and NO1-CB-74144 with the Division of Cancer Biology and Diagnosis, National Cancer Institute, Department of Health, Education and Welfare. Grants have also been received from the Swedish Cancer Society.

[13] *E. Klein* - p. 8

REFERENCES

[1] SJÖGREN H.O., « Progr. Exp. Tumor Res. », *6*, 289 (1965).

[2] KLEIN E. and SJÖGREN H.O., « Cancer Res. », *20*, 452 (1960).

[3] WINN H.J., « J. Immunol. », *86*, 228 (1961).

[4] BALDWIN R.W., GLAVES D. and VOSE B.M., « Int. J. Cancer », *13*, 135 (1974).

[5] STEELE G.J. and SJÖGREN H.O., « Int. J. Cancer », *14*, 435 (1974).

[6] HELLSTRÖM K.E. and HELLSTRÖM I., « Adv. Immunol. », *18*, 209 (1974).

[7] TAKASUGI M., MICKEY M.E. and TERASAKI P.I., « Cancer Res. », *33*, 3898 (1973).

[8] SKURZAK H., STEINER L., KLEIN E. and LAMON E., « Natl. Cancer Inst. Monogr. », *37*, 93 (1973).

[9] JONDAL M. and PROSS H., « Int. J. Cancer », *15*, 596 (1975).

[10] DE VRIES J.E., MEYERUNG M., VAN DONGREN A. and RÜMKE P., « Int. J. Cancer », *15*, 301 (1975).

[11] KIESSLING R., KLEIN E. and WIGZELL H., « Eur. J. Immunol. », *5*, 230 (1975).

[12] HERBERMAN R.B., NUNN M.F. and LAVRIN D.H., « Int. J. Cancer », *16*, 230 (1975).

[13] BECKER S. and KLEIN E., « Eur. J. Immunol. », *6*, 892 (1976).

[14] VOSE B.M., VANKY F., ARGOV S. and KLEIN E., « Eur. J. Immunol. ». In press. (1977).

[15] BECKER S., FENYÖ E.M. and KLEIN E., « Eur. J. Immunol. », *6*, 882 (1976).

[16] HALLER O., KIESSLING R., ÖRN A., KÄRRE K., NILSSON K. and WIGZELL H., « Int. J. Cancer », *20*, 93 (1977).

[17] HANSSON M., KÄRRE K., BAKÁCS T., KIESSLING R. and KLEIN G., To be published.

[18] KIESSLING R., PETRÁNYI G., KLEIN G. and WIGZELL H., « Int. J. Cancer », *15*, 933 (1975).

[19] BECKER S., KIESSLING R. and KLEIN G., To be published.

[20] PROSS H.F. and BAINES M.G., « Int. J. Cancer », *18*, 593 (1976).

[21] KLEIN E. and ÅSJÖ B., To be published.

[22] ARGOV S. and KLEIN E., To be published.

[23] STJERNSWÄRD J., « J. Natl. Cancer Inst. », *35*, 885 (1965).

[13] *E. Klein* - p. 9

[24] STUTMAN O., « Science », *183*, 534 (1974).

[25] SULIT H.L., GOLUB S.H., IRIE R.F., GUPTA R.K., GROOMS G.A. and MORTON D.L., « Int. J. Cancer », *17*, 461 (1976).

[26] DE VRIES J.E. and RUMKE Ph., « Int. J. Cancer », *17*, 182 (1976).

[27] TAKASUGI M., KOIDE Y., AKIRA D. and RAMSEYER A., « Int. J. Cancer », *19*, 291 (1977).

[28] HERSEY P., EDWARDS A., EDWARDS J., MILTON G.W. and NELSON D., « Int. J. Cancer », *16*, 173 (1975).

[29] BAKÁCS T., GERGELY P., CORNAIN S. and KLEIN E., « Int. J. Cancer », *19*, 441 (1977).

[30] BAKÁCS T., GERGELY P. and KLEIN E., « Cellular Immunology », *32*, 317 (1977).

[31] PETER H.H., KNOPP G. and KALDEN J.R., « Z. Imm. Forsch. », *151*, 263 (1976).

[32] WEST W.H., CANNON G.B., KAY H.D., BONNARD G.D. and HERBERMANN R.B., « J. Immunol. », *48*, 355 (1977).

[33] BAKÁCS T., KLEIN E., GERGELY P. and STEINITZ M., « Z. Imm. Forsch. ». In Press. (1977).

[34] PETER H.H., EIFE R.F. and KALDEN J.R., « J. Immunol. », *116*, 342 (1976).

[35] TAKASUGI M., KOIDE D., AKIRA D. and RAMSEYER A., « Int. J. Cancer », *19*, 291 (1977).

[36] PERLMANN P., PERLMANN H., WAHLIN B., and HAMMARSTRÖM S., *Proceedings of the 7th Int. Symp. of Immunopathology.* In Press. (1977).

[37] ARGOV S. and KLEIN E., To be published.

[38] ENGERS H.D. and MacDONALD R., *Contemporary Topics in Immunobiology.* « Plenum Press, New York », *5*, 145 (1976).

[39] POROS A. and KLEIN E., To be published.

[40] KLEIN E., To be published.

[41] DREW S.I., TERASAKI P.I., BILLING R.J., BERGH O.J., MINOWADA J. and KLEIN E., «« Blood », *49*, 715 (1977).

[42] ZINKERNAGEL R.M. and DOHERTY P.C., « J. Exp. Med. », *141*, 1427 (1975).

[43] SHEARER G.M., « Eur. J. Immunol. », *4*, 527 (1974).

[44] TING C.C. and LAW L.W., « J. Immunol. », *188*, 1259 (1977).

[45] SVEDMYR E. and JONDAL M., « Proc. Natl. Acad. Sci. », *72*, 1622 (1975).

[46] BAKÁCS T., SVEDMYR E. and KLEIN E., Cancer letters, in press (1978).

[47] KLEIN E., BECKER S., SVEDMYR E., JONDAL M. and VÁNKY F., « Ann. N.Y. Acad. Sci. », *276*, 207 (1976).

[48] BAKÁCS T. and KLEIN E., Cancer letters, in press (1978).

[49] VÁNKY F. and STJERNSWÄRD J., In: *In vitro methods in cell mediated and tumor immunity.* B. Bloom and J.R. David, eds. Vol. II, 597-606 (1976).

[50] VOSE B.M., VÁNKY F. and KLEIN E., « Int. J. Cancer », *20*, 512 (1977).

DISCUSSION

ROSENBERG

You mentioned that the NK killing is effective against tissue culture cells but not against the fresh cells, and this is a common finding for NK killers. Is there some analogy to some of the findings I discussed yesterday in which we could not find embryonic antigen expression on any fresh adult cell but any normal cell we put in tissue culture did express these embryonic antigens? Is is possible that the receptor for NK killing — that is the target antigen — is an embryonic antigen?

EVA KLEIN

The cold target inhibition with fresh embryonic cells was done in the mouse system. There was no indication that embryonic antigen is the target of the NK cell. However, since it is important to use the right stage of the embryo, when such antigens are expressed, it is possible that its detection was missed, since the studies were not performed systematically, taking embryo tissue from various ages. Inhibition tests with anti sera against fetal antigens were not done.

ROSENBERG

Are fresh embryonic cells susceptible to NK killing?

EVA KLEIN

I am not aware whether this was tested. Depending on the test conditions explanted cells may be sensitive. However, I would like to stress again that there is a wide range of difference in sensitivity among various cells, even cell lines. We may state as a rule that the highly sensitive cells are those which have been carried in culture, but not all such cells are sensitive. We may also state that tumor derived cell lines are sensitive, this fact is apparent if one compares lymphoblastoid cell lines derived from tumors or transformed from lymphocytes of healthy human donors by EBV.

MATHÉ

What is the effect of immunity adjuvants on NK cells?

EVA KLEIN

Injection of BCG, interferon and interferon inducers, inoculation of tumor cells to mice augments temporarily the NK potential of the spleen population. Infection with bacteria and viruses will also booster. The mechanism behind this action is not known.

BARCINSKI

Is the expression of the NK cells in any sense macrophage dependent?

EVA KLEIN

That is difficult to say because we do not know how many macrophages remain, but in all our experiments our first step is to deplete for macrophages.

NOSSAL

I wonder whether you have tried the following sort of experiment. Peripheral blood is an interesting tissue which contains, as well as effector cells, some cells on their way to their lodging place that, for example, type as null cells but turn into B cells a day or two later.

Have you done the following experiment in the human: taken the cell, done your fractionation, got your population out, matured them for 24 hours, then removed cells that had developed T or B cell markers (I am sure many would) and then asked whether the ones that are still negative are NK? and do they now have any other recognizable characteristics?

[13] E. Klein - p. 12

EVA KLEIN

Such experiments were not done.

NOSSAL

I was really thinking of something like a 24 hour culture before fractionation of the cells. 24 hours is quite enough for a null cell to display Ig receptors, for example.

EVA KLEIN

Lymphocytes cultivated alone in autologous serum have low or no NK activity. There is good cell survival, and cell surface marker analysis shows that the composition of the population is similar to that of fresh lymphocytes. In fact addition of K562 cells after 5 days to such lymphocyte cultures will generate cytotoxic cells.

NOSSAL

I would be a little worried that the phenomenon studied at the end of five days is what I have in mind.

OETTGEN

Dr. Nossal, could it also be that this assumed non-differentiated cell is in fact a highly differentiated cell whose markers we do not know and cannot test for?

NOSSAL

Well, that is precisely what I was probing for: if you get rid of all the others, maybe you are left with some cell that you *can* identify.

EVA KLEIN

We have tried to fractionate the null cell population. We have depleted Fc receptor positive cells by EA rosetting, but we did not eliminate the NK effect. Also, we removed low affinity E receptor carrying cells — which are present in the null fraction if no special measure is taken to remove them together with the majority of T cells — and the residual population was still highly active.

We have also characterised the cultures in which lymphocytes were cocultivated with K562. The cytotoxic effect was not confined to a particular subset. Compared to fresh lymphocytes there was a difference in that the active cells aquired the property to adhere to nylon wool. Similar to fresh lymphocytes the cells readily rosetting with SRBC, i.e. having high avidity E receptors, were not cytotoxic.

TERRY

The discovery of NK cells arose from *in vitro* tumor immunology experiments. The biology of these cells has therefore been pursued in the context of tumor immunology. Do we know anything, or are you prepared to speculate, about the broader biological significance of this category of cells? Do we know anything about the relationship of such cells to infectious processes or to immune phenomena other than those relevant to cancer cells?

EVA KLEIN

We know little about the biological significance of these cells. As I mentioned before, infection with bacteria and viruses boosters NK activity. On the other hand, nude mice which have a perfectly functioning NK system are highly susceptible to infection.

G. KLEIN

There are some remarkable parallels between the properties of the NK cells and the properties of cells that mediate hybrid resistance on the Cudkowicz type against bone marrow grafts. I would also like to mention the study by Lopez from Sloan-Kettering, who found that the natural resistance of mice to herpes simplex infections is mediated by cells with the same properties as the NK cells. Presumably, NK cells have quite a wide range of reactivity.

[13] *E. Klein* - p. 14

Eva Klein

The A mouse which is low in NK activity does not show any remarkable difference in sensitivity to oncogenic C type viruses.

G. Klein

I think that it would be necessary to develop congenic mouse strains with high and low NK reactivity, respectively, to answer some of these questions, since genetic variation of other loci will otherwise have a profound and unknown influence on the comparison.

IMMUNOLOGICAL TOLERANCE
AND THE CANCER PROBLEM

G.J.V. NOSSAL and BEVERLEY L. PIKE

The Walter and Eliza Hall Institute of Medical Research
Melbourne, Victoria 3050, Australia

In both human cancer and in many experimental models, it is common to find that immune responsiveness, and more particularly function of the T lymphocyte system, is depressed during the later stages of the disease. Furthermore, there have been a number of claims that specific immune responses against tumor-associated antigens are mounted by the host during early cancer, but disappear later. It is thus most important to understand the control loops which govern immunological reactivity in situations where antigen persists chronically within the body in gradually increasing concentrations.

Detailed study of such control loops, and particularly of immunological tolerance, in tumor models is rendered difficult by our restricted knowledge of the structure and extracellular fluid concentrations of the important tumor antigens. For this reason the main emphasis of studies has been on pure antigens in simpler model systems. From these, it has become clear that a number of separate mechanisms, initiated by the introduction of antigen into the body, can suppress both antibody formation and cell-mediated immunity. As these have recently been reviewed elsewhere [1, 2], the purpose of this paper will be to describe two sets of recent results from our Institute relevant to tolerance induction. In particular, we wish to highlight certain technical advances which should help materially in clarifying the cellular and molecular basis of tolerance. Both examples will be shown to be relevant to key problems in tumor immunology.

The Concept of Clonal Abortion as applied to B cells

One immunoregulatory loop is the phenomenon of clonal abortion [3-6] of B lymphocytes. The two key elements are that immature B cells can be switched off by extremely low concentrations of antigen, and that the important variable is the immaturity of the differentiation stage of the B cell rather than of the whole animal. Thus, many bone marrow B cells recently born in an adult animal behave just like the immature spleen B cells from a newborn animal [4, 7]. We prefer the term clonal abortion to that of clonal deletion because the former carries the implication of the destruction of an entity not yet fully formed or developed. It is now clear that immature B cells differ in a number of respects from the bulk of mature virgin and memory B cells in the mouse. In particular, they "cap" their Ig receptors much more readily after antiglobulin treatment [8]; they are susceptible to apparently irreversible modulation of such receptors if the treatment is prolonged [8, 9]; and they lack readily detectable amounts of IgD, an immunoglobulin class present on the surface of the majority of mature B cells [10]. It seems probable that one or more of these hallmarks of immaturity is causally related to the unusual behavior of the B cells when confronted with antigen. It is also possible to induce immunological non-reactivity in mature B cells [1, 2], which in general involves higher concentrations and higher degrees of multivalency of the antigen in question. It would be preferable to reserve the concept of clonal deletion to such processes. It must be stressed that the question of whether the tolerogenic event involves an actual physical destruction of the progenitor B cell (as the words abortion and deletion imply), or simply a long-term physiological silencing, is still entirely open. Another new and exciting finding has opened the possibility that the mature cell may not irreversibly have lost its capacity for ready tolerance induction. It appears that if the IgD receptor is digested away by mild papain-mediated cleavage [11] or is blocked or modulated by the use of specific anti-δ anti-serum

[14] *Nossal, Pike* - p. 2

[12], the formerly phenotypically mature B cell now becomes susceptible to tolerance induction by low antigen concentrations. Therefore, it has become a matter of considerable importance to define the tolerance-susceptible B cell subsets with greater precision.

Use of hapten-specific B cell populations to study tolerance induction.

So far, our studies of clonal abortion have relied on the enumeration of clonable precursors of anti-hapten plaque forming cells (PFC) in spleen [5] or bone marrow [6] populations pre-cultured in bulk suspension. This two-stage culture system has the merit of great precision in the read-out step. However, it suffers from the problem that the pre-cultured starting population is an extremely heterogeneous mixture of cells at various stages of maturity. Even in the neonate, a few cells with IgD receptors may be present, (i.e a few mature cells amongst the large pool of immature); and amongst the immature cells, some are clearly more differentiated than others. Furthermore, using this mixture of cells, impressive degrees of tolerance could not be achieved in under 48 hr. These constraints made it difficult to pinpoint exactly the target cell for tolerance induction.

As a next approach to this question, we have sought to isolate from the heterogeneous mixture of spleen cells those B cells with receptors specific for the antigen to be used for tolerance induction. The results to be presented address the question with respect to both adult and neonatal mouse spleen cells.

Two-stage approach to the preparation of hapten-specific B cells

In previous work, we had made extensive use of the hapten-gelatin method of preparing hapten-specific B cells [13, 14]. This depends on allowing a lymphoid cell population from an unimmunized animal to adhere at 4° to a monolayer of hapten covalently coupled to gelatin. After nonadherent cells, about 99.95 per cent of the total, are washed away, the gel is melted by addition of excess warm medium; the bound cells are recovered by centrifugation

[14] Nossal, Pike - p. 3

and the adherent antigen is removed by collagenase treatment. Such cells can be antigenically stimulated in microcultures containing 2×10^6 thymus "filler" cells. Hapten coupled to polymerized flagellin (POL) is used to induce individual clones of anti-hapten PFC. When limit dilution analysis is performed on unfractionated adult spleen cells, using the dinitrophenyl (DNP) or nitroiodophenyl (NIP) haptens, the frequency of clonable precursors of anti-hapten PFC is 1 to 2×10^{-4}. In contrast, following DNP — or NIP — gelatin fractionation, it rises to 2 to 4×10^{-2}, that is an approximate 200-fold enrichment is achieved.

In theory, the fluorescence-activated cell sorter (FACS) is ideally suited for the preparation of antigen-specific B cells, and it has in fact been used for this purpose [15, 16]. However, the speed of sorting (maximum 5000 cells/sec) is a limiting factor. We explored the question of whether high cloning efficiencies could result from using the already-enriched, hapten-gelatin fractionated cells as an input for the FACS. For this purpose, we switched to fluoresceine (FLU) as a hapten, FLU-sheep erythrocytes as the plaque-revealing cells and FLU-POL as the stimulating antigen. Following FLU-gelatin fractionation and collagenase treatment, the cells were relabelled either with FLU-POL or with FLU-GEL and sorted on FACS. Batches of cells were collected according to their relative fluorescence intensity and cultured. Some relevant results are given in Fig. 1 and Table 1.

The first point to note is that FACS was able to achieve a further enrichment of the cells. When adult FLU-gelatin pre-fractionated cells were subdivided into sets according to their relative fluorescence intensity, that cohort of cells which represented the 10 percentile with the most intense fluorescence yielded antibody-forming clones with a frequency varying from 1 in 6 to 1 in 10 (mean 1 in 8.7), nearly 5-fold higher than the hapten-gelatin enriched starting population (Table 1). Progressively less intensely fluorescent cells gave lower cloning frequencies, Fig. 1 showing a typical experiment. Going up still higher in binding affinity, e.g. to the top 3 or 5% of fluorescence intensity, did not further increase the proportion of anti-FLU precursors. Separate experiments (not shown) revealed that highly fluorescent cells made antibody of higher avidity than unfractionated cells. In other words, the combined technologies

[14] *Nossal, Pike* - p. 4

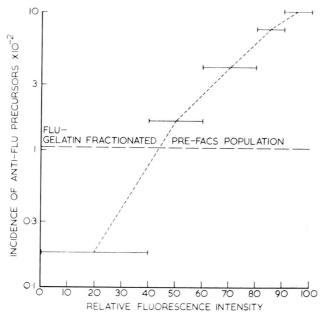

FIG. 1 — Comparative cloning efficiences of FACS-separated cells of various fluorescence intensities, using as input cells pre-fractionated on FLU-gelatin.

of hapten-gelatin fractionation and FACS-sorting provided a population of highly efficient precursor cells for *in vitro* stimulation experiments.

A closer look at Table 1 provides further interesting information. With adult cells, the polyclonal B cell activator, E. coli lipopolysaccharide (LPS) stimulates approximately the same number of cells as does the antigen FLU-POL. However, LPS which stimulates B cells regardless of the specificity of their Ig receptors, slightly out-performs antigen for unfractionated cells, but for the subset with the most highly avid receptors, antigen out-performs LPS by a small factor.

Against this background, the situation with neonatal cells is noteworthy. First, we see that both the hapten-gelatin and the combined technique are very successful in achieving enrichment. Secondly, it appears that LPS is substantially more effective a trigger

TABLE 1 - *Frequencies of anti-FLU precursor B cells using LPS or FLU-POL[1].*

| | FREQUENCIES × 10^{-4} | | | | | |
| | 8 to 10 WEEK CBA | | | 5 DAY CBA | | |
	LPS	FLU-POL	RATIO LPS:FLU	LPS	FLU-POL	RATIO LPS:FLU
Unfractionated spleen	3.3	2.35	1.4	1.23	22	5.62
FLU-gelatin Fractionated spleen	206	237	0.87	345	187	1.84
Most highly fluorescent 10-15% of FLU-gelatin fractionated spleen [b]	754	1153	0.65	922	529	1.74

[*] Cells were placed in microcultures of 200 µl volume containing 2×10^6 anti-Ia-treated thymus filler cells, stimulated with 0.1 µg/ml of FLU-POL or 20 µg/ml of LPS, and 3 days later positive clones were identified through detection of hapten-specific PFC. Frequencies were determined through Poisson analysis.
[b] An analytical FACS run was first performed to show the fluorescence distribution. Then channel gates were set accordingly for a preparative run.

than antigen for newborn spleen cells, though this advantage diminishes with increasing median affinity of cells for antigen. This at least raises the possibility that antigen, even though attached to the highly immunogenic carrier POL, may be inducing tolerance in a proportion of the specific immature cells. In contrast, LPS, which triggers cells through some mechanism independent of the Ig receptors, stimulates the fractionated immature cells with as high an efficiency as in the case of mature cells. This working hypothesis is under detailed study at present.

Tolerance Induction in Fractionated Hapten-Specific Cells

Unfortunately, we have not yet been able to explore the question of tolerance induction in fractionated hapten-specific immature cells in any depth. However, preliminary results have indicated that the immature enriched cells can be rendered tolerant more rapidly and more completely than the bulk population of unfractionated neonatal spleen. The results from one preliminary experiment are summarized in Table 2. Cells were incubated at limit dilution in thymus filler cells for one day in the presence or absence of various concentrations of the tolerogen FLU_4-human gamma globulin (FLU-HGG). Then the microcultures were challenged with an immunogenic concentration of FLU-POL, and after two further days, were assayed for the incidence of clones of anti-FLU PFC. Consistent with previous experience, this relatively short tolerization period did not affect adult unfractionated spleen cells, and caused a barely detectable reduction in clone frequency amongst unfractionated neonatal spleen cells, though we know that longer treatment would have shown up marked tolerance in the newborn cells. However, when the FLU-gelatin, hapten enriched cells were treated at 5 µg tolerogen/ml, a tenfold reduction in clone frequency was observed and even at 0.05 µg/ml, most of the B cells were tolerized. Two possible explanations can be offered for these results. First, it is certain that the cells with receptors of high avidity for the tolerogen would have bound more antigen than those with low avidity, and as the FLU-gelatin binding cells are probably of higher median avidity than the totality of clonable anti-FLU precursors, the actual dose of tolerogen captured on their surface would have been higher than average. Secondly, amongst the unfractionated cells, there would have been some Ig^{-ve} pre-B cells which,

TABLE 2 - *Per cent reduction in clonable Anti-FLU precursors as a result of 24 hr preincubation with FLU-HGG[1].*

Adult whole spleen,	5 µg	0
Newborn whole spleen,	5 µg	16
Newborn FLU-gelatin enriched cells,	5 µg	90
	0.5 µg	79
	0.05 µg	79

[1] Following 24 hr tolerogenesis of cells placed in thymus filler microcultures at limit dilution, the tolerogen was removed and replaced with 0.1 µg/ml FLU-POL. Cultures were harvested 48 hr later and clones of PFC detected as before.

not bearing Ig receptors, would not have "seen" the tolerogen. These could have matured into B cells with receptors in the post-tolerogenesis phase and have engendered small clones. Again, the resolution of these questions is the object of current work. It will be of particular relevance to study the tolerizability of FACS-sorted neonatal cells of even higher median avidity than the hapten-gelatin fractionated cells.

Possible Mechanisms of Clonal Abortion Tolerogenesis

In many respects, the effects of antigen on immature B cells resemble the effects of anti-μ antiserum, and one wonders whether a prominent factor in clonal abortion may not be the permanent modulation of the cell's surface Ig receptors through repeated cycles of patching, capping and endocytosis. In a previous study [17], we have shown that circumstances which can cause tolerance in adult B lymphocytes, such as the attachment of *large* quantities of hapten-POL to surface receptors, also lead to apparently irreversible modulation of the receptors. Perhaps the capacity for a B cell to be switched off through these intensive cycles of receptor-ligand interactions persists throughout the whole differentiation pathway, as even antbody secretion can be stopped in active plaque-forming cells through exposure to high concentrations of multivalent ligands, a phenomenon we have termed effector cell blockade [18, 2]. In other words, the differences between the different B cell maturation stages may be ones of degree rather than of kind. If so, receptor modulation may be one final common pathway of B cell tolerogenesis. Because of some peculiarity of lipid viscosity or Ig receptor tethering, the immature B cell may be especially susceptible to capping and receptor modulation, though we know nothing about the molecular feedback loops which engender receptor resynthesis under some circumstances but not under others. The mature B cell, on the other hand, may require much higher concentrations of attached antigen to achieve the irreversible modulation. In any event, if a B cell is so altered as to fail to express its Ig receptors, it has lost its possibility to function. It may well be that *in vivo* some mechanism exists to ensure its early death.

[14] *Nossal, Pike* - p. 8

Though we believe modulation to be very important, we think it is not the only key event in tolerogenesis. This is because of a recent observation which suggests that a powerful negative signal can be given to immature B cells by quite a short exposure to anti-μ antibody (and by implication to antigen). The findings come from a different B cell cloning system, namely the agar colony generating system of Metcalf [19]. In this system, B cells from newborn or adult mice can be stimulated by mitogens contained in the agar to divide and form large colonies of activated lymphocytes. Mercapto-ethanol is essential for the phenomenon, and one or more co-mitogens, ideally derived from added macrophages, is required for optimal growth. Using this system, we have noted (Table 3) that a brief exposure (1 hr, 37°) to anti-μ antibody either does not affect or actually slightly stimulates the growth of B cell colonies. However, B cells from 5 day old mouse spleens are severely inhibited, even by low concentrations acting over such a short time. The finding is especially noteworthy as the mitogenic signal to the B cell exerted by the agar mitogens acting as polyclonal B cell activators probably

TABLE 3 - *Effect of anti-μ antibody (1 hr, 37°) on B lymphocyte colony formation by mouse spleen cells*[a].

Concentration of anti-μ (μg/ml)	Per Cent of Control Response Adult	Neonate
Nil	100 ± 9	100 ± 13
10	94 ± 14	27 ± 3
30	147 ± 4	12 ± 3
60	112 ± 4	7 ± 2
100	101 ± 6	3 ± 2

[a] The cloning system used involved placing the cells in agar gel cultures in the presence of 2-mercaptoethanol and sheep erythrocytes. After one week's culture, the erythrocytes were lysed with acetic acid and colonies counted at × 20 magnification. Pool of 2 experiments, 4 cultures per group, each experiment normalized to its control.

[14] *Nossal, Pike* - p. 9

does not flow via the Ig receptors. Clearly a negative signal has been given to the cells via the IgM receptors of the immature cells which the agar mitogens could not override.

Progress in the study of suppressor T cells

Interesting though the tolerization or blockade of B cells may be, the cancer researcher may well be even more concerned with mechanisms of tolerance involving lymphocytes. Thus, we wish to end this brief review of recent work by mentioning some data from the Experimental Pathology Unit of our Institute obtained by TANIGUCHI and MILLER [20]. We have seen how much greater precision of knowledge can be gained in the case of B-lymphocytes through working with fractionated, pure populations capable of reacting with only one antigen. Now TANIGUCHI and MILLER have taken the first step towards providing pure populations of antigen-specific T suppressor cells. Using deaggregated HGG to raise carrier-specific suppressor T cells in adult mice, they have used two simple principles to devise a method for the approximate 100-fold enrichment of suppressors. The first is that antibody sticks readily and firmly to plastic. The second is that receptors for antigen are exposed on suppressor cells at 25° but apparently not at 0°. Spleen cells from de-HGG-injected mice were first placed on petri dishes at 25° to which an anti-mouse globulin had been attached. Most of the B cells adhered firmly, and most T cells could be recovered in the supernatant. Next, these T cell-enriched populations were placed on dishes to which HGG had been attached. A small proportion of T cells adhered and the rest were washed away. Finally, the dishes were brought to 0°. Spontaneously, many T cells came off the dishes. These were compared in an adoptive immune assay for their capacity to suppress a B cell response to hapten-HGG. As a rough comparison, 3×10^5 of these enriched suppressors were as effective as 3×10^7 unfractionated cells. The enriched cells carrying the suppressor properties were Thy-1$^+$, Ig$^-$, Ly2$^+$, Ly1$^-$, and I-J$^+$, thus exhibiting all the classical features of suppressor T cells. The population of cells is not yet entirely specific, as T cells of other phenotypes also adhere and only about 30 per cent of the recovered

[14] Nossal, Pike - p. 10

cells carry the above phenotype spectrum. Nevertheless, the availability of the enriched cells markedly facilitates further research into the nature of suppressor cell action and the chemistry of soluble factors derived from suppressor T cells.

Significance of tolerance induction to the cancer problem

If we assume that at least some human tumors bear on their surface specific tumor antigens which can signal the immune system, it is clear that some of this material must enter the circulation as the tumor progresses. Some degree of shedding and metabolic turnover of cell surface macromolecules must occur, and particularly in the later stages, some necrosis of tumor cells is common. This antigen would in part be degraded by serum enzymes and by phagocytic cells, but many opportunities for the creation of multivalent antigenic aggregates also present themselves. First, if some serum antibody is present, soluble complexes might form and at late stages of the disease would be in the zone of antigen excess. It is well known that such complexes can exert a severe suppressive effect on both B and T cells [21], perhaps through the modulation mechanisms just described. Secondly, membrane fragments from damaged or dead cells could present multivalent antigen. Thirdly, matrix-generating mechanisms exist through the activity of antigen-trapping cells [22]. In all cases, the multivalent antigen could, under the appropriate circumstances, activate the receptor modulation cycle. Of course, the net effect on the whole immune system would depend on the integration of stimulatory and suppressive events. For the mature cell, it appears that low concentrations of multivalent antigen are immunogenic provided that appropriate co-mitogens from T cells and/or macrophages are present. For immature cells, low concentrations are tolerogenic. Therefore during earlier stages of tumor growth, one might anticipate an active immune response, but, as the tumor grows, the entry of new immunocompetent T and B cells from the thymus and bone marrow into the reactive cell pool might be prevented through the clonal abortion pathway. If the tumor is not rejected early, the odds become progressively more stacked against the immune system. High doses of complexed or multivalent antigen could suppress even the mature cells. High doses of soluble, monomeric antigen would activate suppressor T cells and would also therefore tend to lower immunological reactivity.

All the classical adjuvants of immunology act to prevent this suppressive scenario. Antigens given absorbed to or incorporated in adjuvants are released slowly, and opportunities for soluble complex formation or high concentrations of soluble antigen causing suppressor T cell activation are minimized. Adjuvants cause macrophage division and activation, influences which favor antigen degradation and the lowering of extracellular fluid antigen concentrations. Adjuvants also promote the release of a variety of lymphokines and co-mitogenic factors from macrophages and T cells, which militate against tolerogenesis. Thus, the simple model systems which the cellular immunologist employs can give insights relevant both to the failure of specific immunity in late cancer and to some of the rationale behind cancer immunotherapy.

However, the main factors limiting the rate of progress of the cellular immunologist are the great heterogeneity of the cells of the immune system and the complexity of the interactions occurring between them. In this paper, we have placed emphasis on techniques which facilitate the study of immune phenomena through the identification and isolation of subsets of relatively homogeneous and highly active cells. The opportunities provided will eventually provide information valuable to the student of tumor immunology.

Summary

This paper has drawn attention to the fact that antigen-activated mechanisms of immunosuppression, such as tolerance induction or suppressor T cell induction, may be most important in late cancer. These phenomena are best studied in simple model systems employing pure antigens.

The paper describes a new method for isolating antigen-reactive B cells in pure and relatively homogeneous form using a combination of an affinity adherence procedure plus the fluorescence-activated cell sorter. Such cells can be induced to form antibody in microcultures with a cloning efficiency of 10 to 16 per cent. The method can also be applied to cells from newborn mice with only slightly lower

[14] *Nossal, Pike* - p. 12

efficiency. The antigen-specific cells from neonatal but not from adult mice can be rendered tolerant through 24 hr exposure to very low antigen concentrations. The method can be used to investigate possible mechanisms of tolerogenesis at the single cell level. Some evidence suggests that receptor modulation is an important mechanism, but other evidence shows that powerful negative signal can be delivered to immature B cells by relatively brief treatments not capable of permanently modulating the Ig receptors.

Knowledge of the detailed role of T cells in tolerance phenomena is less advanced. For this reason it becomes very important to isolate and study the subset of suppressor T cells. Brief reference is made to a new method developed by TANIGUCHI and MILLER which affords a substantial enrichment of carrier-specific, activated suppressor T cells based on principles of adherence to antigen.

ACKNOWLEDGMENTS

We are grateful to Ms. K. CRUISE and E. CAIN for expert technical assistance. This work was supported by the National Health and Medical Research Council, Canberra, Australia; and by Grant No. AI-03958 from the National Institute for Allergy and Infectious Diseases, U.S. Public Health Service.

REFERENCES

[1] Nossal G.J.V., *Principles of immunological tolerance and immunocyte receptor blockade.* « Adv. Cancer Res. », *20*, 93 (1974).

[2] Abbas A.K. and Klaus G.G.B., *Antigen-receptor interactions in the induction of B lymphocyte unresponsiveness.* « Curr. Top. Microbiol. Immunol. », (in press).

[3] Nossal G.J.V. and Pike Beverley L., *New concepts in immunological tolerance.* In: « Immunological Aspects of Neoplasia ». Ed. E.M. Hersh and M. Schlamowitz, Baltimore, Williams and Wilkins, p. 87-101 (1975).

[4] Nossal G.J.V. and Pike Beverley L., *Evidence for the clonal abortion theory of B lymphocyte tolerance.* « J. Exp. Med. », *141*, 904-917 (1975).

[5] Stocker J.W., *Tolerance induction in maturing B cells.* « Immunol. », *32*, 283-290 (1977).

[6] Nossal G.J.V., Shortman K., Howard M. and Pike B.L., *Current problem areas in the study of B lymphocyte differentiation.* « Immunol. Rev. », *37*, 188-210 (1977).

[7] Metcalf E.S. and Klinman N.R., *In vitro tolerance induction of neonatal murine B cells.* « J. Exp. Med. », *143*, 1327-1340 (1976).

[8] Raff M.C., Owen J.J.T., Cooper M.D., Lawton A.R., Megson M. and Gathings W.E., *Differences in susceptibility of mature and immature mouse B lymphocytes to anti-immunoglobulin suppression in vitro.* « J. Exp. Med. », *142*, 1052 (1975).

[9] Sidman C.L. and Unanue E.R., *Receptor-mediated inactivation of early B lymphocytes.* « Nature », *257*, 149 (1975).

[10] Goding J.W. and Layton J.E., *Antigen-induced co-capping of IgM and IgD-like receptors on murine B cells.* « J. Exp. Med. », *144*, 852 (1976).

[11] Cambier J.C., Vitetta E.S., Kettman J.R., Wetzel G. and Uhr J.W., *B cell tolerance. III. Effect of papain-mediated cleavage of cell surface IgD on tolerance susceptibility of murine B cells.* « J. Exp. Med. », *146*, 107 (1977).

[12] Scott D.W., Layton J.E. and Nossal G.J.V., *Role of IgD in the immune response and tolerance I. Anti-delta pretreatment facilitates tolerance induction in adult B cells in vitro.* « J. Exp. Med. », *146*, 1473 (1977).

[13] Haas W. and Layton J.E., *Separation of antigen-specific lymphocytes. I. Enrichment of antigen-binding cells.* « J. Exp. Med. », *141*, 1004 (1975).

[14] Nossal G.J.V. and Pike Beverley L., *Single cell studies on the antibody-forming potential of fractionated, hapten-specific B lymphocytes.* « Immunol. », *30*, 189 (1976).

[14] *Nossal, Pike* - p. 14

[15] JULIUS M.H., JANEWAY C.A. Jr. and HERZENBERG L.A., *Isolation of antigen-binding cells from unprimed mice II. Evidence for monospecificity of antigen-binding cells.* « Eur. J. Immunol. », 6, 288 (1976).

[16] JULIUS M.H. and HERZENBERG L.A., *Isolation of antigen-binding cells from unprimed mice.* « J. Exp. Med. », 140, 904 (1974).

[17] NOSSAL G.J.V. and LAYTON J.E., *Antigen-induced aggregation and modulation of receptors on hapten-specific B lymphocytes.* « J. Exp. Med. », 143, 511 (1976).

[18] SCHRADER J.W. and NOSSAL G.J.V., *Effector cell blockade - a new mechanism of immune hyporeactivity induced by multivalent antigens.* « J. Exp. Med. », 139, 1582 (1974).

[19] METCALF D., WARNER N.L., NOSSAL G.J.V., MILLER J.F.A.P., SHORTMAN K. and RABELLINO E., *Growth of B lymphocyte colonies in vitro from mouse lymphoid organs.* « Nature », 255, 630 (1975).

[20] TANIGUCHI M. and MILLER J.F.A.P., *Enrichment of specific suppressor T cells and characterization of their surface markers.* « J. Exp. Med. », 146, 1450 (1977).

[21] FELDMANN M. and NOSSAL G.J.V., *Tolerance, enhancement and the regulation of interactions between T cells, B cells and macrophages.* « Transplant. Rev. », 13, 3 (1972).

[22] NOSSAL G.J.V. and ADA G.L., *Antigens, Lymphoid Cells and the Immune Response.* New York and London, Academic Press. (1971).

DISCUSSION

Weiss

I like the model you presented, and your statement of the clonal deletion view of specific immunological tolerance. I should like to ask, however, how is it possible, then, to interpret the findings of different investigators over recent years, which suggest that specific tolerance is a positive rather than a negative phenomenon. Do such positive states of tolerance require an additional, alternative explanation?

Nossal

The answer to your question is very clear-cut. Those of us who have been puzzling about tolerance for years were much enriched by the papers of Gershon and Kondo, and of McCullogh, and by the subsequent work demonstrating the presence of suppressor T cells. I am sure that there are many situations, both in real life and in our laboratory models where the suppressor T cell is the explanation of the failure of antibody production to antigens. Clonal abortion has distinct molar thresholds. For the sort of antigens that I am talking about, this is around 10^{-9} molar. With respect to many of the proteins that we have in our cells, which never reach the extra-cellular fluid in reasonably detectable amounts, I am sure that we do *not* have B cell tolerance of clonal abortion type. For example, in the case of thyroglobulin we have competent B cells, ready to make anti-thyroglobulin antibodies in our own bodies; and if we now want to have some mechanism for stopping that from happening, we have to have some other mechanism. I think of the suppressor T cells as a failsafe, I think of clonal abortion as the primary self-recognition mechanism, and I think of both suppressor T cell activation and the antigen antibody complex mediated tolerance as two very powerful and very effective failsafes should the cell slip by clonal abortion for some reason. Everything has to be qualified by the affinity parameter. There is no doubt, I think, from what we have presented here, that high affinity cells are tolerized more easily and at lower molar concentrations of antigens than low affinity cells, as you would predict on the clonal selection theory. We probably have got low affinity cells even against some serum proteins. We have got to stop those being activated in some way, and suppressor T cells, I think, are one such way.

SELA

You described this nice technique of selecting suppressor T cells. Do you have absolute and experimental proof that these are still suppressor cells? How do you know that you have selected suppressor T cells, or is it really a mixture of suppressors, helpers and effectors?

NOSSAL

The answer to your question is very simple. The fact that they are T cells has been proved by studying the classical markers-Thy-1, Ig etc. In fact the prefractionation step for removing the B cells is pretty effective, we have only about 1% of B cells left. However, not all of the cells are of the Ly 2-3 phenotype or are I-J positive. In fact, only 30% are of the phenotype typical of suppressor cells. The other 70% of cells are IJ negative. It is possible that refinements of this technique will provide purer suppressor T cells. Let me just say one more thing: the technique unfortunately does not work for helper cells — not so far; whether there is something complex about helper T cells receptor expression, whether you have to bind these to antigens hooked on to macrophages or something like that we do not know, but operation of this technique does not work for helpers.

TERRY

I would like to push you to make a closer association between this very basic immunology and the tumor situation. If you believe that the evolution of a tumor depends in part upon immunologic tolerance, how do you explain the presence of antigen-antibody complexes that apparently are present in tumor bearing animals? If antibody is being produced, there is no tolerance.

[14] *Nossal, Pike* - p. 18

NOSSAL

Well, I can conceive this, perhaps a little bit simplistically, in progressive terms. Let us suppose you have a tumor, it gets to the size of a few thousand or a few million cells — I would imagine there is a threshold that needs to be reached before the immune system is signalled at all. When the immune system is signalled, it starts to make killer T cells and antibodies. I suspect that there are many situations where that attack is enough to oppose the further growth of that tumor, because fundamentally I am a believer in immunological surveillance, at least in some situations. But supposing that for whatever reason (either the quantitative amount of antibodies made or the particular division propensities of that tumor) that early phase is passed and the tumor is not destroyed but continues to grow, then I can conceive that antigen will be present in excess, tolerogenic amounts, particularly if antigen-antibody complexes are formed, in slight antigen excess. Now, I could well imagine a kind of balanced dynamic equilibrium situation for a long time. Those complexes would exert a powerful negative feedback effect limiting the escalation of antibody production. If you did not have the complexes, you might get much antibody formed, but as the complexes are there and are acting as a negative controlling force on the immunocytes, you have got a limit to the antibody production. I think in many situations that limit will not switch off the immune attack completely — I think it would be too much to expect that you would bounce right back into a total blockade. Now, supposing this goes on for long enough, I could conceive that eventually you might have a true tolerance and a failure of antibody production, and as some of the early papers of Martin Lewis suggest, a situation in which antigens predominate, no antibodies present, the immune system fails and the whole thing switches off. But that is clearly an oversimplified view.

RAPP

I am vitally interested in tumor specific transplantation antigens, but I think it is a mistake to consider them the *sine qua non* of tumor immunotherapy. Your point of view derives mainly from xenogeneic systems in which the differences on a chemical basis between antigens and recipients are relatively great, so that the kinds of reactions you get, at least on a quantitative level, are going to be very different from those that you get against an allograft or in autoimmunity. And if we look at tumor immunity as something just this side of auto-immunity, that is still another situation. Immunologists need to be reminded that they advised clinicians against trying to transplant kidneys, and yet a way was found to do it successfully. So I think that tumor immunology may be a new subject which cannot be approached completely by trying to apply what we have learned in allogeneic or xenogeneic systems; and maybe we need new basic information to assure progress in tumor immunology. Now before you respond to that, can I ask you one real question: Have you ever seen any mutual influences if you mix adult cells with newborn cells?

NOSSAL

Thank you very much for your comments. Not only do I profoundly agree with all that you have said, but you have taken about five minutes of my summary tomorrow morning. But to respond to your real question, we *have* done these experiments, obviously influenced by the concept of suppression or infectious tolerance and the answer always has been that mixtures of adult and newborn cells behaved exactly as you would predict. So to this tolerance confined to immature B cells, there is no infectious parameter, there is no suppression. I should aso add that the most critical experiments on the B cell tolerance have been done with nude mice, eliminating the T cell question.

MATHÉ

With chemotherapy, we can break tolerance or kill suppressor cells; and one knows that in some experimental or even clinical conditions, one can, with chemotherapy, restore immunity or increase immunity, even specific. You said that the paralysable cells are in G-1. Thus one is tempted to use drugs which are working in G-1 to inhibit them. My question is: can you break tolerance with cytostatics working in G-1? My second question is: can you extrapolate from B cells to T cells? In other words, are paralysable T cells in G-1?

[14] *Nossal, Pike* - p. 20

NOSSAL

I reply to your first question, we have not done that; I think it is a very intriguing suggestion — I think the drugs could help us very much to analyze this tolerance further. In reply to your question about T cells: do these same tolerance mechanisms also work with T cells? I can tell you that together with Jacques Miller we tried very hard indeed to answer that question and we have been foiled so far by the complicating expression of the second phenomenon, namely the induction of suppressor T cells. It is a really curious thing that the very mechanisms which we have used for inducing tolerance of clonal abortion type in B cells are also the mechanisms that seem to raise the suppressor T cells, and we have so far not been able to dissect the two. I think with the LY and IJ phenotypes of the T cells now becoming clear, it should be possible to dissociate the phenomena. My bias would be to say that clonal abortion works for T cells as well, but I have no evidence for that.

DE DUVE

I have two questions: one immunological and one biochemical. The first one: how do you or can you distinguish between transient and permanent paralysis? The biochemical question is: what is a gelatin monolayer?

NOSSAL

Well, the first question, I would say the following: that in these short-term tissue culture experiments, what one actually sees *in vitro* is the continued persistence of receptorless B lymphocytes, cells which are blinded, cells which cannot see — you have done something to them that takes away their capacity to redevelop their receptors and to mature toward this normal "IgM and IgD positive" step. You will ask me — I have not seen deletion as such *in vitro*, in the test tube. Now you will ask me what is the likely fate of such a cell in the body — is it going to swim around like the Ancient Mariner in a lonely, lost sort of way looking for an antigen when it can no longer see, (without its Ig receptors) or will the body have developed some mechanism for getting rid of it?   And while I cannot answer, by experiment, my bias would be to say that such a cell probably would not live for very long.   But in the test tube it has to be freely admitted that we have *not yet* got any evidence for a physical deletion of the end result of this modulation phenomenon.   To your second question, perhaps thin layer is a better description than monolayer.

ROSENBERG

Do you think there is any experimental evidence that immunologic tolerance as you have defined it plays any role in cancer defense mechanisms?

NOSSAL

I think the answer to that is "no" because there is no system in which the tumor antigens and their relations to T and B cells in animals are yet sufficiently defined.   I am looking for someone like Dr. Baldwin to construct the systems that are analyzable in the sorts of terms that I have described.

BALDWIN

Just to make some comments, Gus, to put it into practical terms, we know chemically induced hepatomas and chemically induced sarcomas, but when you plant something like a million cells, the first thing you can see in the serum is a rapid distribution of antigens into circulation; the next event you see is immune complexes, and in untreated tumors the terminal event is death. Now when you do the other model experiment, of giving immune stimulation at implantation sites, you do not get this distribution of antigens into circulation and the tumor does not grow.

NOSSAL

Well, of course that is the type of thing that one would very much like to be able to analyze in quantitative terms for both B cells and T cells.   There certainly are relevant experiments with model antigens, the work of Geoffrey Asherson, for example.   I am afraid you are very close to convincing me that in the tumor models that we have at hand there is not going to be much tolerance.

BALDWIN

No, I think all you have to do is tell us how to do your very elegant techniques with these very crude tumor associated antigens.

WEISS

Two brief comments.   For one, I should like to cite an observation made more than twenty years ago in Oxford by the late A. Q. Wells and myself which suggests a role of immunological adjuvants in the context of responsiveness-unresponsiveness equilibria.   We attempted to induce specific tolerance to various tubercle bacillus entities in guinea pigs, by injecting the materials into the fetal animals, *in utero*, several days to weeks before birth.   It turned out that mycobacterial entities which have strong adjuvant properties, such as intact killed bacilli and MER, failed to induce tolerance to tuberculoproteins even when introduced as early as four to six weeks before birth, and, to the contrary, facilitated maturation of immunological responsiveness.   On the other hand, injection of soluble tubercle bacillus proteins, with no general immunomodulator properties, elicited significant degrees of specific tolerance.   Thus, a facilitated maturation of immunocyte functions early in life, and perhaps throughout life in the chain of differentiation from precursor cells, might be a central mechanism of nonspecific immunomodulator effects.

My other comment pertains to the exchange between Drs. Rosenberg and Baldwin.   It was demonstrated, in a series of investigations conducted by both Dr. Don Morton and myself in the 1960's, that mice of strains not infected at birth or prenatally with the mammary tumor viruses (MTV and NIV) develop strong transplantation immunity to mammary carcinoma cells infected with the agents and expressing virus-associated antigens, upon specific immunization.   In contrast, mice infected early in life with the viruses showed, in most instances, marked impairment in the acquisition of such immunity.   When mice of substrains free of the viruses were foster-nursed on infected mothers, resistance ability later in life was abrogated; conversely, when newborn animals from infected strains were given foster mothers free of the viruses immediately after birth, strong tumor resistance could be produced in adult life by specific sensitization. Thus, presence or absence of the living MTV and NIV early in life are a determining factor in this system. Moreover, it was found that in some strains, tolerance with regard to transplantation resistance against the syngeneic mammary carcinomas was not necessarily accompanied by a failure to produce free antibody to the virion and/or to virus-associated antigens. It might be possible, then, to analyze tolerance induction differentially for cellular and for humoral immunological reactivities in these models.

NOSSAL

Thanks very much for those two models. I cannot make any useful comment on the second; but as regards the first, I entirely agree with you, that polyclonal B cell activators and lymphokines can counteract tolerogenic signals under some circumstances, as Weigle's group has shown very clearly. Cells that would otherwise be tolerized can be rescued from tolerance through polyclonal B cell activators.

OETTGEN

You indicated that the macrophage could possibly aid in circumventing some of the problems that arise from tolerance. We know that LPS-activated adult macrophages prevent the antibody-induced suppression of antibody formation, and facilitate B cell differentiation. Do you have any information on the functional state of the macrophage in the newborn spleen? Is it part of the system in the newborn spleen that permits tolerance? Is it functionally different from the adult macrophage?

NOSSAL

I agree, Dr. Oettgen, to your three functions of macrophages. As you know, we also, with John Schrader, have been studying the co-mitogenic factors coming from macrophages. As regards the newborn, there is no question that what you say is correct — the newborn is deficient in its antigen capturing and processing function. The first work on this was done in 1957 by Frank Dixon and colleagues, who documented the poor

[14] *Nossal, Pike* - p. 24

capacity of the newborn mouse to sustain adoptive immunization; that was soon confirmed by us and was later extended by the late Werner Braun, who pinned it down to a defect in the macrophages. So there is a lot of evidence to support the immaturity of the RES being one of the factors pushing the newborn towards immune tolerance and incapacity to immunize — it is only one of the factors.

RAPP

I would like to describe an observation related to the findings of others and ask you whether any of your ideas or findings might be applicable to it. If a mixture of living BCG or the BCG cell wall vaccine with living tumor cells is injected into a healthy non-tumor-bearing animal, the growth of the tumor cells is invariably suppressed; but if a tumor is growing on one side and a mixture of tumor cells plus BCG is injected on the other side, in a significant number of animals that challenge dose or that vaccinating dose of tumor cells grows right out of the mixture of BCG.

NOSSAL

That is a tough one because it is going in the opposite direction of what Dr. North told us yesterday. I cannot give you a quick answer to it except perhaps to raise the question of whether in the latter case a ceiling level of anti-tumor immunoreactivity had already been reached and even the nonspecific immunity phenomena could not induce extra tumor suppression.

WESTPHAL

A purely technical question: if your fluorescent antigen reacts with antibody or receptors, can you differentiate between specific reaction and non-specific absorption?

NOSSAL

Yes, we have asked ourselves that a number of times, but we have not done any experiments to approach this question. In all cases we

[14] *Nossal, Pike* - p. 25

have used multivalent antigens with free haptenic groups to label the cells prior to fluorescence sorting. My prediction would be from the work of Eisen and others that we would get quite significant shifts if haptens were used. The problem is that a hapten labeling of B cells is so easily reversible, particularly if the B cell is metabolizing. So I think the experiments could be technically difficult, nonetheless enormously interesting.

[14] Nossal, Pike - p. 26

ANTI-TUMOR
EFFECTS OF BACTERIAL ENDOTOXIN
(LIPOPOLYSACCHARIDES, LIPID A)
AND SYNTHETIC LYSOLECITHIN ANALOGUES

OTTO WESTPHAL, URSULA WESTPHAL, RAINER ANDREESEN
and PAUL G. MUNDER

Max-Planck-Institut für Immunbiologie
Freiburg - Germany

ENDOTOXIN

Human and animal cancer may spontaneously undergo regression, especially under conditions of concomitant infectious fever. These observations promted various heroic approaches of clinical cancer therapy by inducing artificial infections or artificial fever. Already in 1774 a case was reported by a physician in Paris [1]. The Protocol says:

> *Case Schwenke.* — Female adult, inoperable mammary carcinoma; patient had been treated by all the most effective remedies then in use... without effect. Having lost all hope of cure she ceased treatment... (Artificial suppuration, accompanied by fever, was then induced by local injections of pus into one leg). As suppuration became more abundant, cancer diminished, then disappeared. Against advice patient allowed ulcer to heal; cancer at once recurred; new "issue" then opened at site of former abscess on leg; when suppuration was well established breast cancer gradually disappeared.

The famous physiologist François MAGENDIE (Paris) demonstrated in 1823 that the intravenous injection of pus and putrid fluids caused shots of high fever together with toxic effects in dogs [2].

After the isolation of pure bacterial cultures, due to Robert
Koch's pioneering work, F. FEHLEISEN (Würzburg) in 1882 described the treatment of human cancer with artificial *Erysipelas*
(streptococcal) infections [3].

He was followed by William B. COLEY (New York) who,
since 1893-1898 replaced live bacteria by a mixture of killed
Streptococci and *B. prodigiosus (Serratia marcescens)* in successful
treatment, mainly of sarcoma [4, 5]. His preparation was used
over decades in cancer treatment under the name of "COLEY's
toxin" or "COLEY's vaccine". Later in the forties, M. J. SHEAR
(Bethesda/USA) demonstrated that the tumor-hemorrhaging principle of Gram-negative bacteria, such as *Serratia marcescens*, is identical with their Endotoxin [6, 7]. Already in 1894 E. CENTANNI
(Bologna) had shown, that the endotoxic and pyrogenic principles
of bacteria cannot be separated; and this is why CENTANNI called
his extraction products "pirotoxina bacterica" [8]. As to the
history of the subject see the review by O. WESTPHAL *et al.* [9].

All efforts to develop a therapy of cancer by clinically applying
the tumor hemorrhage-producing principle of bacteria failed because
of the toxic components exerted by endotoxin. Thus, since the
times of M. J. SHEAR no further clinical trials have been unter-
taken so far.

During the last 25 years, endotoxin was extracted from many
bacteria, especially *Enterobacteriaceae*, highly purified and thoroughly analyzed. From these investigations we know that endotoxin is retained in the *lipopolysaccharide* which — in contrast to
typical bacterial *exotoxins* — is firmly bound to the outer bacterial
membrane (cell wall) [10]. In the lipopolysaccharide (LPS) the
polysaccharide carries the serological O- and R-specificities of the
species, while the lipid component — called *Lipid A* — is responsible for endotoxic activities, such as fever etc. [10]. Injection
of pure LPS into experimental animals (rabbits, dogs, horses —
and the same is true for man) causes quite a series of typical endotoxic reactions, a whole syndrome, and it was shown that even
pure lipid A, in high dispersion [11], will still exert *many* endotoxic manifestations, as shown in *Table I* [9, 12].

Criteria for the standardization of LPS (and lipid A) preparations are being developed [13], and with such reproducible and

[15] *O. Westphal, U. Westphal, Andreesen, Munder - p. 2*

TABLE I — *Typical Endotoxic Reactions given by Bacterial Lipo-polysaccharide and its Lipid A Component.*

Pyrogenicity	Activation of Macrophages
Leucopenia followed by Leucocytosis	
Immune Modulation	Induction of Colony-stimulating Factor (CSF)
Mitogenicity (for B Lymphocytes)	Induction of Prostaglandin Synthesis
Induction of IgG Synthesis in new-born Mice	Induction of Interferon Synthesis
Activation of Complement	Activation of Hagemann Factor
Plasminogen Activation	Induction of Endotoxin (pyrogenic) Tolerance
Non-Specific Resistance to Infections	Limulus Lysate Test (Geletion)
Induction of Tumor Necrosis *	

* There is a difference between the action of Lipopolysaccharide and Lipid A (see this article).

structurally well analyzed materials many biological activities are being investigated in detail [14]. These studies led also to a reinvestigation of the tumor-necrotizing activity of LPS, using the methylcholanthren-induced fibrosarcoma (Meth A tumor) of CBF_1 mice [15].

The tumor cells can be grown as ascites in CBA or CBF_1 mice. For therapeutic tests $1-5 \times 10^5$ Meth A tumor cells are injected intradermally; within 7-10 days a solid tumor develops to a size of about 7×7 mm. Generally, the 7th-10th day is the best time for the onset of treatment. With no treatment the tumor grows gradually to sizes of more than 20×20 mm, and eventually after 4-6 weeks all animals (controls) will die. Under normal laboratory conditions, i.p. injections of 10-100 µg of pure LPS (standard LPS of *Salmonella abortus equi*, Na^+ salt form [10, 13]) will cause hemorrhage of the tumor within 2-3 days followed by rejection of the hemorrhagic tumor mass and healing within another 7-10 days. Once the animals have undergone successful LPS treatment they can be shown to be fully resistant toward a secondary or third inoculation of the original or even greater number of Meth A tumor cells.

[15] *O. Westphal, U. Westphal, Andreesen, Munder* - p. 3

This transplantable Meth A tumor proved to be a good model for a general screening of several questions:

1) What is the relation of fever to tumor regression and hemorrhage?

2) Is acute toxicity necessarily related to the effect of LPS on tumors?

3) If not, can "heroic" (toxic) side effects of LPS tumor treatment be inhibited or reduced by any means?

These questions appeared reasonable after it was shown that many, if not all, endotoxic reactions are due to the stimulation and/or release of *endogenous mediators*. The pyrogenic action of LPS or lipid A in endotoxin-sensitive animals and man is, thus, mediated by an endogenous pyrogen, the so-called leukocyte or secondary pyrogen [16] which is released from granulocytes and macrophages. In more recent years it was shown that prosta-glandins of the E type mediate fever [17]. As to the action of endotoxin on various tumors the group of Lloyd OLD *et al.* at the Sloan-Kettering Institute for Cancer Research in New York found that in normal animals a "tumor-necrotizing factor" (TNF) will be released into the blood stream after high doses of endotoxin [18]. TNF release by LPS was found to be considerably enhanced in animals presensitized by BCG or *Corynebacterium parvum*. Sera rich in TNF proved to be nontoxic — indicating that TNF may be an endogenous mediator, induced by BCG or *C. Parvum* and re-leased by LPS.

In a big review L. DELMONTE [19] collected all data on the anti-tumor effects of endotoxin suggesting that the sensitivity of a given tumor (Meth A) to LPS — in other words: the dose by which 50 or 100 per cent of the tumor-bearing animals undergo hemorrhage and tumor rejection — depends on the relative sen-sitivity of the *host* to endotoxin. Thus, a Meth A tumor of C_3H. HeJ mice, an LPS-resistent mutant of C_3H [20], is also resistant to LPS treatment. It is known that the sensitivity of mice to the lethal effect of endotoxin very much depends on the actual environ-mental temperature [21]. The LD_{50} figures estimated at 10-15°C can be > 100 times higher as compared to those estimated at 30-

[15] O. *Westphal, U. Westphal, Andreesen, Munder* - p. 4

35°C. We, therefore, tested the LPS sensitivity of a standard Meth A tumor in groups of female CBF₁ mice which were kept at different environmental temperatures for about 12-16 hrs prior to LPS injection. *Table II* shows that "warm" mice reacted to considerably lower doses of LPS than "cold" ones.

This finding clearly indicates that the relative sensitivity of the animal is essential with regard to the *dose* of endotoxin that exerts tumor hemorrhage. However, it does not open new therapeutic possibilities.

The next series of experiments aimed at the question whether any of the typical endotoxic manifestations (comp. Table I) can be shown *not* to be involved in tumor necrosis and rejection. Years ago, E. EICHENBERGER [22] demonstrated that the activation of the fibrinolytic system by pure endotoxin (LPS) in man, which leads over a plasminogen activator as mediator [23], is not inhibited if antipyretic drugs are used to selectively reduce the fever

TABLE II — *LPS-Induced Necrosis of the Meth A Fibrosarcoma of CBF₁ Mice in Relation to Endotoxin Sensitivity of the Host.*

NUMBER OF MICE	DAY			LPS i.p. 8	CURED 23
	1	7-8			
10			20°C	10 µg	7/10
10	5×10⁵ Meth A Cells i.d.	Tumor Size: 0.6-0.8 cm ∅		1 µg	2/10
10			30°C	10 µg	10/10
10				1 µg	6/10
10				0.1 µg	2/10
10		20 or 30°C		— (Control)	0/10

[15] *O. Westphal, U. Westphal, Andreesen, Munder* - p. 5

response. Today we know that most antipyretic drugs are prostaglandin synthease inhibitors [24]. We, therefore, tried whether
such drugs influence the tumor action of LPS. For our studies we
used Indometacin, which is known as powerful antipyretic principle and clinically recommended in conditions of endotoxin shock.

It should be added that after the injection of LPS mice do not react with
fever (hyperthermia), but with *hypothermia* [25] which is inhibited also by
Indometacin.

Groups of female CBF₁ mice, 10 each, with standard Meth A
tumor of a size of about 7 × 7 mm, received 200 µg Indometacin
i.v. alone, 10 µg of LPS i.p. (*S. abortus equi* LPS, Na⁺ salt) alone,
and 200 µg Indometacin followed 1hr later by 10 µg LPS. A control group of the same tumor-bearing mice received only buffer
(PBS). The results are shown in *Table III*.

As can be seen, Indometacin not only does not interfere with
the tumor action of LPS, it even enhances its effect. Indometacin
alone has a slight effect on the Meth A tumor, but lower or higher
doses (up to 250-300 µg per mouse) will not show any more pronounced tumor effect. In similar experimental set ups we were

TABLE III — *Combined Action of Indometacin and LPS on the
   Meth A Fibrosarcoma of CBF₁ Mice.*

NUMBER OF MICE	DAY			CURED ANIMALS
	1	8	8	25
10	5×10⁵ Meth A Cells i.d.	Tumor Size: 0.6-0.8 cm ⊘	10 µg LPS i.p.	7/10
10			200 µg Indometacin i.v. 10 µg LPS i.p.	10/10
10			200 µg Indometacin i.v.	1/10
10			— (Control)	0/10

[15] O. *Westphal*, U. *Westphal*, *Andreesen*, *Munder* - p. 6

able to show that the dose of endotoxin (LPS), given after Indometacin, can be reduced, compared to LPS alone, to reach the same therapeutic result.

It is known that repeated injections of endotoxin into animals will cause *endotoxin tolerance* effects [26]. In our Institute, in cooperation with the group of D. W. WATSON in Minneapolis, it was demonstrated by E. Th. RIETSCHEL and Ch. GALANOS that pyrogenic tolerance is due to specific immune reactions against structures of the lipid A component of endotoxin [27]. The question, therefore, arose wether the action of LPS on the Meth A tumor would also be subject to tolerance after repeated LPS injections. I.p. injections of various LPS, lipid A, or chemical LPS derivatives were given to tumor-bearing animals in doses below the threshold of induction of tumor hemorrhage. Several days later an otherwise effective dose of LPS was injected i.p. It was found that various "endotoxic" preparations *conditioned* the animals in a way that the later challenge with LPS was very effective and at the same time generally *better tolerated* as the same LPS dose alone — as, for example, judged by following the loss of body weight of the animals after the relatively high doses of LPS. Non-pretreated Meth A-bearing animals will lose 12-18 per cent body weight and show rather severe diarrhea after 100 μg of LPS (i.p.), while the conditioned animals show weight losses between 3-8 per cent and no, or very mild diarrhea only. Two endotoxic preparations were found to be quite effective in conditioning the animals: Lipid A (triethylamine salt [11]) in doses of 1-10 μg; phthalylated LPS [28] (Na$^+$ salt) in doses of 10 μg i.p.

Lipid A, interestingly, differs from LPS in that it causes tumor *enhancement* over a wide dose range (1-100 μg i.p.); see Figure 1, but it conditions the animals favorably for the later LPS challenge. Phthalylated LPS is almost nontoxic and has little or no effect on the Meth A tumor in doses up to 500 μg i.p.; but 10 μg, given 3-5 days before 50-100 μg of LPS, condition the animals for better toleration of LPS with 100 per cent tumor hemorrhage and cure and almost no signs of untoward side effects (see Figure 2).

For the Meth A tumor system of CBF$_1$ mice we may conclude: (1) Mice react to LPS injections with a drop in body temperature

[15] *O. Westphal, U. Westphal, Andreesen, Munder* - p. 7

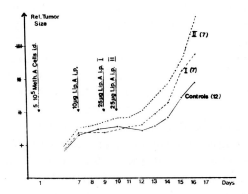

Fig. 1 — Effect of Lipid A i.p. on the Meth A Fibrosarcoma of CBF₁ Mice. 10 µg of Lipid A was given at day 7; 25 µg of Lipid A followed on day 9 (I) and day 10 (II) respectively.

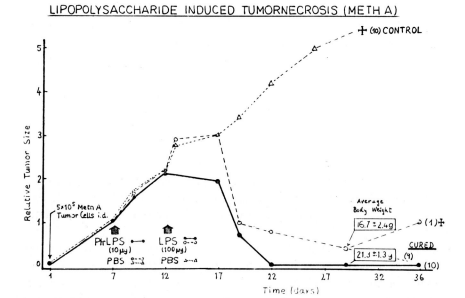

Fig. 2 — Lipopolysaccharide Induced Tumor Necrosis (Meth A) with and without Pretreatment of phthalylated LPS (10 µg i.p. at day 7) followed by 100 µg LPS on day 12.

[15] *O. Westphal, U. Westphal, Andreesen, Munder* - p. 8

(hypothermia), and this effect is counteracted by prostaglandin syn-
thetase inhibitors, such as Indometacin. (2) The acute toxicity of
bacterial endotoxin (LPS) can be discriminated from its Meth A
tumor-necrotizing activity by (a) suppressing acute LPS toxicity
with Indometacin, or (b) by conditioning the tumor-bearing animals
with either small amounts of lipid A or of LPS derivatives, such
as phthalylated LPS.

These observations offer new possibilities for a more sophisticated therapy of those tumors which are sensitive to endotoxin.
Clinical trials with dogs carrying authochtonic tumors are being set
up in cooperation with Drs. OETTGEN and HARDY of the Sloan-
Kettering Institute for Cancer Research, New York, to answer the
question wether our findings are applicable to species different from
mice. It may be recalled that dogs react to LPS with *hyper*thermia,
which can be inhibited by Indometacin.

At present the optimal treatment of Meth A sarcoma-bearing
mice consists of pretreating them at day (around) 6 to 8 with
1-10 μg of lipid A or 10 μg of phthalylated LPS i.p. followed 3 to
5 days later by a combination of 100-200 μg Indometacin (i.v.)
and, 1 hr later, 50-100 μg of the *S. abortus equi* LPS (Na^+ form)
i.p. Under these conditions, even tumors of bigger size — such
as 12 mm in diameter — will react favourably with almost no sub-
jective toxic side effects and in most instances with 100 per cent
cure.

Animals, treated in this way, can be challenged within 3-4
weeks with 5×10^5 or 10^6 Meth A cells without tumor growth.
This challenge can be repeated several times and with increasing
tumor load. In our Institute it was found that after several such
challenges peritoneal macrophages can be isolated from the animals
which are highly cytotoxic against Meth A tumor cells *in vitro* if
endotoxin is added to a co-culture of these cells [30]. Following
this observation, it was found by P. G. MUNDER and E. Th. RIET-
SCHEL [31] (see also [33]) that in such *in vitro* system pure LPS
is active in quantities as low as 1-10 picograms/ml (see Figure 3)!

This finding also offers the possibility of elaborating a new
sensitive test for endotoxin (LPS).

It is known that *macrophages* are the source of many mediators of endotoxin action, such as endogenous pyrogen, prostaglan-

[15] *O. Westphal, U. Westphal, Andreesen, Munder* - p. 9

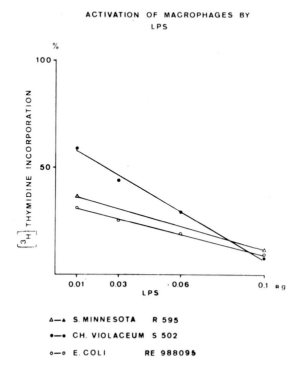

FIG. 3 — *Activation of macrophages by LPS*. 10-12 day old bone marrow macrophages, cultivated as described (see Figure 7), were incubated with Meth A sarcoma cells in a ratio of 5 : 1 in the presense of lipopolysaccharides (LPS). 24 hours later the tumor cells were filled into microtiter wells in quadruplicate and pulsed with [³H] thymidine for 3 hours. The results are epressed as the percentage of thymidine incorporation as compared to the control culture containing only macrophages and Meth A sarcoma cells.

dins, colony-stimulating factor (CSF) and probably also the tumor-necrotizing factor (TNF). In C₃H-HeJ mice, bearing a Meth A tumor, which are insensitive to endotoxin, tumor hemorrhage can be restored by infusing macrophages from endotoxin-*sensitive* lines of C₃H mice, indicating that the defect in C₃H-HeJ mice is on the macrophage level [20, 32]. Recent publications by J. H. HIBBS *et al*. [33] have shown that macrophages and their state of activation play a crucial role in the microenvironment of the tumor during LPS-induced tumor necrosis.

[15] *O. Westphal, U. Westphal, Andreesen, Munder* - p. 10

We are following at present the concept that the local production of mediators by macrophages in the vicinity of a solid tumor (Meth A) can be *selectively* influenced *pharmacologically* (Indometacin etc.) and/or *by conditioning* the animals (pretreatment with phthalylated LPS etc.). Using our test system, we are screening various types of immune modulators for their ability to act as TNF "inducer", including also synthetic lysolecithin analogues (see following chapter).

In this context it may well be that BCG or *C. parvum* pretreatment of animals for optimal production of TNF by endotoxin [18] might be replaced by TNF "inducers", like phthalylated LPS, which only sensitize the animal for local TNF production, but at the same time induce tolerance to toxic side effects. We feel that by further following these aspects new interest in tumor therapy with bacterial endotoxin may arise.

Lysolecithin Analogues

The fact, that many immunopotentiators like the above mentioned BCG or *C. parvum* are phagocytozed by macrophages and lead, if given systematically, to a remarkable increase in the host defense mechanisms against bacterial infections as well as tumors, prompted an extensive biochemical study in which the metabolism of these host defense cells was studied in the presence of immunopotentiators [34, 35, 36].

The most significant finding was that almost all of the immunopotentiators, like complete Freund's adjuvant, BCG, *C. parvum*, silica and others, are able to activate a phospholipase A in macrophages which degrades 3-sn-phosphatidylcholine and 3-sn-phosphatidylethanolamine to the corresponding lyso-compounds [36].

This finding led to the question whether the continuous endogeneous formation of lyso-compounds in granulomas induced by the immunopotentiators might be one of the common denominators to explain how substances which have chemically nothing in common may exert such a profound effect on host defense mechanisms. Lysophosphatidylcholine then should act as a adjuvant itself. This has indeed been found to be true: it increases or modulates the humoral and the cellular immune response [37]. Due to the fact that lysophosphatidylcholine — a highly surface-active natural principle — is rapidly metabolized by at least two so called "safety enzymes" [38] it was decided to synthesize lysophosphatidylcholine analogues which have almost identical physico-chemical characteristics but are not as easily metabolized as the physiologically occurring parent substance. Several modifications have been substantiated. So far the biological activity of two such chemical variations have been studied: the replacement of the acyl-bond in sn-1 of the glycerol backbone by an alkyl bond and the substitution of the OH group in sn-2 of this molecule. The following three compounds were hitherto found to be the most effective ones in stimulating the immune response *in vivo* and *in vitro*:

Racemic 1-Octadecyl-2-methyl-glycero-3-phosphocholine (ET-18-OCH₃);

Racemic 1-Octadecyl-glycero-3-phosphocholine (ET-18-OH), and

1-Octadecyl-propanediol-3-phosphocholine (ET-18-H).

When we studied the effect of these alkyl-lysophospholipids on the immune system, a surprising observation was made. These compounds do not only stimulate or modulate humoral or cellular immune responses, they also have a remarkable anti-tumor effect *in vivo*, as demonstrated in several tumor models of mouse and rat [37, 39]. The most extensively investigated model was the Meth A sarcoma in CBF_1 mice (Fig. 4 and Table IV).

Figure 4 demonstrates the therapeutic effect of ET-18-OH when given daily i.v.

From Table V it can be seen that ET-18-OCH₃ is also effective by *oral* application. Provided that not more than 2×10^5 tumor cells were injected, significant retardation or even complete inhibition of tumor growth and regression can be observed. Concentrations as low as 50 µg/mouse/day were found to be effective as can be seen from Table V. In contrast, natural lysophosphatidylcholine and synthetic 1-Acyl-compounds were ineffective.

In similar experiments concentrations as low as 5 — 10 µg/mouse/day showed a significant retardation of tumor growth. A

[15] *O. Westphal, U. Westphal, Andreesen, Munder* - p. 12

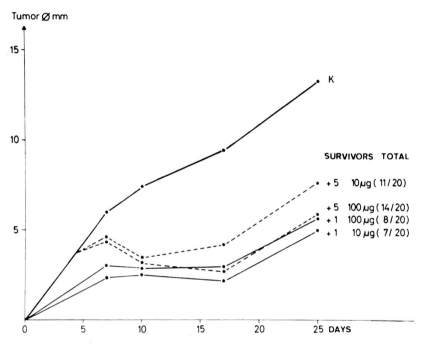

THE INFLUENCE OF ET-18-OH ON THE SUBCUTANEOUS GROWTH OF METH-A SARCOMA

(I.V. APPLICATION)

FIG. 4 — *The influence of ET-18-OH on the subcutaneous growth of Meth A sarcoma (i.v. application).* 10^5 Meth A sarcoma cells were injected i.c. in (Balb/c × C57Bl/6)F₁ female mice. 1 or 5 days later 10 or 100 µg of ET-18-OH were injected i.v. in 0.2 ml PBS. The control mice received only PBS. Tumor growth was determined by measuring 2 diameters in each animal twice a week. The animals were observed up to 8 weeks after the primary tumor transplantation.

direct cytotoxic action on tumor cells by alkyl-lysophospholipid appeared rather unlikely, although, some accumulation of the alkyl-lysophospholipids was found in the tumor tissue [40]. Therefore, we looked for an amplifying cellular mechanism. A first indication that macrophages might be the activated cell type came from studies in which alkyl-lysophospholipids were injected intraperitoneally. Four days later 10^4 cells of a highly malignant subline of Ehrlich ascites tumor was injected i.p. The pretreatment by alkyl-lysophospholipids resulted in a complete protection of the animals

TABLE IV — *Tumor Growth Inhibition in vitro by Alkyl-lysophos-phatidyl-activated Macrophages.*

LLA	DAY −4	DAY −1	−6 HRS
1.0 mg	17 *	50	116
0.5 mg	2	29	110
0.25 mg	0	74	129
0.05 mg	31	117	105
CONTROL	100	100	100

* Growth inhibition as compared to inhibition by normal macrophages — measured by 3_H thymidine incorporation.

TABLE V — *Growth * of 10^5 Meth A Sarcoma Cells i.d. in (Balb/c × C 57/Bl/(6)F₁ Mice during oral Treatment with Lysoleci-thin and Synthetic Analogues.***

	DAYS				SURVIVORS/
	7	14	21	28	TOTAL
CONTROL	4.0	11.1	26.3	133.2	0/10
LYSOLECITHIN	3.4	5.1	15.4	83.5	0/10
ET-12-H	0.9	1.6	3.8	24.5	6/10
ET-18-OCH₃	1.0	0.9	1.04	6.0	7/10

* Total tumor volume in 10 mice (group) in cm^3.
** 0.05 mg/mouse were given daily for 15 days.

[15] O. Westphal, U. Westphal, Andreesen, Munder - p. 14

lasting for more than 30 days during which the tumor load could be raised 10,000-fold.

When peritoneal cells were collected from alkyl-lysophospholipid-treated mice and incubated with Meth A sarcoma cells in a syngeneic situation, tumor growth was almost completely inhibited as shown in Table IV.

Thus, alkyl-lysophospholipids induce in the peritoneal cavity a highly tumorcidal population of cells. When macrophages were removed from this population by appropriate techniques (iron-magnet-treatment, adherence techniques) the tumorcidal capacity of the peritoneal cells was abolished.

We then studied whether normal peritoneal cells can be activated after *in vitro* incubation with alkyl-lysophospholipids together with Meth A sarcoma cell as target. As shown in Table VI, normal peritoneal macrophages are unable to kill Meth A sarcoma cells. When ET-18-OCH$_3$ was added in sublytic amounts a dose-dependent increase in tumorcidal capacity of these normal cells could be elicited. 2-Lysophosphatidylcholine (natural lysolecithin) had no activating effect.

These experiments, however, did not rule out the possibility that the application of alkyl-lysophospholipids would liberate mediators from the admixed peritoneal lymphocytes which in turn would activate macrophages. This could be excluded when bone marrow macrophages were incubated with alkyl-lysophospholipids. 12-14 Day old bone marrow macrophages cultured *in vitro*, and free of T and B lymphocytes and granulocytes can be activated by alkyl-lysophospholipids to a highly significant degree as shown in Fig. 5.

Although the effect is most pronounced when the alkyl-lysophospholipids are present during the effector-target cell interaction, both cell types can also be incubated separately, washed and then co-cultured again. Under such condition a significant increase in tumorcidal capacity of pure bone marrow macrophages could still be observed.

Figure 5 demonstrates also a slight inhibition of tumor cell proliferation by the alkyl-lysophospholipid alone. We have studied this phenomenon in more detail. Indeed, it was found that many established murine tumor cell lines are more or less sensitive to a slow, progressive cellular destruction by alkyl-lysophospholipids.

[15] O. Westphal, U. Westphal, Andreesen, Munder - p. 15

TABLE VI — *In vitro activation of normal peritoneal macrophages by alkyl-lysophospholipids.*

LYSOPHOSPHOLIPID	μg/ml	% ^{3}H-THYMIDINE UPTAKE OF METH A SARCOMA CELLS AFTER	
		24 HOURS	48 HOURS
- - - - - - - -	- -	99	108
LYSOPHOSPHATIDYL	10	102 ± 13	101 ± 12
CHOLINE	5	98 ± 11	97 ± 12
	3	107 ± 16	101 ± 10
ET-12-H	20	92 ± 8	65 ± 7
	10	80 ± 24	106 ± 23
	5	110 ± 16	127 ± 27
ET-18-OCH₃	5	32 ± 13	16 ± 7
	3	43 ± 8	39 ± 13
	2	67 ± 14	54 ± 16

Peritoneal macrophages were collected from the peritoneal cavity of CBF_1 mice and incubated in a ratio of 2.5 : 1 macrophages : Meth A sarcoma cells in the presence of lysophospholipids.
Final volume: 5 ml Dulbecco's modified Eagle's medium + 10% fetal calf serum. The thymidine incorporation of the Meth A sarcoma cells was measured in quadruplicate, cultured in microtiter plates.

This direct cytotoxic effect of alkyl-lysophospholipids on tumor cells has nothing to do with the surface activity of these substances but is rather due to an anti-metabolic effect affecting specifically neoplastic cells.

Together with our colleagues at the Medical Department of the University Hospital of Freiburg (Prof. Dr. G. Löhr) more than 80 different human leukemias have been found to be sensitive. As shown in Figure 6 the proliferation of human leukemic cells is strongly inhibited by alkyl-lysophospholipids. ET-18-OH which can be acylated to 1-alkyl-2-acyl-phosphatidylcholine has no cytotoxic effect [41].

[15] *O. Westphal, U. Westphal, Andreesen, Munder* - p. 16

IN VITRO ACTIVATION OF BONE MARROW MACROPHAGES

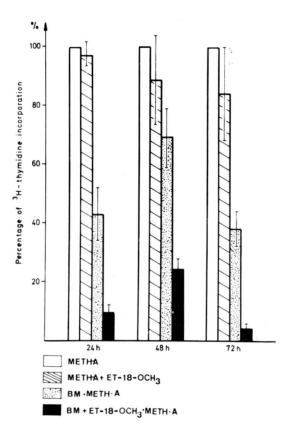

FIG. 5 — *In vitro activation of bone marrow macrophages.* Bone marrow macrophages of $(Balb/c \times C57Bl/6)F_1$ female mice were cultivated in Dulbecco's modified Eagle's medium + 10% fetal calf serum (FCS) + 30% conditioned medium obtained from the supernatant of L929 fibroblasts. 2×10^6 bone marrow cells were filled into 100 ml culture bags made from Teflon. After 10-12 days $10-15 \times 10^7$ pure macrophages can be collected. The bone marrow macrophages were washed and incubated with syngeneic Meth A sarcoma cells in a ratio of macrophages: tumor cells of 2.5 : 1 in the presence or absence of the alkyl-lysophospholipid ET-18-OCH₃ (5 μg/ml). The cells were cultivated in a final volume of 5 ml and every day 1 ml cell suspension was withdrawn, filled in quadruplicate into microtiter plates and pulsed for 6 hours with [³H] thymidine and then collected with a multisample harvester on glass fiber filters. Afterwards the radioactivity was counted in a scintillation counter. In addition, the number of trypan blue positive tumor cells was counted and found to be in close parallel to the decrease of [³H] thymidine incorporation.

[15] *O. Westphal, U. Westphal, Andreesen, Munder* - p. 17

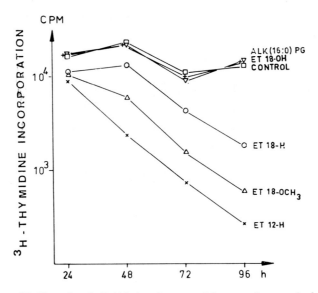

Fɪɢ. 6 — *Alkyl-lysophospholipid-induced cytotoxicity on human leukemic cells.*
The cells from a patient with a chronic myelocytic leukemia were freshly collected
and separated over a Ficoll gradient, removing granulocytes and erythrocytes. The
remaining leukemic cells were incubated with the indicated alkyl-lysophospholipid
in a concentration of 5 µg/ml/1×10⁶ leukemic cells. The cell suspensions were
incubated in microtiter plates in a final volume of 0.2 ml and pulsed for 24 hours
on 4 consecutive days.

Other tumors, like glioblastoma and ovarian carcinoma, are
presently under study and were found to be sensitive to most of
the alkyl-lysophospholipids tested. The only exception we encountered so far are melanomas. Table VII summarizes our results.

Alkyl-lysophospholipids then activate macrophages for tumor
killing and at the same time induce a slow progressive tumor cell
destruction. These two biological manifestations could be explained by experiments shown in Figure 7.

The proliferating tumor cells (Meth A sarcoma) adsorb much
more alkyl-lysophospholipids than peritoneal cells (PC). On the
other hand, peritoneal cells metabolize alkyl-lysophospholipids with
increasing rate by an activated enzyme system whereas the tumor
cells appear to be unable to do so. Normal cells have a 1-O-alkyl-

[15] *O. Westphal, U. Westphal, Andreesen, Munder* - p. 18

TABLE VII — *Sensitivity of human neoplastic cells to alkyl-lyso-phospholipid induced cell destruction.*

CELLS	SOURCE	24 H [³H] THYMIDINE UPTAKE AFTER 2 DAYS IN CULTURE		
		CPM	% OF THE CONTROL ET-12-H	ET-18-OCH³
I. *Leukemias*				
AML	Blood	14,000	1	3
AMML	Blood	35,000	9	7
ALL	Blood	3,500	2	56
ALL Established Line (ALL-20)		93,000	1	2
ALL-Childhood Leukemia	Blood	4,600	3	1
AUL-Relapse	Blood	23,200	1	3
AUL-Remission	Blood	3,300	3	6
Smoldering Leukemia	Blood	19,000	10	10
CGL	Blood	31,000	78	4
	Bone Marrow	24,400	12	4
CGL-Acute Blastic Crisis	Blood	32,000	1	1
CLL	Blood	1,400*	4	6
	Lymph Node	1,700	2	3
II. Centrocytic Lymphoma	Blood	1,050	3	2
Immunoblastic Lymphoma	Blood	1,500	8	25
	Lymph Node	36,000	1	5
Multiple Myeloma	Bone Marrow	5,900	10	6
Polycythemia Vera	Blood	1,100	7	30
EBV-Transformed Lymphoblastoid Cells		40,800	8	15
III. Glioblastoma	Tissue Specimen	5,600	n.t.	1
Long Term Culture **		1,200	n.t.	100
Ovarian Carcinoma	Pleural Effusion	1,140	27	48
Long Term Culture **		22,000	31	73
Malignant Melanoma	Lymph Node	7,300	82	100
Established Line (EI)		41,000	n.t.	100
HELA		60,000	100	100

Abbreviations:

AML	acute myelocytic leukemia
AMML	acute monocytic myelocytic leukemia
ALL	acute lymphocytic leukemia
AUL	acute undifferentiated leukemia
CLL	chronic lymphocytic leukemia
CGL	chronic granulocytic leukemia

* ³H-Uridine Uptake.
** More than 4 weeks in culture.

[15] O. Westphal U. Westphal, Andreesen, Munder - p. 19

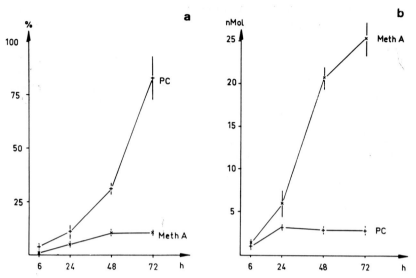

Fig. 7 — *Adsorption and cleavage of* [³H]-ET-18-OCH₃ *by peritoneal cells* (PC) *and Meth A sarcoma cells* (*Meth A*). 1×10⁵ peritoneal or Meth A sarcoma were incubated with 25 nmol [³H] ET-18-OCH₃ in a final column of 5 ml in Dulbecco's modified Eagle's medium in the presence of 10% fetal calf serum. At the time indicated 1 ml of the cell suspension was centrifuged and the radioactivity determined in the supernatant or in the cells. Diagram (a): After separation and washing of the cells the phospholipids of the cells were extracted and separated by thin layer chromatography. The separated phospholipid and lipid Scraped off into scintillation vials shaking for 48 hours and after the addition of appropriate scintillation cocktail the radioactivity measured in a scintillation counter. Diagram (b) gives percentage of adsorption of the [³H] ET-18-OCH₃ by the two cell types.

cleavage enzyme [42] which can apparently be activated by its complementary substrate. Many tumor cells do not display this enzymatic activity [43, 44]. Taking into account that tumor cells have a rather high content of alkyl-lipids [43] due to the absence or low level of the 1-O-cleavage enzyme, our findings can be summarized by the following concept: The addition of alkyl-lysophospholipids seems to activate the O-alkyl-cleavage enzyme in host defense cells, like macrophages. This activated enzyme system will attack alkyl-lipids in the tumor cell membrane after both cell types have come into close contact. On the other hand, if tumor cells

[15] *O. Westphal, U. Westphal, Andreeseń, Munder* - p. 20

are incubated with alkyl-lysophospholipids they accumulate these surface active compounds, as there is no enzyme for their immediate degradation.

Recent biochemical studies in our laboratory have shown that alkyl-lysophospholipids act as specific anti-metabolites of the phospholipid metabolism in tumor cells. They inhibit the de-novo-synthesis of phospholipids and also interfere with the acylating-deacylating Lands pathway of phospholipid metabolism [45]. The resulting severe alteration in the dynamic structure of the lipid bilayer of the plasma membrane may lead to a break-down of the permeability barrier in sensitive cells. In addition, changes in the lipid composition near the plasma membrane bound enzymes may occur. The activity of these enzymes has been shown to depend on this lipid "microenvironment" [46, 47, 48, 49, 50]. It is, therefore, conceivable that an alkyl-lysophospholipid-predamaged neoplastic cell will be of considerably higher sensitivity to activated, and even normal macrophages. We are following this concept in our present studies [51-55].

[15] O. Westphal, U. Westphal, Andreesen, Munder - p. 21

REFERENCES

[1] DE LISLE DUPRE, *Traité du Vice cancereux*. Couturiers Fils, Paris (1774).

[2] MAGENDIE F., *Remarques sur la notice précédente (de Dupre) avec quelques expériences sur les effets des substances en putréfaction et putrides, sur la vaccine etc.* « J. Physiol. (Paris) », *3*, 81-88 (1823).

[3] FEHLEISEN F., *Über die Züchtung der Erysipel-Kokken auf künstlichen Nährböden und die Übertragbarkeit auf den Menschen.* « Deutsch. Med. Wochenschr. », *8*, 553 (1882). For review see H. LEHNHARTZ: *Erysipel, die septischen Erkrankungen*, in H. NOTHNAGEL (edit.) Spezielle Pathologie und Therapie III, 2/1, pg. 1-78, H. HOLDER, Vienna (1903).

[4] COLEY W.B., *The treatment of malignant tumors by repeated inoculations of Erysipelas; with a report of original cases.* « Am. J. Med. Sci. », *105*, 487-511 (1893). COLEY W.B., *The treatment of inoperable sarcoma with the mixed toxins of Erysipelas and Bacillus prodigiosus.* « J. Am. Med. Assoc. », *31*, 389-95 (1898).

[5] COLEY W.B., *The treatment of inoperable sarcoma by bacterial toxins.* « Proc. Roy. Soc. Med. London », *1909*, 1-48.

[6] SHEAR M.J. and TURNER F.C., *Chemical treatment of tumors. V. Isolation of the hemorrhage-producing fraction from Serratia marcescens (Bac. prodigiosus) culture filtrates.* « J. Natl. Cancer Inst. », *4*, 81-97 (1943).

[7] HARTWELL J.L., SHEAR M.J. and ADAMS J.R., *VII. Nature of the hemorrhage-producing fraction from Serratia marcescens (Bac. prodigiosus) culture filtrates.* « J. Natl. Cancer Inst. », *4*, 107-22 (1943).

[8] CENTANNI E., *Untersuchungen über das Infektionsfieber - Das Fiebergift der Bakterien.* « Deutsch. Med. Wschr. », *20*, 148 (1894).

[9] WESTPHAL O., WESTPHAL U. and SOMMER T., *The History of Pyrogen Research.* « Microbiology », *1977*, 221-238. Am. Soc. Microbiol., Washington (1977).

[10] GALANOS CH., LÜDERITZ O., RIETSCHEL E. TH. and WESTPHAL O., *Newer aspects of the Chemistry and Biology of bacterial lipopolysaccharides, with special reference to their lipid A component.* « Biochemistry of Lipids II », Vol. *14*, 238-336, University Park Press, Baltimore - London - Tokyo (1977).

[11] GALANOS CH. and LÜDERITZ O., *Electrodialysis of lipopolysaccharides and their conversion to uniform salt forms.* « Europ. J. Biochem. », *54*, 603-10 (1975). See also GALANOS CH. and LÜDERITZ O., *The role of the physical state of lipopolysaccharides in the interaction with complement.* « Europ. J. Biochem. », *65*, 403-08 (1976).

[12] WESTPHAL O., *Bacterial Endotoxin. The 2nd Carl Prausnitz Memorial Lecture, Copenhagen 1974.* « Int. Arch. Allergy appl. Immunol. », *49*, 1-43 (1975).

[15] *O. Westphal, U. Westphal, Andreesen, Munder* - p. 22

[13] GALANOS CH., LÜDERITZ O. and WESTPHAL O., *Preparation and properties of a standardized lipopolysaccharide from* Salmonella abortus equi *(Novo-Pyrexal).* « Zbl. Bakt. I Orig. », (1978), in press.

[14] Chapter IV - *Bacterial Antigens and Host Response.* I. *Endotoxins and other cell wall components of Gramnegative bacteria and their biological activities.* « Microbiology », 1977, 239-297. - II. *Genetic and cellular aspects of host response to endotoxin.* « Microbiology », 1977, 298-329.

[15] The tumor line was introduced by Dr. LLOYD OLD *et al.* at the Sloan-Kettering Institute for Cancer Research, New York.

[16] ATKINS E., *Pathogenesis of Fever.* « Physiol. Rev. », 40, 580-646 (1960). - DINARELLI C.A., GORDIN N.P. and WOLFF S.M., *Demonstration and characterization of two distinct human leukocytic pyrogens.* « J. Exp. Med. », 139, 1369-81 (1974).

[17] FELDBERG W., *Body temperature and fever: Changes in our views during the last decade* (The Ferrier Lecture 1974). « Proc. Roy. Soc. London B », 191, 199-229 (1975).

[18] CARSWELL E.A., OLD L.J., KASSEL R.L., GREEN S., FIORE N. and WILLIAMSON B., *An endotoxin-induced serum factor that causes necrosis of tumors.* « Proc. Natl. Acad. Sci. (USA) », 72, 3666-670 (1975). - GREEN S., DOBRJANSKY A., CARSWELL E.A., KASSEL R.L., OLD L.J., FIORE N. and SCHWARTZ M.K., *Partial purification of a serum factor that causes necrosis in tumors.* « Proc. Natl. Acad. Sci. (USA) », 73, 381-85 (1976).

[19] DELMONTE L. (Sloan-Kettering Institute for Cancer Research, New York): *Antitumor effects of endotoxin - a review.* In press (1978).

[20] SULTZER B.M., *Genetic control of host responses to endotoxin.* « Infect. Immun. », 5, 107-113 (1972). - SULTZER B.M. and GOODMAN G.W., *Characteristics of endotoxin-resistant low-responder mice.* « Microbiology », 1977, 304-09.

[21] KASS E.H., ATWOOD R. and PORTER P.J., *Observations on the locus of lethal actions of bacterial endotoxin.* In Bacterial Endotoxins (ed. by M. Landy and W. Braun), New Brunswick, Rutgers Institute of Microbiology, 1964, 596-601. - ATWOOD R.P. and KASS E.H., *Relationship of body temperature to the lethal action of bacterial endotoxin.* « J. Clin. Invest. », 43, 151-54 (1964).

[22] EICHENBERGER E., *Fibrinolyse nach intravenöser Injektion bakterieller Pyrogene.* « Acta Neurovegetativa », 11, 201-06 (1955). - EICHENBERGER E. et al., *Effets biologiques d'un pyrogène rigoureusement purifié (lipopolysaccharide) provenant de* Salmonella abortus equi. « J. Suisse Med. », 85, 1190, 1213 (especially the chapter: Influence sur la coagulation du sang) (1955).

[23] UNGAR G., *Biochemical mechanisms of the allergic reaction (Review).* « Int. Arch. Allergy appl. Immunol. », 4, 258-81 (1953). - DEUTSCH E. and ELSNER P., *The mechanism of fibrinolysis induced by bacterial pyrogens.* « Thromb. Diath. haem. », 3, 286-96 (1959).

[24] VANE J.R., *Inhibitors of prostaglandin, prostacyclin, and thromboxane synthesis, in Advances in Prostaglandin and Thromboxane Research* (ed. by COCEANI F. and OLLEY P.M.) Vol. 4, 27-44 (1978).

[15] *O. Westphal, U. Westphal, Andreesen, Munder* - p. 23

[25] GREER G. GORDON and RIETSCHEL E. TH., *Lipid A-induced tolerance and hyperreactivity to hypothermia in mice*. « Infect. Immun. », *19*, 357-68 (1978). - *Inverse relationship between the susceptibility of lipopolysaccharide (lipid A)-pretreated mice to the hypothermic and lethal effect of lipopolysaccharide*. « Infect. Immun. », *20*, 366-74 (1978).

[26] BEESON P.B., *Development of tolerance to typhoid bacterial pyrogen and its addition to reticulo-endothelial blockade*. « Proc. Soc. exp. Biol. Med. », *61*, 248-50 (1946).

[27] RIETSCHEL E. TH. and GALANOS CH., *Lipid A antiserum-mediated protection against lipopolysaccharide and lipid A-induced fever and skin necrosis*. « Infect. Immun. », *15*, 34-49 (1977).

[28] MCINTIRE F.C., HARGIE M.P., SCHENCK J.R., FINLEY R.A., SIEBERT H.W., RIETSCHEL E. TH. and ROSENSTREICH D.L., *Biologic properties of nontoxic derivatives of a lipopolysaccharide from* Escherichia coli K 235. « J. Immunol. », *117*, 674-78 (1976).

[29] TASKOV H. and LOHMANN-MATTHES M.L., in preparation (1978).

[30] FISCHER H., LOHMANN-MATTHES M.L. and RITTER J., *The amplification of specific macrophage cytotoxicity by nonspecific stimulants*. In: Activation of Macrophages, Workshop Conferences Hoechst, Vol. *2*, 318-22 (1974).

[31] MUNDER P.G., PAHLKE and RIETSCHEL E. TH., in preparation (1978).

[32] ROSENSTREICH D.L., GLODE L.M., WAHL L.M., SANDBERG A.L. and MERGENHAGEN S.E., *Analysis of the cellular defects of endotoxin-unresponsive C3H-HeJ mice*. « Microbiology », *1977*, 314-20, especially pg. 319.

[33] HIBBS J.H., TAINTOR R.R., CHAPMAN H.A. and WEINBERG J.B., *Macrophage tumor killing: Influence of the local environment*. « Science », *197*, 279-282 (1977).

[34] MUNDER P.G., FERBER E., MODOLELL M. and FISCHER H., *The influence of various adjuvants on the metabolism of phospholipids in macrophages*. « Int. Arch. Allergy », *36*, 117-128 (1969).

[35] MUNDER P.G., MODOLELL M., FERBER E. and FISCHER H., *The relationship between macrophages and adjuvant activity*. In: Mononuclear phagocytes, R. van Furth (Ed.), pp. 445-460, Blackwell Scientific Publications, Oxford and Edinburgh, 1970.

[36] MUNDER P.G. and MODOLELL M., *The influence of Mycobacterium bovis and Corynebacterium parvum on the phospholipid metabolism of macrophages*. « Recent Results in Cancer Research », *47*, 244-250 (1974).

[37] MUNDER P.G., WELTZIEN H.U. and MODOLELL M., *Lysolecithin Analogs: a new class of immunopotentiators*. In: Immunopathology VII. Int. Symposium, P.A. Miescher, (ed.) pp. 411-424, Schwabe & Co. Publishers, Basel/Stuttgart, 1976.

[38] MULDER E., and VAN DEENEN L.L.M., *Metabolism of red cell lipids*. III. *Pathways for phospholipid renewal*. « Biochim et Biophys. Acta », *106*, 348-356 (1965).

[39] MUNDER P.G., FISCHER H., WELTZIEN H.U., OETTGEN H.F. and WESTPHAL O., *Lysolecithin analogs: a new class of immunopotentiators with anti-tumor activity*. « Proc. Am. Assoc. Cancer Res. », *17*, 174 (1976).

[15] *O. Westphal, U. Westphal, Andreesen, Munder* - p. 24

[40] ARNOLD B., REUTHER R. and WELTZIEN H.U., *Distribution and Metabolism of synthetic lysophosphatidylcholine analogs in mice.* « Biochim et Biophys. Acta », in press (1978).

[41] ANDREESEN R., MODOLELL M., WELTZIEN H.U., EIBL H., COMMON H.H., LÖHR G.W. and MUNDER P.G., *Selective destruction of human leukemic cells by alkyl-lysophospholipids.* « Cancer Research », 38, 3894-3899 (1978).

[42] PFLEGER R.C., PIANTADOSI C. and SNYDER F., *The biocleavage of isomeric glyceryl ethers by soluble liver enzymes in a variety of species.* « Biochim. et Biophys. Acta », 144, 633-648 (1967).

[43] SNYDER F., *Ether-linked lipids and fatty alcohol precursors in neoplasma.* In: Snyder, F. (ed.) Ether Lipids, Chemistry and Biology, pp. 273-296, Academic Press, New York/London, 1972.

[44] SOODSMA J.F., PIANTADOSI C. and SNYDER F., *The biocleavage of alkyl glyceryl ethers in Morris hepatomas and other transplantable neoplasms.* « Cancer Res. », 30, 309-311 (1970).

[45] VAN DEN BOSCH H., *Phosphoglyceride metabolism.* In: Annual review of biochemistry, 43, 243-277, E. Snell, P.D. Boyes, A. Meister and C.C. Richardson (eds.), Annual Rev. Inc. Palo Alto, 1974.

[46] HUNG St. C. and MELNYKOVYCH G., *Increase in activity of partially purified alkaline phosphatase after treatment with Mg^{2+}, Zn^{2+} and lysolecithin,* « Enzyme », 22, 28-34 (1977).

[47] HUNG St. C. and MELNYKOVICH G., *Alkaline phosphatase in HeLa cells. Stimulation by phospholipase A_2 and lysophosphatidylcholine.* « Biochim. et Biophys. Acta », 429, 409-420 (1976).

[48] O' DOHERTY P.J.A., *Steric requirements for the stimulation of glycosyltransrerase activity by lysophosphatidylcholine.* « Reprinted form Lipids », 13, 297-300 (1978).

[49] ZWILLER J., CIESIELSKI-TRESKA J. and MANDEL P., *Effect of lysolecithin on guanylate and adenylate cyclase activities in neuroblastoma cells in Culture.* « FEBS Letters », 69, 286-290 (1976).

[50] DUPPEL W. and ULLRICH V., *Membrane effects on drug monooxygenation activity in hepatic microsomes.* « Biochim. et Biophys. Acta », 426, 399-497 (1976).

[51] TARNOWSKI G.S., MOUNTAIN I.M., CHESTER STOCK C., MUNDER P.G., WELTZIEN H.U. and WESTPHAL O., *Effect of lysolecithin and analogs on mouse ascites tumors.* « Cancer Res. », 38, 339-344 (1978).

[52] MUNDER P.G., JANSEN A., ANDREESEN R. and MODOLELL M., *Synthetic lysophosphatides as inducers of macrophage cytotoxicity.* Proceedings of the XII. Int. Cancer Congress, Buenos Aires, Vol. 1, p. 166, (1978).

[53] ANDREESEN R., MODOLELL M., COMMON H.H. and MUNDER P.G., *Parameters influencing leukemic cell destruction by alkyl-lysophospholipids.* Cancer Research, submitted for publication, 1978.

[54] MODOLELL M., ANDREESEN R., BRUGGER U. and MUNDER P.G., *Disturbance of phospholipid metabolism during the selective destruction of tumor cells induced by alkyl-lysophospholipids.* Cancer Research submitted for publication, 1978.

[55] ANDREESEN R., OEPKE G., RUNGE M., MUNDER P.G., *Sensitivity of various human neoplastic cells to alkyl-lysophospholipid induced cell destruction.* In preparation.

DISCUSSION

CLERICI

Dr. Westphal, I would like you to clarify one point for me. Salmonellae can be serologically classified following the Kaufmann-White scheme and then they can be reclassified according to 16 (or more) chemiotypes. The first chemiotype is the simplest one, because it corresponds to the R_I or R_{II} structure of Salmonellae. I did not understand clearly whether the polysaccharides you are talking about correspond to the first chemiotype, plus the lipid moiety, or only to the lipid moiety plus the KDO terminus. If the second case is the correct one, how do you split the hexosophosphates chain from the KDO terminus? This is my first question.

And now my second question. The European snake's venom is a lysolecithinase. If somebody is bitten by a snake, the enzyme removes one fatty acid residue from lecythine of red cell membranes, so that a dramatic hemolitic anemia is produced. I was wondering whether you could incubate *in vitro* macrophages with snake's venom so that compounds similar to lysophosphatide analogues would be created inside the cells, instead of accumulating from outside, as you suggested in order to explain the increased killing capacity for tumor cells of macrophages from mice treated with synthetic lysophosphatide analogues.

WESTPHAL

When you speak of *in vitro* experiments, this has not been done, but could be done. But I think this would rather be a step backwards. Firstly, it is rather difficult to control the enzymatic activity of phospholipase A_1 or A_2 if added to a macrophage culture. Degradation of cellular phospholipids by these enzymes will lead to cell destruction. Secondly, as macrophages have no 1-alkyl-2-acyl-phospholipid, the enzymatic degradation by phospholipase A_2 does not lead to alkyl-lyso-phospholipids which would activate macrophages *in vitro* and *in vivo*.

WEISS

As you know, Dr. Westphal, we have been testing in our laboratories for the past 18 months a number of the lysolecithin and endotoxin compounds which you sent us, for effects on macrophage functions. The agents are administered to mice, and their peritoneal, and other, macrophages derived subsequently are tested *in vitro* for a variety of enzymatic, phagocytic, and antibacterial activities. So far, none of the materials which we have examined has appreciable potentiating action on lysozomal hydrolytic enzyme activity. On the other hand, some of the compounds do heighten macrophage phagocytic and antibacterial capacities, but only when the donor animals are treated repeatedly. In comparison, single injection of MER to donor mice leads to pronounced amplification of both enzymatic and phagocytic and antibacterial macrophage capacities.

Neither the compounds you sent us nor MER exert such effects consistently when they are added to macrophages in culture. However, when we incubate T lymphocytes with MER *in vitro* and then take the culture supernates and add them to macrophage cultures, potentiated activities by the latter become evident. The macrophage, then, may not be the primary target cell for the action of some immunomodulators, but may require the agency of mediator(s) produced by lymphoid cells under the influence of the adjuvants. We are now pursuing these observations with a variety of agents, and expect to extend them to *in vivo* test systems, incubating various immunocyte populations with the test agents in diffusion chambers and then assaying various host immunocyte populations for reactivity.

WESTPHAL

I quite agree with your statement.

MATHÉ

The best way to distinguish the cytostatic effect and the immune effect in the global efficiency of an agent is to use immunoprophylaxis tests; for example, BCG and other adjuvants work when given before tumor implantation. Have you tried such a test?

[15] *O. Westphal, U. Westphal, Andreesen, Munder* - p. 28

WESTPHAL

Well, the first slide showed results of experiments with Ehrlich ascites tumor growing i.p. — Lysophospholipids given 5-20 days before the i.p. inoculation of Ehrlich ascites tumor cells protect mice against a 10,000-fold higher tumor load which would kill 100 per cent of non-pretreated mice. In the first screening experiments we tried to correlate biological activity and chemical structure of the synthetic lysophospholipids. But we felt that prophylaxis was, of course, not so interesting. We therefore concentrated later on the more therapeutic approach by treating already established tumors.

MATHÉ

And it worked?

WESTPHAL

It worked, yes.

WOLFF

Two brief questions: (1) when you talk about lipopolysaccharide, you said a great deal about the biology and the toxicity; when you talked about your analogues you did not. Have you looked at the toxicity of the analogues in terms of fever, in terms of those sorts of things, and are there differences between them? (2) When you talk of tumor necrosis, you have cures down there; are these animals in fact cured and the tumors do not come back?

WESTPHAL

First, the synthetic lysolecithin analogues are well tolerated. We have treated mice for 20 days with 1 mg of alkyl-lysophospholipid daily i.v., complexed to isologous serum, without observing any serious signs of toxicity. There was no weight loss nor any change of body temperature. However, in some animals signs of transient liver irritation were observed on histological examination. But, these doses are 10-100-fold higher

[15] O. Westphal, U. Westphal, Andreesen, Munder - p. 29

than the therapeutically efficient doses. Secondly, all animals in which the tumor had completely disappeared due to lysophospholipid-induced tumor regression, remained free of tumor. These animals are immune against this MethA tumor. They will not take a 10-100-fold higher tumor load. After several challenging injections of tumor cells, a large number of cytotoxic macrophages appear in the peritoneal cavity and, in addition, antibodies against MethA tumor cells can be detected in the serum of the challenged mice.

TERRY

Are there any additional tumor systems other than the one that you described today, where you have used these materials and where it either does or does not work?

WESTPHAL

We tested the substances in two s.c. growing myelomas, on several other methylcholanthren-induced fibrosarcomas and on the Lewis lung carcinoma. They worked in all systems particularly when the substances were administered orally. When we tested our compounds on Lewis lung carcinoma, we usually saw no effect on the primary tumor, but the development of metastases in the lung was either completely inhibited or greatly retarded.

OETTGEN

I wonder if you would care to discuss a third aspect of lysolecithin analogue action? You mentioned that they turn on the macrophage and turn off the tumor cell. Could you also comment on their ability to liberate immunogenic cell surface components from tumor cells?

WESTPHAL

Well, this is of course a slightly different aspect. If one incubates MethA or other tumor cell suspensions *in vitro* with higher concentrations of synthetic lysolecithins having a shorter aliphatic chain in position 1, like ET$_{12}$-H, the plasma membranes and microsomes are solubilized, but

[15] O. Westphal, U. Westphal, Andreesen, Munder - p. 30

the nuclei stay intact. After several purification steps, performed with the supernatant of the lysate, one gets a uniform protein fraction with a molecular weight of about 48,000 dalton. Interestingly, some ET_{12}-H stays complexed with this material, and the associated ET_{12}-H seems to be necessary for optimal protection. 1-10 µg of this material will protect mice against the methylcholanthren-induced sarcoma from which the material was extracted.

NOSSAL

My question is a little bit in the direction of David Weiss's. As you recall, you were kind enough to send us some lysolecithin analogues for testing in various *in vitro* systems, including systems aimed at studying antibody production and various T-cell helper effects *in vitro*. To our disappointement, after you had these clear-cut *in vivo* activities in the mouse we failed to show any effects *in vitro*. Now at that time I was uncomfortable about solubility, and I ask you: have you encountered any difficulty in the solubilization of these materials, any batch variations, and have you had occasion to go back to some of these experiments? You know of course that LPS worked well *in vitro*.

WESTPHAL

Synthetic lysolecithin analogues with a long aliphatic substituent at position 1, of 16-18 C atoms, tend to fall out from aqueous solution and at low temperature. But if you warm up such dispersions to 37°C or above, concentrations as high as 0.1-0.5 mg/ml form clear solutions. If these substances are, however, injected i.v. or added to serum-containing medium, the compounds will quickly bind to plasma proteins. In fact, certain proteins and lipoproteins act as carriers for these substances, from which they are exchanged onto the cellular plasma membranes [1]. That the lipid portion of lipoproteins might, indeed, play an important role in inhibiting or enhancing — in other words, regulating — antitumor

---

[1] See BELL F. P.: *Lipoprotein-lipid exchange in biological systems.* In C. E. Day and R. S. Levy (editors), Low density lipoproteins, pg. 111-26. Plenum Press, London/New York, 1976.

[15] *O. Westphal, U. Westphal, Andreesen, Munder* - p. 31

effects of macrophages, has recently been suggested by I.B. HIBBS *et al.* (²⁻ ³). We think that the ordered slow transfer of our synthetic analogues onto macrophages and tumor cells is a necessary step in mediating the effects we have observed *in vivo* and *in vitro*. In the past we thought that binding to serum would largely inactivate the synthetic lysolecithin analogues. The contrary seems to be true. Nevertheless, we still have to learn much more about this exchange reaction facilitated by aid of lipoprotein carrier systems, for which we are now using radiolabelled compounds.

(²) HIBBS J.B., TAINTOR R.R., CHAPMAN H.A. and WEINBERG J.B.: *Macrophage Tumor Killing - Influence of the Local Environment*. « Science », 197, 279-82 (1977).

(³) CHAPMAN H.A. and HIBBS J.B.: *Modulation of Macrophage Tumoricidal Capability by Components of Normal Serum - A Central Role of Lipid*. « Science », 197, 282-84 (1977).

[15] *O. Westphal, U. Westphal, Andreesen, Munder* - p. 32

NATURALLY OCCURRING DOUBLE STRANDED POLYRIBONUCLEOTIDES: BIOLOGICAL ACTIVITIES OF POTENTIAL ANTITUMOUR SIGNIFICANCE

JANET M. DEWDNEY and ROBERT C. IMRIE

I. Introduction

There has been considerable interest in the biological effects of polyribonucleotides since the discovery that antiviral activity observed with culture filtrates derived from Penicillium species resided in the double-stranded RNA of viruses infecting the fungal hosts. Since then, a number of double-stranded polyribonucleotides have been isolated from natural sources or prepared synthetically.

In our laboratories the properties of BRL 5907, a dsRNA extracted from virus infecting *Penicillium chrysogenum* have been studied in detail. BRL 5907 has a sub-unit structure as shown in Fig. 1. It is essentially analogous in structure to dsDNA and differs substantially only with respect to the 2′ hydroxyl groups on the ribose moieties which influence both the secondary and tertiary structure of the molecule. The two purine bases, adenine and guanine and the two pyrimidine bases, cytosine and uracil are present in equimolar amounts. Hydrogen bonding between the base pairs gives a structure of high T_m which is relatively resistant to both pancreatic and serum ribonucleases. It has a sedimentation coefficient of 12.5 $s_{20, w}$ and when subjected to polyacrylamide gel electrophoresis separates into three molecular weight bands within the $1.9 - 2.2 \times 10^6$ dalton range. This degree of homogeneity is

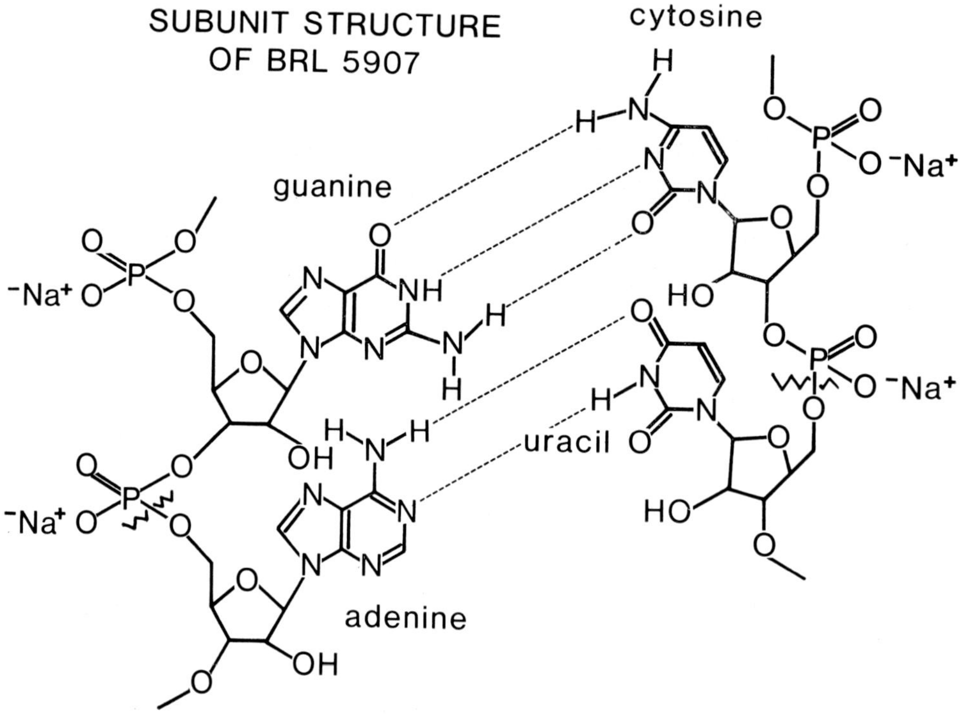

FIG. 1 — *BRL 5907. Subunit Structure.*

significantly greater than that of the semisynthetic duplexed poly-ribonucleotides such as Poly I · Poly C and some alternative natur-ally derived dsRNA's. Details of the production, characterisation and properties of the material have been reported and reviewed previously (BANKS *et al.*, 1969 and reviews by DEWDNEY, 1977 and PLANTEROSE, 1977).

This paper brings together experimental data which show that BRL 5907 can act as an antitumour agent in a variety of test systems and analyses in some detail the biological properties of BRL 5907 which might contribute to the overall antitumour effect. An important objective of the paper is also to highlight the possibility that dsRNA or close analogue might be of value in the control of clinical conditions which can accompany malignant diseases such as virus infections and anergy.

[16] *Dewdney, Imrie* - p. 2

II. ANTITUMOUR STUDIES

PILCH and PLANTEROSE (1971) were the first to demonstrate antitumour properties of BRL 5907 against murine Friend virus leukaemia. This model has been used extensively in the study of other polyribonucleotides (WHEELOCK *et al.*, 1974) and the results obtained with BRL 5907 were similar.

BRL 5907, administered by the intraperitoneal route at a dose of 5 mg/kg during the phase of rapid proliferation of Friend cells in the spleen, which in the mouse strain used was between the 7th - 11th day post infection, gave a highly significant inhibition of splenomegaly and the recovery of normal spleen structure. Alternate day dosing at 2.5 mg/kg was equally effective. This erythroleukaemia is usually rapidly fatal but remissions of duration in excess of 10 weeks were obtained although by this time 70% of infected mice had relapsed. The effects observed were dependent upon the time of dosing relative to day of infection. Prophylactic administration of BRL 5907 or treatment on the first 6 days after infection exacerbated the splenomegaly.

The discrepancy observed between the effects of prophylactically and therapeutically dosed mice has been a feature of a number of other antitumour studies with double-stranded polyribonucleotides. PARR *et al.* (1973) showed quite clearly that the administration of BRL 5907 before inoculation of either lymphoma cells or cells derived from chemically-induced fibrosarcomata was without effect whereas its administration after a palpable tumour mass was present led to antitumour effects. For example, 5 mg/kg BRL 5907 given intraperitoneally in repeated doses commencing 7 days after implantation of L5178Y into syngeneic DBA/2 mice led to permanent regression (3 months' survival) in two of five mice and temporary regression in a further three mice. HEYES *et al.* (1974) in our laboratories found essentially similar results in the L5178Y model in which dosing before Day 8 did not produce regression of tumours. From these initial studies, it was established therefore that better efficacy could be achieved by later administration of BRL 5907 and this led to a number of studies in which the agent was injected directly into an established tumour mass. Direct intratumour administration of BRL 5907 to mice carrying either L5178Y or FS6 tumours resulted in tumour regression; multiple and rather high level dosing was required to achieve permanent regression of FS6 tumour (PARR et al., 1973; HEYES et al., 1974). The concept of topical administration of BRL 5907 was taken a step further by HEYES and CATHERALL (1974) who evaluated its activity when administered by aerosol to mice bearing FS6 fibrosarcomata in their lungs and to mice with metastatic Lewis lung carcinoma. Significant antitumour effects were achieved in both models; the timing of the major effects were in accord with reported efficacy of BRL 5907 after the establishment of the tumour mass. PIMM and BALDWIN (1976) also found that introduction of BRL 5907 into the pleural and peritoneal cavities of rats can similarly control tumours at these sites.

A second observation made by PARR et al. (1973) was that the effectiveness of BRL 5907 was greater in the more immunogenic tumours; for example, greater effects were demonstrated against the strongly immunogenic L5178Y in DBA/2 mice and SL2 lymphoma compared with a range of other lymphomata and similar correlations were found using several different fibrosarcomata.

PIMM et al. (1976) also studied this aspect of the activity of BRL 5907. They selected a range of tumours in rats which varied very widely in their intrinsic immunogenicity. Systemic administration of BRL 5907 was without significant effect but the injection of BRL 5907 together with tumour cells led to significant suppression or retardation of tumour growth and the most pronounced effects were against tumour cells derived from the highly immunogenic methylcholanthrene-induced sarcomata and hepatoma D23. An additional point of interest arose in these studies. Unlike the situation when mycobacterial preparations were used in similar experiments, tumour immunity was not established and neither did the dsRNA prevent tumour growth at a distant site.

It is clear then that under certain circumstances, BRL 5907, in common with other dsRNA's, can achieve antitumour effects in mice and rats. Some of the requirements for optimum effectiveness have been indicated by the studies reviewed above. It is by no means a universally active antitumour agent. It differs very significantly from bacterial products, for example, BCG and C. parvum and is only in some respects similar to bacterial endotoxin in its

TABLE 1 — *Characteristics of the antitumour activity of BRL 5907.*

MOST EFFECTIVE AGAINST ESTABLISHED TUMOURS.

NON ACTIVE, OR EXACERBATES, IF GIVEN PRIOR TO TUMOUR CELLS.

INTRATUMOUR AND OTHER TOPICAL ROUTES OF ADMINISTRATION IMPROVE EFFICACY.

MOST EFFECTIVE AGAINST IMMUNOGENIC TUMOURS AND INTACT HOST IMMUNOLOGICAL RESPONSIVENESS NECESSARY.

CONTACT ADJUVANT ADMINISTRATION EFFECTIVE BUT TUMOUR SPECIFIC IMMUNITY NOT DEMONSTRATED.

SUGGESTED MODES OF ACTION INCLUDE INTERFERON-INDUCTION MACROPHAGE-MEDIATED EFFECTS AND DAMAGE TO TUMOUR SUPPORTING VASCULATURE.

antitumour profile. Some of these characteristics are shown in Table 1 and more complete comparisons are given by BAST *et al.* (1976) and ALEXANDER (1974). There is sufficient activity to warrant investigative work into possible mechanisms by which these antitumour properties are achieved and this work is reviewed in the following section.

III. MECHANISMS OF ACTION. BIOLOGICAL PROPERTIES OF BRL 5907 WHICH MIGHT CONTRIBUTE TO ANTITUMOUR EFFECTS

A. *Interferon Induction*

A readily demonstrable biological effect of dsRNA is the induction of interferon leading to its appearance in the circulation. High levels of interferons in serum are produced in mice 4-6 hours after the administration of BRL 5907 in doses within the range 0.05-0.5 mg/kg by the intravenous or intraperitoneal route (BUCK *et al.*, 1971; SHARPE *et al.*, 1971; PLANTEROSE, 1977). These doses are in excess of 10-fold lower than those required in the same species to demonstrate antitumour effects. It is in fact a general

TABLE 2 — *Dose ranges for biological activity of BRL 5907 in mice.*

BIOLOGICAL ACTIVITY	DOSE REQUIRED i.v. OR i.p. ROUTE (mg/kg)
INTERFERON INDUCTION	0.05 - 0.5
ANTIVIRAL PROTECTION	0.05 - 0.5
ANTITUMOUR EFFECTS	2.5 - 5.0
MACROPHAGE ACTIVATION	2.5 - 5.0
ADJUVANCY	5.0
IMMUNOSUPPRESSION	5.0
TOXICITY LD_{50}	12 - 40

finding that substantially higher doses of BRL 5907 are required to demonstrate biological effects other than interferon induction and antiviral protection as reference to Table 2 shows. Other species are in general less responsive to interferon induction by BRL 5907. Cattle and pigs (SELLERS *et al.*, 1973) and man (AOKI *et al.*, 1978) were poorly responsive under the conditions used by these authors and by analogy with studies carried out using other dsRNA's monkeys also produce low levels of serum interferon in response to this type of inducer (BESSEL *et al.*, 1971). Only the rabbit appears to respond as readily as the mouse.

Imrie in our laboratories has shown that one of the reasons for this marked species variation could be the efficiency with which the dsRNA is broken down by host serum ribonucleases; thus, a number of ribonuclease protected dsRNA's prepared in our laboratories (HARNDEN *et al.*, 1973; HEYES *et al.*, 1974) have shown better activity in non-murine species. Other properties are however undoubtedly important. Differential uptake of interferon or indeed of 5907 by cells could be critical in this respect.

To what extent can interferon induction contribute to the antitumour properties of dsRNA? Activity in some tumour models can arguably be regarded as a direct consequence of the ability of interferon to protect cells from infection with oncogenic virus. Some murine virus-induced sarcomata and Friend leukaemia might be regarded as examples. It is not, however, universally true that animal tumours of known viral aetiology are susceptible to the activity of dsRNA's; some, such as SV40 virus in neonatal hamsters or in adults (LARSON et al., 1970) are not and in the Friend leukae-mia model as discussed later in this paper, it is an inadequate expla-nation of activity. For many of the tumour models in which BRL 5907 has shown activity, there is no known or putative viral aetio-logy at all and on balance it seems unlikely that the antiviral attri-butes of BRL 5907 treatment mediated through interferon are of significance in most of the tumour studies.

Interferons are protein molecules which possess a range of biological activity in addition to their contribution to the antiviral state and it might be these properties of interferon which dictate the antitumour properties of BRL 5907. Gresser and his group have studied extensively the effect of exogenous murine interferon in inhibiting the growth of tumours of different types; not only virally-induced but also solid tumours and chemically induced fibro-sarcomata (GRESSER et al., 1969 a, b and Review by OXMAN, 1973). There is no doubt that antitumour effects can be achieved but mode of action is not certain (GRESSER et al., 1972). In part, the reported inhibitory effects of interferon on cell multiplication pos-sibly mediated via inhibition of protein synthesis might be respon-sible. It is now accepted that interferon preparations can inhibit cell multiplication although no interference with synthetic functions in non-dividing cells has been recorded and that the molecular spe-cies responsible for this activity is the same as that responsible for antiviral effects. Experiments in many laboratories, based on the results of separation and purification techniques and on the sensi-tivity of both biological activities to treatment of the preparation with enzymes or heating, support this view, as too does the fact that the same species specificity exists for both activities. None-theless, it is of interest that there is a marked discrepancy between the doses of interferon required to demonstrate anticell effects and those required to protect cells from virus infections; in some cell systems the demonstration of anticell effects requires doses 1,000-

fold higher and there is some evidence now that the anticell activity of interferon is not an essential prerequisite for protection of cells from viruses (KUWATA et al., 1976).

It seems to us improbable that the interferon-inducing properties of BRL 5907 provide an exclusive explanation of its antitumour activity and in fact, we were able to draw a similar conclusion in relation to the antiviral properties of BRL 5907. One of the most persuasive arguments that titres of serum interferon alone are inadequate to explain antiviral effects were results obtained in our laboratories demonstrating that the repeated injection of BRL 5907 rendered mice hyporesponsive with respect to the induction of serum interferon after only the third daily injection but local antiviral protection remained undiminished (SHARPE et al., 1971).

The antiviral properties of BRL 5907 however mediated could benefit the cancer patient and be of particular value in the control of severe viral infection which can threaten the life of patients immunosuppressed by disease or by therapy. The ability of the drug to protect mice and other species against a wide range of viruses has been recorded previously (for reviews: DEWDNEY, 1977; PLANTEROSE, 1977) and ribonuclease-resistant analogues may prove equally effective in man.

B. *Direct Cytotoxicity of BRL 5907*

The effectiveness of BRL 5907 in antitumour situations in which it and tumour cells are given in admixtures, or injected directly into the tumour mass suggests that BRL 5907 may have a directly toxic effect on the tumour cells.

PIMM et al. (1976) in their study in rats reported that hepatoma D23 and sarcoma Mc7 cells incubated *in vitro* with 1 mg/ml BRL 5907, washed and injected into rats subcutaneously, failed to grow into tumours although even at this very high dose, cell viability was not apparently affected. BRL 5907 was also shown by these workers to inhibit the growth of tumour cells *in vitro*; 31% inhibition of growth was obtained of a mammary tumour and 96-100% of sarcoma Mc7.

[16] *Dewdney, Imrie* - p. 8

ALEXANDER and EVANS (1971) also considered the question of the possible cytotoxic effects of dsRNA. Using doses in the 10-50 μg/ml range against lymphoma L5178Y cells, no cytotoxicity was observed in the absence of a macrophage population and this critical aspect is further discussed (ALEXANDER, 1974, 1976). They observed that an apparent cytotoxic effect can be observed in cultures of sarcoma cells established directly from sarcomata, in which the host macrophage population can be as high as 40%. In these primary cultures, the apparent cytotoxicity of BRL 5907 for the tumour cell is more a consequence of its ability to activate macrophages which then inhibit sarcoma growth. Thus, BRL 5907 can indirectly achieve a cytotoxic effect but in most circumstances, direct cytolytic effects cannot be demonstrated. An exception might be that recorded by STEWART *et al.* (1972) who showed that pre-treatment of cells in culture with interferon renders them more susceptible to the toxic effects of dsRNA's and thus in this way, cytotoxicity may explain some of the antitumour effects of BRL 5907.

A full appraisal of the toxicity of BRL 5907 in animals is beyond the scope of this paper but many of the toxic effects might be explained on the basis of a selective toxicity for rapidly dividing cells, as for example of haemopoietic cells and cells of the gastric and intestinal mucosa. This is discussed later in this paper in relation to tumour angiogenesis but it seems probable that at least some of the antitumour activity of BRL 5907 might result from this susceptibility of the rapidly dividing cell.

C. *Tumour Angiogenesis and Vascularisation of Tumours*

It is recognised that at an early stage in their growth, solid tumours must acquire a more efficient method of exchange of nutrients and metabolic products than simple diffusion if growth is to be sustained. This is achieved by the release from the tumour cells of a soluble factor which stimulates nearby blood vessels of the host to send out new capillary buds that grow towards the tumour, become canalised and thus vascularise the tumour. Folkman and his colleagues have studied this tumour-induced angiogenesis phenomenon over many years and have recently reviewed the topic (FOLKMAN, 1974; FOLKMAN and COTRAN, 1976). The vascularisation of a small mass of tumour cells is a critical event for only after its accomplishment is the tumour tissue invasive and detrimental to the host's survival.

In our laboratories we have made a preliminary investigation of tumour angiogenesis, or more precisely, its inhibition or antagonism. If the concepts developed by Folkman are correct, inhibition of tumour angiogenesis would prevent vascularisation and invasiveness and he has suggested four ways in which this might be achieved; one, inhibition of the synthesis or release of tumour angiogenesis factor (TAF) a ribonucleoprotein of molecular weight 100,000, two, antagonism of the factor once released, three, inhibition of its action at the endothelial cell level or four, inhibition of the advance of the newly formed blood vessels towards the tumour.

We considered that BRL 5907 might possibly have tumour angiogenesis inhibitory properties by antagonising directly the ribonucleoprotein moiety of TAF, or by directly inhibiting endothelial proliferation in view of its known activity against rapidly dividing cells. Moreover, as will be discussed later, dsRNA is known to damage endothelial lining cells in tumour blood vessels and such damaged cells might no longer be capable of responding to the mitogenic stimulus of TAF.

TAF was isolated from rat Walker 256 carcinoma cells and its activity tested in rats by a modification of the method of FOLKMAN et al. (1971). TAF was introduced into flexible chambers 10 mm in diameter and 1.5 mm thick held in position in the subcutaneous air sacs by nylon tubing attachment to the dorsal musculature of the rats at sites distant from the point of incision. The walls of the chambers were constructed of membrane filters of 0.1 μpore size.

TAF was shown to stimulate, after 2 days' exposure, a significant degree of neovascularisation which was abolished by preheating TAF at 56°C for 60'. The addition of 300 μg BRL 5907 to TAF containing chambers antagonised the activity of TAF such that minimal neovascularisation was seen. Under these experimental conditions, in which the effect was measured after 3 days' exposure, BRL 5907 itself was devoid of angiogenesis properties. BRL 5907

[16] *Dewdney, Imrie* - p. 10

was shown also to inhibit tumour angiogenesis factor when given systemically; 5 mg/kg/day by subcutaneous injection daily for 3 days resulted in almost complete inhibition of angiogenesis (IMRIE and BEESON, unpublished data).

The way in which TAF or its activity is inhibited by BRL 5907 is not known at the present time. An interesting suggestion has been made by Professor P. Alexander that it might be that BRL 5907 is more toxic to newly formed blood vessels than to established vasculature. It is known that the newly stimulated blood vessels which proliferate under the influence of TAF differ in some respects from other neovasculature, notably in that only rarely do they differentiate into venules and arterioles, a situation quite different from that of the blood vessel ingress in for example, wound healing. It is therefore quite possible that they differ also with respect to sensitivity to dsRNA cytotoxicity at the level of the rapidly proliferating endothelial cell.

This aspect of the antitumour activity of dsRNA and of course also of endotoxin, has engaged the interest of Professor Alexander and his group (ALEXANDER, 1974, 1976). Endotoxin injected locally into a tumour mass was associated within 30′ of blood vessel congestion within the tumour and environs and marked extravasation within 24 hours. Similar effects, although slower in onset were demonstrated with BRL 5907. The haemorrhagic necrosis induced by these two substances can in part be inhibited by heparinisation prior to their administration and the similarities with the Shwartzman reaction are obvious. The action of BRL 5907 on blood vessel integrity has also been observed in our laboratories in experiments in which it was applied to eggs and vessels of the chorioallantoic membrane were seen to increase in fragility.

The importance of haemorrhagic lesions in effecting tumour necrosis must depend upon many different circumstances, including the location of the tumour, its state of vascularisation and apparently also its immunogenicity. Alexander has shown that dsRNA and endotoxin are more active against tumours which are immunogenic and one explanation could be that blood vessel damage and extravasation leads to the concentration of various immunological specific effector cells and molecules within the tumour which might then be capable of tumour rejection. It seems obvious that tumour growth and survival will be impaired by the damage to its blood supply, either as a direct consequence of interference with the supply of nutrients and the removal of waste products or by inhibition of tumour angiogenesis.

D. *Immunogenicity and Adjuvancy of dsRNA*

It is important in a consideration of the biological activities of dsRNA to realise that these polyribonucleotides are intrinsically immunogenic. BRL 5907 is immunogenic when injected into many different animal species and neither adjuvant, nor complexing with a methylated serum protein is necessary for its immunogenicity. This property has been studied in detail in our laboratories (CUN- NINGTON and NAYSMITH, 1975 *a, b*; BUTLIN and CUNNINGTON, 1976; NAYSMITH *et al.*, 1974). In general we have found that animals successfully immunised with BRL 5907 and with demons- trable antibody of dsRNA specificity, still respond to BRL 5907. Thus, immunised animals can be fully protected by BRL 5907 from virus infection (NAYSMITH *et al.*, 1974) and still respond to the adjuvant properties of the molecule.

It may be asked to what extent might the immunogenicity of the dsRNA influence antitumour activity? We have not directly compared the antitumour efficacy of BRL 5907 in immunised and non-immunised animals and it may be necessary to do so under a range of different experimental systems, including both local and systemic routes of administration. Theoretically it does seem pos- sible that immunogenicity might have a bearing on the activity of dsRNA given topically. EVANS and ALEXANDER (1972) have dem- onstrated that interaction of armed macrophages with specific antigen will lead to activation of the macrophages which conse- quently develop non-selective tumour cell cytotoxicity. If this type of dsRNA specific immunological reaction is proceeding within the local environment of the tumour and perhaps within the tumour as the result of vasculature damage, it seems likely that it would make a contribution to the overall state of macrophage activation and tumour cell death (see also Section E).

We have also examined in some detail the ability of BRL 5907

[16] *Dewdney, Imrie* - p. 12

to act as an adjuvant to enhance both antibody responses and cell mediated immunity to different immunogens (CUNNINGTON and NAYSMITH, 1975 a; CUNNINGTON, M.Sc. Thesis University of London, 1976). In essence it was found that BRL 5907 given with or shortly after, thymus dependent antigens enhanced plaque forming cells in the spleen and haemagglutinating antibody and exacerbated delayed hypersensitivity in graft-versus-host in mice or allergic encephalomyelitis in guinea pigs. Administration prior to immunogen invariably resulted in poorer immune responses and this immunosuppression was in most situations a more profound effect than the adjuvancy achieved by later 5907 administration. The role of this adjuvant effect on tumour regression mediated by tumour-specific immune reactions is not known but it seems unlikely to be a significant factor. PIMM and BALDWIN (1976) found that dsRNA in admixture with tumour cells failed to stimulate tumour specific antibody in rats under conditions in which BCG was effective. Moreover, PARR et al. (1973) have presented evidence that dsRNA (and endotoxin) are more effective against immunogenic tumours than against poorly immunogenic tumours. Work in our laboratories has shown clearly that it is under adverse circumstances where, for a variety of reasons, there is a poor immune response that BRL 5907 is most effective as an adjuvant (CUNNINGTON and NAYSMITH, 1975 a). Fig. 2 illustrates this point by demonstrating that adjuvancy is greater in young mice and old mice which have a rather poor immune response to sheep erythrocytes compared with young adult mice (8 weeks old) and is greater also where the normal immune response has been depressed by pretreatment with rabbit anti-lymphocyte serum compared with pretreatment with normal rabbit serum. One might therefore have expected that if tumour specific adjuvancy played a significant part in the antitumour activity of BRL 5907, it would have been more readily demonstrated where the intrinsic immune response to tumour was poor.

The adjuvancy properties of BRL 5907 might however be of more interest seen from another point of view. Depression of immunological functions and responsiveness is characteristic of many patients with malignant disease and may be a consequence either of the disease state or of its therapy with suppressive drugs. It

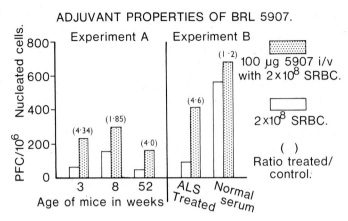

FIG. 2 — *Adjuvant properties of BRL 5907.*

Expt. A: CFLP mice aged 3, 8 or 52 weeks were injected i.v. with sheep erythrocytes and/or BRL 5907 in doses stated. Plaque forming cells in the spleen were measured 72 hours post injection by direct assay. The number in parentheses is the ratio of the number of PFC in animals receiving BRL 5907 compared with controls. *Expt. B*: 0.5 ml rabbit anti-lymphocyte serum or normal rabbit serum given i.p. Days 1, 3, 5 and 7. Sheep erythrocytes and BRL 5907 in doses stated given i.v. on Day 14. PFC assay performed as in Exp. A.

(CUNNINGTON and NAYSMITH, 1975).

could be of very real value to overcome such suppression and in our laboratories we have recently focussed upon this aspect of BRL 5907's activity. The following data are in preparation for publication by IMRIE and CATHERALL. The model we are working on is Friend leukaemia virus infection in mice. BRL 5907 is extremely active in suppressing the erythroleukaemia as noted in Section II and it is known that the infection produces immunodepression manifested in poor antibody responses and probably also defective delayed hypersensitivity (DENT, 1972) which are reversed by treatment with another dsRNA preparation "Statolon" (WHEELOCK *et al.*, 1974). The experimental protocol we are using is as follows. Friend leukaemia virus is injected intravenously into CD1 mice. On Day 8, at a time when there is rapid proliferation of leukaemia cells, sheep erythrocytes are administered intravenously. The mice are finally bled on Day 16, their sera assayed for haemagglutinating antibodies to the sheep erythrocytes and spleen weights recorded.

[16] *Dewdney, Imrie* - p. 14

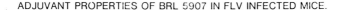

ADJUVANT PROPERTIES OF BRL 5907 IN FLV INFECTED MICE.

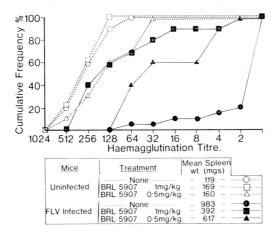

Mice	Treatment		Mean Spleen wt. (mgs)	
Uninfected	None		– 119 –	······○······
	BRL 5907	1mg/kg	– 169 –	·······□·····
	BRL 5907	0·5mg/kg	– 160 –	·····△····
FLV Infected	None		– 983 –	●—
	BRL 5907	1mg/kg	– 392 –	■—
	BRL 5907	0·5mg/kg	– 617 –	▲—

FIG. 3 — *Adjuvant properties of BRL 5907 in FLV infected mice.*
CDI mice were infected with FLV on Day 0. BRL 5907 was given i.p. in the doses stated on Days 4-10 inclusive. Sheep erythrocytes, 2×10^8 i.v. were given on Day 8 and antibody to sheep erythrocytes measured on Day 16. The haemagglutination titre is the reciprocal of the highest dilution causing visible agglutination. Cumulative frequency is a measure of the proportion of mice in each group, expressed as a percentage, with antibody titres equal to or greater than the given value. Spleen weights were measured on Day 16.

Fig. 3 shows that infected mice respond very poorly to sheep erythrocytes compared with uninfected controls. The administration of BRL 5907 at an intravenous dose of 0.5 to 1 mg/kg daily from Day 4 to 10 with respect to infection on Day 0 results in an impressive adjuvant effect.

It can be seen from the data in this Figure, that BRL 5907 under the experimental conditions used, did not increase titres of antibody to sheep erythrocytes in uninfected mice, providing a further example of the better activity of BRL 5907 as an adjuvant under conditions of less than optimal immune responses. Figure 4 summarises data which show the influence of time of administration of the dsRNA on the adjuvant effect achieved. It appears that daily treatment is required, optimally between Days 3 and 10; therapy on alternate days is less effective. Comparison of spleen

[16] *Dewdney, Imrie* · p. 15

ADJUVANT PROPERTIES OF BRL 5907 IN FLV INFECTED MICE. INFLUENCE OF DOSING REGIMEN.

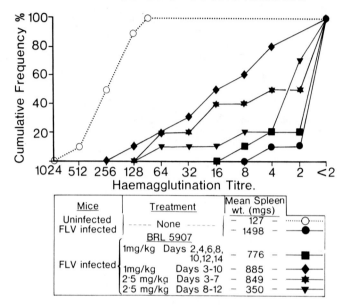

Mice	Treatment	Mean Spleen wt. (mgs)	
Uninfected	----- None -----	– 127 –	·····○·····
FLV infected		– 1498 –	──●──
	BRL 5907		
	1mg/kg Days 2,4,6,8, 10,12,14	– 776 –	──■──
FLV infected	1mg/kg Days 3-10	– 885 –	──◆──
	2·5 mg/kg Days 3-7	– 849 –	──✱──
	2·5 mg/kg Days 8-12	– 350 –	──▼──

FIG. 4 — *Adjuvant properties of BRL 5907 in FLV infected mice: influence of dosing regimen.* Experimental details as Figure 4. BRL 5907 given i.p. at times and doses stated.

weights from these mice is of interest (Figures 3, 4). There is no correlation between optimum schedules for reduction in spleno-megaly and for restoration of the antibody response to sheep eythro-cytes although it is clear from the mean data given in these Figures that the administration of BRL 5907 results in both these events. Analysis of data from individual mice also supports the finding that there is no obvious direct relationship between the efficacy of BRL 5907 in overcoming immune depression and in reduction of spleen weight in infected mice.

In order to understand more fully the activity of BRL 5907 in this model other compounds have been investigated. Clearly the role of interferon warrants evaluation. Preliminary results show that mouse interferon (Litton Bionetics, Maryland U.S.A.) at

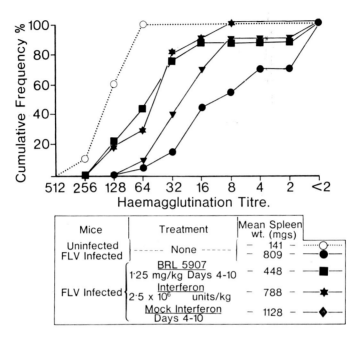

ADJUVANT PROPERTIES OF INTERFERON IN FLV INFECTED MICE.

Mice	Treatment	Mean Spleen wt. (mgs)	
Uninfected	------ None ------	– 141 –	·······○·······
FLV Infected		– 809 –	—●—
FLV Infected	BRL 5907 1·25 mg/kg Days 4-10	– 448 –	—■—
	Interferon 2·5 x 10⁶ units/kg	– 788 –	—★—
	Mock Interferon Days 4-10	– 1128 –	—◆—

Fig. 5 — *Adjuvant properties of interferon in FLV infected mice.* Experimental details as Figure 4. BRL 5907, interferon or mock interferon given i.p. at times and doses stated.

2.5×10^6 units/kg had significant activity in overcoming the immunodepression although effects on spleen weights were only modest (Figure 5). Some immunostimulants including BCG, tilorone and levamisole were without effect. A full report on the effect of these and other drugs in this model is in preparation for publication (IMRIE and CATHERALL).

E. *Macrophage Activation*

The increased interest in the role of the macrophage in tumour control in recent years has derived from studies which have indicated that the macrophage content of tumours is an important determinant of their biological behaviour. Tumours with a high proportion of host macrophages are those which are most immunogenic and least likely to undergo spontaneous metastasis (for Reviews: SIEGAL, 1976; CURRIE, 1976).

One aspect of the effector role of macrophages which has been the subject of studies by Alexander and his group is the ability of dsRNA to cause macrophage activation.

ALEXANDER and EVANS (1971) have demonstrated that exposing non-immune macrophages *in vitro* to 10-50 µg/ml BRL 5907 renders them cytostatic for target L5178Y lymphoma cells and sarcoma tumour cells. Cook in our laboratories has confirmed the ability of BRL 5907 to activate normal mouse syngeneic macrophages such that they non-specifically inhibit growth of TLC5 lymphoma cells; tritiated thymidine uptake as a measure of cell growth was found to be inhibited by 60% of control after incubation of the macrophages with 15 µg/ml 5907 and by 89% at a dose of 30 µg/ml and similar results have been obtained against TLX5 cells (COOK, unpublished data). Interestingly, peritoneal macrophages derived from FLV infected mice 8 days after infection, that is, at a time when BRL 5907 has been shown to inhibit erythroleukaemia (PILCH and PLANTEROSE, 1971) are not themselves cytostatic for TLX5 tumour cells, nor does BRL 5907 at a dose of 25 µg/ml render them so (COOK R. M., unpublished data).

BRL 5907 is also capable of rendering normal mouse macrophages cytostatic to *in vitro* cultured tumour cells when administered intraperitoneally at 100 µg one day prior to macrophage collection (ALEXANDER and EVANS, 1971). This has been confirmed at a dose of 1.25 mg/kg 5907 in our laboratories recently by Cook who extended his studies to the FLV infected mouse. Treatment of FLV infected mice with 1.25 mg/kg BRL 5907 on days 4-7 with respect to infection on Day 0 and macrophage harvest on Day 8 failed to render the peritoneal macrophage cytostatic for tumour cells and the additional application of BRL 5907 in culture was without effect also (COOK, unpublished data). It is difficult to assess the implications of these data. They suggest that the ability of dsRNA to activate macrophages is not exclusively responsible either for its activity in suppressing erythroleukaemia nor for

[16] *Dewdney, Imrie* - p. 18

overcoming the immunodepression which is manifested in a poorer antibody response to sheep erythrocytes. It should be stressed that these are preliminary findings and in a complex biological model the temporal relationships between stage of infection and dsRNA administration may be critical. Moreover, the observations are based on only the peritoneal macrophage cell population and it is not known how representative this population is of the total macrophages of the body.

There are other pieces of evidence which suggest that the activity of dsRNA in the FLV system might be at least in part mediated through the macrophage. It has been shown by WHEE-LOCK et al. (1974) that the efficacy of "Statolon" in suppressing leukaemia in FLV infected mice can be eliminated by prior treatment of the mice with silica and the same group of workers have shown that the phagocytic functions of macrophages are depressed in FLV infected mice and that this depression can be restored by "Statolon" (LEVY and WHEELOCK, 1975). Restoration of macrophage function and reversal of immunodepression were not, however, by themselves sufficient to suppress FLV leukaemia (LEVY and WHEELOCK, 1976).

The collective evidence in different biological systems strongly suggests that the macrophage is an important target cell of BRL 5907, not only in relation to antitumour activity but also in mediating antiviral effects, adjuvancy and immunosuppression and further study is now required to explore in depth the nature of the influence of dsRNA on macrophage function.

F. Conclusions

No single mechanism can be suggested which accounts for the antitumour activity of BRL 5907. Clues to mode of action come from observations that the drug is active only after a tumour mass is established whereas it can exacerbate tumour growth if given before implantation, that it is more active against immunogenic tumours to which the host can respond immunologically and is more active against tumours containing a high proportion of host macrophages. These characteristics lead to ideas which centre around the effects of interference with tumour blood supplies, by damage to vasculature or by interference in tumour angiogenesis. Increased extravasation into the tumour would bathe the tumour mass in immune effector molecules derived from both macrophages and lymphocytes and of these interferon, derived immunologically in this way, or as the direct consequence of the action of dsRNA, has clear merit as a candidate through which some antitumour effects might be mediated. Interference with vascularisation through anti-angiogenesis would prevent tumour growth and metastasis. The role of macrophage arming and activation are discussed. That BRL 5907 activates macrophages in some manner is clear and many of the experimental findings support the view that this is one of the key events in certain antitumour studies.

Whatever the mode of action, BRL 5907 has definite anti-tumour activity which can be exploited more favourably by local administration, a technique which allows high antitumour concentrations of drug with minimum systemic effects on the host. It has merit as a candidate for further study because of its homogeneity and purity compared with other macromolecules in clinical trials. Careful analysis should be made of the pharmacological and toxicological properties of BRL 5907 to determine conditions under which it might safely be administered to man.

Equally important is the fact that it is possible that patients could derive benefit from a dsRNA with respect to the epiphenomena of cancer; that is, the state of anergy and the susceptibility to viral infection. The diversity and potency of the biological effects of dsRNA in mammalian species are striking. In view of this it is interesting to recall in conclusion that mycophages, from which these dsRNA's are derived, are characteristically lacking in pathogenicity in their natural hosts, the fungi, to an extent that their presence went unobserved until their ability to produce interferon in mammalian cells was noted.

[16] *Dewdney, Imrie* - p. 20

REFERENCES

ALEXANDER P. and EVANS R., « Nature New Biol. », *232*, 76 (1971).

ALEXANDER P., « Johns Hopkins Med. J. (Suppl.) », *3*, 321 (1974).

ALEXANDER P., « Ann. Rev. Med. », *27*, 207 (1976).

AOKI F.Y., REED S.E., CRAIG J.W., TYRREL D.A.J. and LEES L.J., « J. Infect. Dis. », *137*, 82 (1978).

BANKS G.T., BUCK K.W., CHAIN E.B., DARBYSHIRE J.E. and HIMMELWEIT F., « Nature (London) », *222*, 89 (1969).

BAST R.C., BAST B.S. and RAPP H.J., « Ann. N.Y. Acad. Sci. », *277*, 60 (1976).

BESSEL C.I., BOLLING N.J., FANTES K.H., LAURSEN A.C., NEWCOMB J.M., PAMPLIN P.O. and SUTHERLAND E.S., Private Communication (1971).

BUCK K.W., CHAIN E.B. and HIMMELWEIT F., « J. Gen. Virol. », *12*, 131 (1971).

BUTLIN P.M. and CUNNINGTON P.G., « Europ. J. Immunol. », *6*, 607 (1976).

CUNNINGTON P.G. and NAYSMITH J.D., « Immunology », *28*, OLE (1975a).

CUNNINGTON P.G. and NAYSMITH J.D., « Immunology », *29*, 1001 (1975b).

CUNNINGTON P.G., M. Sc. Thesis, University of London (1976).

CURRIE G., « Biochimica et Biophysica Acta », *458*, 135 (1976).

DENT P.B., « Prog. med. Virol. », *14*, 4 (1972).

DEWDNEY J.M., In: *Biologically Active Substances. Exploration and Exploitation.* Ed. Hems, D.A. John Wiley & Sons Ltd., p. 149 (1977).

EVANS R. and ALEXANDER P., « Nature », *236*, 168 (1972).

FOLKMAN J., MERLER E., ABERNATHY C. and WILLIAMS G., « J. exp. Med. », *133*, 275 (1971).

FOLKMAN J., « Adv. in Cancer Res. », *19*, 331 (1974).

FOLKMAN J. and COTRAN R., « Int. Rev. Exp. Path. », *16*, 208 (1976).

GRESSER I., COPPEY J. and BOURALI C., « J. Nat. Cancer Inst. », *43*, 1083 (1969a).

GRESSER I., BOURALI C., LEVY J.P., FONTAINE D. and THOMAS M.T., « Proc. Nat. Acad. Sci. », *63*, 51 (1969b).

GRESSER I., MAURY C. and BROUTY-BOYE D., « Nature », *239*, 167 (1972).

HARNDEN M.R., BROWN A.G., SHARPE T.J. and VERE HODGE R.A., 166th Meeting of the American Chemical Society, Chicago, August 27-31 (1973).

HEYES J. and CATHERALL E.J., « Nature », *247*, 485 (1974).

HEYES J., CATHERALL E.J. and HARNDEN M.R., « Europ. J. Cancer », *10*, 431 (1974).

KUWATA T., FUSE A. and MORINAGA N., « J. Gen. Virol. », *33*, 7 (1976).

LARSON V.M., PANTELEAKIS P.N. and HILLEMAN M.R., « Proc. Soc. exp. Biol. Med. », *133*, 14 (1970).

LEVY M.H. and WHEELOCK E.F., « J. Immunol. », *114*, 962 (1975).

LEVY M.H. and WHEELOCK E.F., « J. Reticulo Endothelial Soc. », *20*, 243 (1976).

NAYSMITH J.D., SHARPE T.J. and PLANTEROSE D.N., « Europ. J. Immunol. », *4*, 629 (1974).

OXMAN M.N., In: *Interferons and Interferon Inducers*. Ed. N. Finter. N. Holland Research Monographs. « Frontiers of Biology », *2*. N. Holland/Elsevier (1973).

PARR I., WHEELER E. and ALEXANDER P., « Brit. J. Cancer », *27*, 370 (1973).

PILCH D.J.F. and PLANTEROSE D.N., « J. gen. Virol. », *10*, 155 (1971).

PIMM M.V. and BALDWIN R.W., « Brit. J. Cancer », *331*, (2), 166 (1976).

PIMM M.V., EMBLETON M.J. and BALDWIN R.W., « Brit. J. Cancer », *33*, (2), 154 (1976).

PLANTEROSE D.N., In: *The Interferon System: A Current Review*. « Texas Reports on Biology and Medicine », *35*. Ed. S. Baron and F. Dianzani (1977).

SELLERS R.F., HERNIMAN K.A.J., LEIPER J.W.G. and PLANTEROSE D.N., Vet. Rec., 28th July, 90 (1973).

SHARPE T.J., BIRCH P.J. and PLANTEROSE D.N., « J. gen. Virol. », *12*, 331 (1971).

SIEGAL B.V., « J. Reticulo Endothelial Soc. », *20*, 219 (1976).

STEWART W.E., DE CLERCQ E., BILLRAN A., DESMYTER J. and DE SOMER P., « Proc. Nat. Acad. Sci., USA », (1972).

WHEELOCK E.F., TOY S.T., WEISLOW O.S. and LEVY M.H., In: *Immunology of Cancer*. « Progress exp. Tumor Res. », *19*, 369, Karger, Basel (1974).

DISCUSSION

STRANDER

What kind of serum concentrations of interferons do you get in the animals which you inject, and how much can you get in tissue culture by using double-stranded RNA as inducer?

DEWDNEY

Interferon titres achieved in tissue culture depend on the type of cell used and whether priming and superinduction are used. The use of DEAE dextran can potentiate induction in some cell systems. In mice, titres of several hundred to two or three thousand I.U. can be achieved following intraperitoneal or intranasal injection. Similar levels are achieved in rabbits using different dsRNA's. Other species produce lower levels of interferon; man and other primates give only low titres in response to dsRNA's although it is important to remember that serum interferon does not always correlate with antiviral protection and protection might still be achieved in these species.

WESTPHAL

Is the whole original molecule necessary? Would split products do it?

DEWDNEY

We have degraded BRL 5907 enzymatically using ribonuclease and mechanically by ultrasonication. Antiviral activity, interferon induction and toxicity tend to decrease in parallel as the molecule is reduced in size. Immunogenicity is also diminished with decrease in molecular size but adjuvancy is retained on degradation to a greater extent.

WESTPHAL

You showed the tolerance effect with regard to interferon induction, but of course here one could think that all interferon has been released. Is it really a tolerance to the inducer? Therefore my question: how about pyrogenicity? As far as I remember, you get tolerance to the pyrogenic effect also.

DEWDNEY

Yes. I would like to take the question in two parts. I think there is some degree of tolerance to the material itself in that animals no longer producing serum interferon to dsRNA can be challenged to do so with an unrelated inducer.

We found it difficult to demonstrate tolerance to the toxicity of BRL 5907 although repeated dosing leads to a degree of tolerance (2-3 fold) in pyrogenicity. It may be that the acute toxicity test is insufficiently sensitive to distinguish 2-fold differences.

WOLFF

About eight years ago we were looking at the pyrogenic effects of poly-I poly-C, and in looking in the rabbit it was clearly pyrogenic and we went to look for the release of leukocytic pyrogen in human white blood cells. We found, as you reported here, that there are RNA's in the serum inhibiting the material so that we could not get it to release pyrogen. We looked at about eleven different species of sera and there was considerable variation among the species and we related that to levels of RNA.

DEWDNEY

There are differences in ribonuclease levels in the different species and this is one factor in determining how effective dsRNA's are as inducers and antiviral agents. I do not know of any correlation between pyrogenicity and levels of ribonuclease. In primates it is broken down rapidly but is pyrogenic. In mice I do not think there is significant fever but it is relatively stable in mouse serum so there may be no correlation.

[16] *Dewdney, Imrie* - p. 24

WOLFF

The problem is that in the two species you picked on, the monkey is very resistant to pyrogenic effect, if anything, and the mouse does not get a fever, as Dr. Westphal reported.

DEWDNEY

That is right.

TERRY

Some years ago, Carl Nathan observed in this type of assay using peritoneal cells that the effector cell suppressing the growth of tumor cells appeared to be a non-phagocytic adherent cell (NPAC), a cell having some of the properties of B cells. Have you performed studies that would indicate whether your effectors are really macrophages or would it be more correct to indicate that it is some cell within the adherent population?

DEWDNEY

You are absolutely right; I should have made the point. These are simply unfractionated adherent peritoneal cell populations.

TERRY

Is there any tendency for this material to "home" to tumor cells? That is, when you inject this material *in vivo*, does the material migrate to the tumor cell and does it do anything in terms of altering the expression of antigens on the cell surface? I ask this in the context of the work Lindemann and others have been doing in terms of viral super-infection of tumor cells. The membranes of such cells begin to express viral antigens or viral induced antigens and become more immunogenetic.

DEWDNEY

I cannot answer that because distribution studies have not been done in tumor-bearing animals. In the normal animal there is a tendency for it to accumulate in gastric mucosa, so one is thinking in terms of it being selectively toxic or having a selective action on rapidly dividing cells; using labelled material you find high concentrations of the label in the gastric mucosa and that, I am sure, accounts for some of the toxicity of dsRNA, as one observes stripping of the gut mucosa in some species. (Harris, G., personal communication).

CLERICI

Usually nucleic acids are not immunogenic. So I wonder which is the special feature which makes the double-stranded RNA highly immunogenic in many species.

DEWDNEY

Well, that was exactly the situation when we started to work with this material — we anticipated that we would have to use adjuvants or have to complex it to methylated serum albumin. The reason why it is immunogenic is I think a function of the rigidity of its structure in relation to the hydrogen bonding, because if you take double-stranded RNA or in fact DNA and measure Tm, which is determined by the strength of the bonding, you find there is correlation between immunogenicity and Tm. Some polyribonucleotides, which are much less tightly bonded, are very poor immunogens, whereas BRL 5907 is a very good one. This is not a feature that one would wish to see in a molecule being given to man but it may be of little clinical significance.

OETTGEN

Dr. Dewdney, the clinical trials that were conducted with poly-I:C several years ago in cancer patients were not very encouraging. Looking at your summary slide, I believe that your material resembled poly-I:C in every respect tested. Do you see an advantage of the new product over poly-I:C on the basis of any of the tested criteria?

[16] *Dewdney, Imrie* - p. 26

DEWDNEY

No, I do not see any major advantages, in terms of biology, with respect to both agents' use for anti-cancer. The advantage that I can see for BRL 5907 would be that this is entirely homogeneous and that one can standardize it as one knows its physical chemical properties from batch to batch; one does not see the batch to batch variation that you get with the semi-synthetic dsRNA's. My own view is that there is no way you are going to show anti-tumor properties with this drug by treating terminal patients. I cannot see any activity in animals at all which would lead one to believe that terminal patients could benefit. And that is what the Poly-I Poly-C trial was. So I do not think one would have expected to see activity in the trials you refer to; they were more directed towards establishing safety and tolerance, I believe.

INTERFERON TREATMENT
OF HUMAN OSTEOSARCOMA

ULF ADAMSON,[1] TOMAS APARISI,[2] LARS-AKE BROSTROM,[2]
KARI CANTELL,[5] STEFAN EINHORN,[3] KERSTIN HALL,[1]
SNORRI INGIMARSSON,[3] ULF NILSONNE,[2] HANS STRANDER [3]
and GUNNAR SODERBERG [4]

For osteosarcoma patients with no initial evidence of metastases and given no adjuvant therapy the 5-year survival rate is
20-25 per cent (HANDELSMAN and CARTER, 1975). In recent years
the value of high-dose adjuvant chemotherapy in this disease has
been examined (CORTES et al., 1974; JAFFE et al., 1974). The
short term survival rate for patients given this form of treatment
is reportedly higher than that for patients of earlier series not so
treated (FREI et al., 1977).

At the Karolinska Hospital we are giving exogenous interferon therapy to a consecutive series of osteosarcoma patients presenting no signs of metastases on admission (STRANDER et al., 1977).
The study has now been running for 6 years, during which time
the series has been steadily augmented. This report outlines the
procedure of the trial and the results obtained to date. Various

[1] *Department of Endocrinology,* [2] *Department of Orthopaedic Surgery,* [3] *Radiumhemmet,* [4] *Department of Tumor Pathology,* at the Karolinska Hospital,
S-104 01 Stockholm 60, Sweden.
[5] *Central Public Health Laboratory,* Mannerheimintie 166, SF 00280 Helsinki,
Finland.
Key words: Bone tumour; interferon: leukocytes; neoplastic disease; osteosarcoma; somatomedins.

aspects of the study have been dealt with in previous articles (STRANDER, 1977, 1978; APARISI et al., 1977; STRANDER, 1977; EINHORN and STRANDER, 1977).

Case series

The *interferon group* comprises all the patients so far given interferon therapy, and at present numbers 28. They have been admitted to the Karolinska Hospital since the end of 1971 with a diagnosis of osteosarcoma and no signs of metastases.

The *historical control group* comprises 35 patients that had received treatment from 1952 to 1971. They were obtained from the Hospital registries.

The *concurrent control group* comprises all the osteosarcoma patients aged up to 30 years that were entered in the Cancer Registry at the National Board of Health and Welfare of Sweden during the period 1972-74 and that had received treatment elsewhere than at the Karolinska Hospital. This and the interferon group contained all the patients with osteosarcoma in Sweden that had received treatment during this period.

Pathological features

All the patients entered in the three groups up to May, 1976, were submitted to a detailed examination by a team of independent investigators from the National Cancer Institute, National Institutes of Health, USA. The patients collected since May, 1976, — so far only ones given interferon therapy — have yet to be checked by independent specialists, but all had classical osteosarcoma according to the criteria established by the visiting team and all of them are included in the interferon group. Histological typing was performed by the method of Dahlin (DAHLIN, 1973), according to which grade I and II tumours are well differentiated and grades III and IV tend to be anaplastic. The tumours were assigned to the three groups osteoblastic, chondroblastic and fibroblastic osteosarcoma (APARISI et al., 1977).

Electron microscopy

Opinions differ as to the ultrastructural appearance of osteo-sarcoma cells (GHADIALLY and MEHTA, 1970; KAY, 1971; PASCHALL and PASCHALL, 1975). To extend our knowledge of the morphology, histogenesis, interrelationships and function of various types of such cells a series of studies of the fine structure, and the histochemistry and biochemistry of the cells has been undertaken. These studies are still in the data-collecting stage, and the results will be reported in due course.

Endocrinological study

It has been suggested that hormonal mechanisms may be a factor in the pathogenesis of osteosarcoma and possibly have a bearing on the course of the disease. Among the more notable features of the disease are the following: Its onset most frequently occurs during the pubertal growth spurt and the tumour is usually located close to the zone of bone growth in the metaphyseal region (DAHLIN and COVENTRY, 1967). The disease is more common among tall persons (FRAUMENI, 1967), and among males, for whom the prognosis is also worse than for females (LINDBOM et al., 1961). Furtermore, *in vitro* studies have revealed synergism between oestrogens and progesterons in tumour growth inhibition (SCRANTON et al., 1975; McMASTER et al., 1975), while metabolic studies have disclosed hyperinsulinism, insulin resistance and high plasma levels of somatomedins in patients with osteosarcoma (McMASTER et al., 1975).

During 1976-77 an analysis of specific hormonal and metabolic parameters has been performed for all patients with osteosarcoma at the Karolinska Hospital. Data relating to height and dental development were also collected, the latter by the method devised by FILIPSON (1974). Values were recorded from birth until the onset of the disease with a view to examining whether these factors have any causative significance. Other points under study are: the somatomedin level in the plasma, the possibility of there being a correlation between this parameter and insulin resistance, how surgical and interferon treatment may affect the plasma

[17] *Strander* - p. 3

level of somatomedins, whether this factor affords a means of predicting recurrence of the disease, and whether the somatomedins are released from the tumour or from some organ of the body.

Analysis of the growth rate and dental development have so far been performed in 20 patients. The stature data did not differ appreciably from those for an agematched control group. It is notable, however, just prior to the onset of the disease that 5 of the patients exhibited a higher growth rate than expected. The results obtained so far confirm those reported by other investigators, who found that some persons with osteosarcoma displayed insulin resistance simultaneously with an elevated level of somatomedins A and B in the plasma.

Prognostic factors

A study was undertaken to ascertain whether the three groups of patients — the interferon and the historical and concurrent controls — were comparable from the aspect of prognostic factors and all the patients collected up to May, 1976, were reviewed by a team of pathologists and clinicians. To increase the number of cases the two concurrent groups were combined. At that time the contemporary group numbered 44 patients, and these were compared with the 35 historical ones. Absence of metastases on admission was checked by reviewing radiographs and clinical reports. Only tumours of the long bones or the pelvis were considered. The prognostic factors examined were sex, age, signs and symptoms, tumour size and site, and histological type (APARISI et al., 1977).

The two groups displayed practically no differences in age or sex ratio, both of them being typical of osteosarcoma patients in general, with a mean age of 18 years and containing about 65 per cent of males. Pain and swelling were the most frequent manifestations of the disease. The incidence of the various symptoms was higher for the historical group. For both groups the duration of the signs and symptoms prior to admission was about 3 months. About 70 per cent of the tumours were located in the region of the knee; the historical group contained more tumours above this level than did the contemporary group. Tumour size was determined on radiographs taken at the time of the diagnosis; the tumours were, on average, larger in the historical than in the contemporary group, the mean greatest diameters being 13 and 9 cm, respectively. Furthermore, the historical group also contained a clear preponderance of grade IV and osteoblastic tumours.

To summarize: the tumours of the historical group were, on average, more malignant and larger than those composing the contemporary group, and the tumours tended to be located more proximally. These factors have all been considered to have a bearing on the prognosis (LOCKSHIN and HIGGINS, 1968). In the light of the results of this analysis it is pertinent to question whether historical groups are acceptable as controls in current studies concerned with ascertaining the efficacy of various forms of treatment for osteosarcoma. At the moment the historical group cannot be regarded as an acceptable control for the interferon group. The series is at present too small for a meaningful statistical analysis, but the results of the prognostic study underline the importance of a careful analysis of prognostic factors in investigations where no prospective randomization can be performed, and especially in those concerned with rare diseases (APARISI et al., 1977).

Interferon preparations

The procedure for preparing the human leukocyte interferon used in this study is based on more than 10 years' experience at the Central Public Health Laboratory in Helsinki (for references see CANTELL and STRANDER, 1977). Briefly: 13 ml of buffy coats are collected from centrifuged fresh blood bags. They are pooled and stored overnight at 4°C. The leukocytes are purified by treatment with ammonium chloride and suspended in a suitable medium, with 10^7 viable cells per millilitre. The cells are incubated in suspension cultures at 37.5°C. The cultures are primed with 100 standard interferon units/ml, and, 2 h later, the formation of interferon is induced with 150 HA units of Sendai virus per millilitre. After incubation for 20 h and low-speed centrifugation the crude interferon is harvested in the supernatant. The latter contains about 40,000 units/ml and about 2.5 mg of protein per millilitre.

Human leukocyte interferon is precipitated in the presence of 0.5 M potassium thiocyanide at pH 3.5. The interferon is dissolved in about one-thirtieth of the original volume of phosphate buffered saline, with full recovery of activity. Such concentrates (C-IF) have been used in clinical studies since 1971 (STRANDER et al., 1973). More recently, a procedure for partial purification of interferon has been developed in which the potassium thiocyanide precipitate is dissolved in cold acid ethanol, and the impurities are selectively precipitated by raising the pH (CANTELL et al., 1974 a; CANTELL and HIRVONEN, 1978). The interferon is precipitated at around the neutral point, and may be concentrated by further precipitation with potassium thiocyanide. With this procedure a roughly one-hundredfold purification and 50 per cent recovery are achieved. Such partly purified preparations (P-IF) contain 10-20 million units per millilitre.

Both C-IF and P-IF preparations are very stable (MOGENSEN and CANTELL, 1977), storage for at least a year at 4°C being possible without significant loss of activity (KAUPPINEN et al., 1977). No stabilizing additives are needed.

The fibroblast interferon, used in some of the in vitro studies, was prepared by the method of HAVELL and VILCEK (1972).

"In vitro" studies

That interferon can inhibit cell multiplication is well established (PAUCKER et al., 1962; see GRESSER, 1977) and we found it of interest to examine whether osteosarcoma cells are sensitive to this property of interferon.

In a study with this purpose 9 established osteosarcoma cell lines were tested for their sensitivity to the CMI (cell multiplication inhibitory) activity of human leukocyte interferon (STRANDER and EINHORN, 1977). An inhibition of growth was recorded for all 9 cell lines, and the degree of inhibition was dose-dependent. The dose of interferon that was required to produce a 50 per cent inhibition in 2 weeks in the various cell lines ranged from 10 to 300 units/ml. Concentrations of the same range have been recorded in the serum of patients treated with interferon (CANTELL *et al.*, 1974 *b*).

In an attempt to select cells resistant to interferon the osteo-sarcoma cell lines were grown in the presence of interferon for a period of 8 weeks. Over this interval there was no appreciable change in sensitivity to interferon.

The CMI activity of human leukocyte and fibroblast inter-feron was compared on 2 osteosarcoma cell lines (EINHORN and STRANDER, 1977). Fibroblast interferon was found to exert a stronger CMI effect on these cell lines than leukocyte interferon. In a comparison performed in parallel tests 2 Burkitt's lymphoma cell lines were found to be more sensitive to leukocyte interferon than to fibroblast interferon (EINHORN and STRANDER, 1977). This suggests that to some extent the effect of interferon might be tissue or tumour specific.

Administration of interferon

The interferon was supplied according to a standardized sche-dule (STRANDER *et al.*, 1977). Over a period of one month in hospital a daily dose of 3×10^6 standard interferon units was given by intramuscular injection. The interferon was then given on an ambulatory basis — 3×10^6 interferon standard units 3 times weekly for a further 17 months. Two interferon preparations were used, namely, the concentrated interferon, C-IF, and the more highly purified interferon, P-IF (see above).

Side effects of interferon

An examination for side effects of interferon has so far been conducted in 27 of the osteosarcoma patients. The total follow-up time for these patients was 340 months. In the course of the interferon therapy 12 distinct symptoms and signs were recorded, between 1 and 5 of which were experienced by each of 24 patients. Three patients did not report any discomfort at all. It should be borne in mind that one symptom can elicit another: fever can give rise to perspiration, for example. All the symptoms reported were registered in this study. The concentrated form of interferon (C-IF) was always given first, and if side effects became trouble-some it was replaced by the partly purified type (P-IF). This mo-dification of the therapy usually sufficed to eliminate the side ef-fects, and in those cases where they persisted it was generally with a lower intensity. The 6 most commonly encountered side effects recorded during the C-IF therapy were fever (59 per cent of the patients), local pain at the injection site (44 per cent), shivers (38 per cent), transient hair loss (28 per cent), itchy erythema (14 per cent) and coryza (14 per cent).

While some of the symptoms — fever, shivers, coryza and slight and transient hair loss — were not completely abolished by the change-over to P-IF, there was no report of these giving rise to major discomfort. All the patients could be given interferon on an ambulatory basis, and in no case was it necessary to abandon the treatment because of the side effects.

Immunological findings

Before, during and after the interferon therapy peripheral lymphocytes from the interferon group were tested for their res-ponse to various mitogens, and for their sensitivity to interferon *in vitro*. It was found that prolonged treatment with exogenous interferon did not change the peripheral lymphocyte counts *in vivo* or the mitogenic response of the lymphocytes *in vitro*. Nor did the interferon sensitivity of the lymphocytes alter during the therapy.

Infections

It is well established that persons suffering from malignant diseases are more prone than others to contract infections diseases (BODEY, 1973). An impression of the incidence, duration and severity of acute infections in osteosarcoma patients during inter-feron therapy was obtained from monthly questionnaires. For comparison the incidence of infections among members of the patients' households was also noted. The household members, numbering 37 to date, composed the control group, while all the patients receiving interferon but clinically free from tumour diseases, numbering 13, constituted the experimental group. A preliminary account of the incidence of infections has been given elsewhere (STRANDER et al., 1975). The total follow-up time for the two groups combined is at present 410 months.

The incidence of infections was lower in the experimental group (the patients receiving interferon) than in the control group. The recorded difference might be on the low side because some of the symptoms, especially coryza and fever, may have been elicited by the interferon therapy (see above). The approximate mean duration of symptoms typical of acute viral infections was 17 days for the control group against 7 days for the interferon group; this suggests that the infections in the control group were of a more severe kind. The number of days of bed rest per period of illness was greater in the control than in the interferon group. Although the recorded symptoms are ones that are typical of acute viral infections some of the infections may have been caused by non-viral infectious agents. To identify the type of infection blood samples were collected at regular intervals from the two groups for serological analysis. The results of these tests will be reported in due course.

Irradiation therapy

Prior to operation high-dose irradiation of the primary site (≥ 4500 rad) was performed in 21 per cent of the patients comprising the interferon group, and low-dose irradiation (1000-4500 rad) in 14 per cent. None of the interferon group has been given preoperative irradiation therapy during the last 3 years, and it is intended to discontinue this form of treatment. Of the concurrent control group 44 per cent were given high-dose and 4 per cent low-dose irradiation. Irradiation prior to operation appears not to be a significant prognostic factor in osteosarcoma (FRIEDMAN and CARTER, 1972).

Surgical treatment

The form of surgical treatment for osteosarcoma has almost invariably been amputation. Whereas this was earlier performed as disarticulation at the level of the joint immediately above the lesion, more recently the amputation has been made through the affected bone, leaving a safe margin.

We have preferred a local tumour resection when this is anatomically practicable, and in the present series this procedure was used in 11 patients (39 per cent). Owing to extensive involvement of the soft tissues by the tumour amputation could not always be avoided, and it was resorted to in 17 cases. Where the diaphyseal or adjoining metaphyseal region was involved a block resection was performed, the defect being replaced by an autogenous bone graft.

When the tumour was localized to the metaphyseal region or encroached on the epiphysis, the block resection also took in the joint surface compartment. For the reconstruction, autogenous grafts or artificial implants were used. In 2 patients with osteosarcoma of the tibial condyle the joint surface was replaced by the autogenous patella. In another case an autogenous fibula was used for reconstruction after resecting the proximal part of the humerus. In a patient with quite an extensive osteosarcoma which involved the distal part of the femur a specially designed endoprosthesis was used. In pelvic osteosarcoma, too, local resection could occasionally be performed.

In 2 cases a local recurrence necessitated subsequent amputation. In one patient there was soft tissue recurrence of the osteosarcoma, which was resected. In one case where a local resection was performed pulmonary metastases developed but no evidence of local tumour growth was found at autopsy.

Metastases and survival rate

A comparison of the interferon and the concurrent groups with respect to development of metastases and the survival rate was performed. The historical group could not be used for such a comparison for the reasons mentioned above in connection with the prognostic analysis.

The primary form of treatment for the two groups was irradiation, surgery or both. None of the patients in either group was given chemotherapy. In all the patients where only irradiation was performed metastases developed during or after the treatment and an operation was originally intended. On detection of the metastases selective surgery, irradiation, high-dose chemotherapy or some other form of treatment was tried (3 patients in each group). Some of the prognostic factors — sex, age, duration of symptoms and tumour site — occurred to the same extent in the two groups. The tumour size differed somewhat, however, with a tendency for the tumours in the interferon group to be somewhat larger (10 cm against 8 cm mean larger diameter). Grade IV tumours were slightly more frequent in the concurrent group. Local resection was performed in 39 per cent of the interferon group, but in only one patient in the control group.

According to life table analysis (PETO et al., 1977) 64 per cent of the patients given interferon should still be free from metastases after $2\frac{1}{2}$ years, compared with only 30 per cent of the concurrent control group. A similar analysis of survival shows that 73 per cent of the interferon group should still be living after $2\frac{1}{2}$ years, against 35 per cent of the concurrent control group.

As regards prognostic factors the two groups do not differ appreciably. There are clear numerical differences between the groups as regards the development of metastases and the survival rate, but the follow-up period is at present too short to warrant any definitive inferences. The study is being continued, and the groups are constantly being added to.

Summary

This paper outlines relevant parameters and the results obtained to date in a clinical trial whose purpose is to examine the efficacy of exogenous leukocyte interferon therapy for osteosarcoma patients.

Interferon therapy has a low toxicity, and preliminary results of this study indicate that most, if not all, of the side effects of the treatment will disappear on further purification of interferon.

For this reason, among others, large scale production of human interferon would seem to be justified.

The incidence of metastases and the survival rate have been determined in the consecutive interferon series and a group consisting of the remaining osteosarcoma patients in Sweden. The results obtained so far are better for the interferon group — although not significantly so — notwithstanding the fact that in more than one third of the patients treated with interferon resection was performed in preference to amputation or disarticulation.

ACKNOWLEDGEMENTS

This study was supported by the Swedish Cancer Society, the Cancer Society of Stockholm, and Dagmar Hasselgren's Fund.

[17] *Strander* - p. 12

REFERENCES

APARISI T., BROSTRÖM L.-A., INGIMARSSON S., LAGERGREN C., NILSONNE U., STRANDER H. and SÖDERBERG G., *Prognostic factors in osteosarcoma. Can historical controls be used in current clinical trials?* « Intern. J. Rad. Oncol. Biol. Phys. », in press (1977).

BODEY G. P., *Infections in patients with cancer.* In: « Cancer medicine ». J. F. Holland and E. Frei (Eds.). Philadelphia, Lea and Febiger, 1973, p. 1135.

CANTELL K. and HIRVONEN S., *Preparation of human leukocyte interferon for clinical use.* « Texas Rep. Biol. Med. », 35, 138 (1978).

CANTELL K., HIRVONEN S., MOGENSES K. E. and PYHÄLÄ L., *Human leukocyte interferon: production, purification, stability and animal experiments.* « In Vitro », 3, 35 (1974 a).

CANTELL K., PYHÄLÄ L. and STRANDER H., *Circulating human interferon after intramuscular injection into animals and man.* « J. gen. Virol. », 22, 453 (1974 b).

CANTELL K. and STRANDER H., *Human leukocyte interferon for clinical use.* In: « Conference on blood leukocytes - Function and Use in Therapy ». C.F. Hogman, K. Lindahl-Kiessling and H. Wigzell (Eds.). Uppsala, 1977, p. 73.

CORTES E. P., HOLLAND J. F., WANG J. J., SINK L. F., BLOM J., SENN H., BANK A. and GLIDEWELL O., *Amputation and adriamycin in primary osteosarcoma.* « N. Engl. J. Med. », 291, 998 (1974).

DAHLIN D. C., *Bone Tumours - General Aspects and Data on 3987 Cases.* Illinois, Springfield, Charles C. Thomas, 2nd ed., 1973.

DAHLIN D. and COVENTRY M., *Osteogenic sarcoma. A study of 600 cases.* « J. Bone Joint Surgery », 49A, 101 (1967).

EINHORN S. and STRANDER H., *Is interferon tissue specific? Effect of human leukocyte and fibroblast interferons on the growth of lymphoblastoid and osteosarcoma cell lines.* « J. gen. Virol », 35, 573 (1977).

EINHORN S. and STRANDER H., *Interferon therapy for neoplastic disease in man -* in vitro *and* in vivo *studies.* In: « Production of Human Interferon and Investigations of Its Clinical Use ». A Symposium Workshop. W. Alton Jones Cell Science Center, Lake Placid, USA, May 19-20, in press 1977.

FILIPSON R., *Eruption Curve of the Permanent Teeth.* A Method for Evaluation of Somatic Development in Children. Thesis, Stockholm, 1974.

FRAUMENI J., *Stature and malignant tumors of bone in childhood and adolescense.* « Cancer », 20, 967 (1967).

Frei III E., Jaffe N., Skipper H. E. and Gero M. G., *Adjuvant chemotherapy of osteogenic sarcoma: progress and perspectives.* In: « Adjuvant Therapy of Cancer ». S. E. Salmon and S. E. Jones (Eds.). Amsterdam, Elsevier North-Holland Biomedical Press, 1977, p. 49.

Friedman M. A. and Carter S. K., *The therapy of osteogenic sarcoma: current status and thoughts for the future.* « J. Surg. Oncol. », *4*, 482 (1972).

Ghadially F. N. and Mehta P. N., *Ultrastructure of osteogenic sarcoma.* « Cancer », *25*, 1457 (1970).

Gresser I., *Antitumor Effects of Interferon.* In: « Cancer. A Comprehensive Treatise ». F. Becker (Ed.), in press (1977).

Handelsman H. and Carter S. K., *Current therapies in osteosarcoma.* « Cancer Treatm. Rev. », *2*, 88 (1975).

Havell E. A. and Vilcek J., *Production of high titered interferon in cultures of human diploid cells.* « Antimicrob. Ag. Chemother. », *2*, 476 (1972).

Jaffe N., Frei III E., Traggis D. and Bishop Y., *Adjuvant methotrexate and citrovorum-factor treatment of osteogenic sarcoma.* « N. Engl. J. Med. », *291*, 994 (1974).

Kay S., *Ultrastructure of an osteoid type of osteogenic sarcoma.* « Cancer », *28*, 437 (1971).

Kauppinen H.-L., Myllylä G. and Cantell K., *Large scale production and properties of human leukocyte interferon used in clinical trials.* In: « Production of Human Interferon and Investigations of its Clinical Use ». A Symposium Workshop. W. Alton Jones Cell Science Center, Lake Placid, USA, May 19-20, in press (1977).

Lindbom A., Söderberg G. and Spjut J., *Osteosarcoma. A review of 96 cases.* « Acta Radiol. », *56*, 1 (1961).

Lockshin M. D. and Higgins I. T. T., *Prognosis in osteogenic sarcoma.* « Clin. Orthop. Related Res. », *58*, 85 (1968).

McMaster J., Scranton P. and Drash A., *Growth and hormone control mechanisms in osteosarcoma.* « Clin. Orthop. », *106*, 366 (1975).

Mogensen K. E. and Cantell K., *Production and preparation of human leukocyte interferon.* « Pharmacol. Ther. C. », *1*, 369 (1977).

Paschall H. A. and Paschall M. M., *Electron microscopic observations of 20 human osteosarcomas.* « Clin. Orthop. », *111*, 42 (1975).

Paucker K., Cantell K. and Henle W., *Quantitative studies on viral interference in suspended L cells. III. Effect of interfering viruses and interferon on the growth rate of cells.* « Virology », *17*, 324 (1962).

Peto R., Pike M. C., Armitage P., Breslow N. E., Cox D. R., Howard S. V., Mantel N., McPherson K., Peto J. and Smith P. G., *Design and analysis of randomized clinical trials requiring prolonged observation of each patient. II. Analysis and examples.* « Br. J. Cancer », *35*, 1 (1977).

Scranton P., McMaster J. and Diamond P., *Hormone suppression of DNA synthesis in cultured chondrocyte and osteosarcoma cell lines.* « Clin. Orthop. », *112*, 340 (1975).

Strander H., *Interferons: anti-neoplastic drugs?* « Blut », *35*, 277 (1977).

STRANDER H., *Anti-tumour effects of interferon and its possible use as an anti-neoplastic agent in man*. « Texas Rep. Biol. Med. », *35*, 429 (1978).

STRANDER H., CANTELL K., CARLSTRÖM G., INGIMARSSON S., JAKOBSSON P.-Å. and NILSONNE U., *Acute infections in interferon-treated patients with osteosarcoma. Preliminary report of a comparative study*. « J. Infect. Dis. », *133*, Supplement A, 245 (1976).

STRANDER H., CANTELL K., CARLSTRÖM G. and JAKOBSSON P.-Å., *Systemic administration of potent interferon to man*. « J. Natl. Cancer Inst. », *51*, 733 (1973).

STRANDER H., CANTELL K., INGIMARSSON S., JAKOBSSON P.-Å., NILSONNE U. and SÖDERBERG G., *Interferon treatment of osteogenic sarcoma: a clinical trial*. « Fogarty Intern. Center Proc., Washington D.C. », *28*, 377 (1977).

STRANDER H., CANTELL K., JAKOBSSON P.-Å., NILSONNE U. and SÖDERBERG G., *Exogenous interferon therapy of osteogenic sarcoma*. « Acta Orthop. Scand. », *45*, 958 (1974).

STRANDER H. and EINHORN S., *Effect of human leukocyte interferon on the growth of human osteosarcoma cells in tissue culture*. « Int. J. Cancer », *19*, 468 (1977).

DISCUSSION

NOSSAL

Dr. Strander, this question may sound impolite and perhaps not appreciated after such a beautiful and exciting demonstration six years after you started the trial; but when you started in 1971, what reason did you have to think that this would work so well that you did not start a randomized trial? It is very hard for me to understand that. You had to show about 25 slides in order to convince us that your historical and contemporary controls are of some value. I mean there are so many things that enter into the treatment and diagnosis of a cancer patient — some of them measurable, some of them subliminal: the quality of chemotherapy, the quality of diagnosis, the selection of patients because they are coming to you, because they know something special is going on — the extra-motivation of patients — a hundred and one variables. Can you please explain to us now, even though you have been justified, or apparently have been justified, why was not a randomized trial performed?

STRANDER

Well, first of all, I think it is very easy for us *now* to draw these conclusions. All trials going on at that time in osteosarcoma were never randomized. For example, there is not a single chemotherapeutic trial where randomization was made. The reason for this was that every clinic all over the world had the same miserable results without adjuvant therapy. Secondly, in our case it was a rather small matter, I think, which made us decide not to randomize — and that was the successful treatment of the first patient who had osteosarcoma. In that case, the surgeon just made a curettage. He could not remove the tumor completely. We started interferon treatment, and after six months the patient still did not have pulmonary metastases. This led to the idea of doing resections and giving interferon therapy. The surgeons then refused to do local resections if the patients did not receive adjuvant interferon therapy. It is very difficult then at a clinic to amputate some patients and to resect some others. The patients talk to each other and would wonder why some have to be amputated. It is also an ethical question for the surgeons.

MATHÉ

What about nonviral infection? Have you looked for the frequency of nonviral infections?

STRANDER

We have only so far asked the patients — we have had questionnaires filled every month and we have talked to the parents and patients and collected symptoms. Not a single serological test has been done on these patients, except for the virus side, where it was obvious to do it. But since a complement-fixation inhibitor is present, and since there are so many things one can think of doing, the sera are very precious. We think they still should be kept frozen and untouched.

MATHÉ

Do you still have the patients for tests?

STRANDER

Yes, we have only tested the sensitivity of the lymphocytes to antigens and mitogens. We have considered doing other tests but we have really not known what kind of immunological tests we should do on the patients. There have been discussions about it.

TERRY

What is your minimal followup now on the patients in the trial in both the concurrent and the treatment group?

STRANDER

Well, in the treatment group I have here 28 patients and they have been followed between eight months and 5½ years, and they are scattered through this time period. They are fairly evenly distributed between 8 months and 5½ years. I could give you the precise number at any point but I have to look it up.

TERRY

You say that you are accruing about four patients a year into your treatment group?

STRANDER

Yes, that would be right.

TERRY

I assume that those rather impressive looking curves you showed us were actuarial curves.

STRANDER

Yes.

TERRY

And what is the statistical evaluation of those curves at this time?

STRANDER

If we want to have some statistical significance, let us put it this way: I think we would need about 40-45 patients in the treated group and in the concurrent control — if it would go on, the same way as it has up to now. We have not analyzed the concurrent cases from '75 and '76, but we have of course collected the data. If anything, they might be worse off than the concurrent cases collected up to that time; on the other

[17] *Strander* - p. 19

hand they might be worse off in prognostic factors — it is difficult for me to say. But if it would go on as before, it would be, I think, somewhere between 40 and maybe up to 45 patients required in each group.

ROSENBERG

Does your answer to that last question mean that it is not statistically significant now?

STRANDER

Yes.

ROSENBERG

Did you mention that interferon showed that you got *in vitro* killing with osteosarcoma lines *in vitro*?

STRANDER

No, it is only inhibition of growth.

ROSENBERG

Okay, on the inhibition of growth. What do you see when you test under similar conditions, normal lines from those same patients? Do you see a difference between the osteosarcomas and the normal lines?

STRANDER

What we have done so far is only to send biopsy material to Uppsala, where they have a big tissue culture lab; but the lines we have tested in Stockholm are osteosarcoma lines which have been well characterized, we have received them from Houston, New York and Uppsala because it is very difficult to primarily grow osteosarcoma cell lines. One has to do a lot of tests and characterize them very properly. I think there are very few lines which are available.

[17] *Strander* - p. 20

ROSENBERG

Have you any reason to believe that the osteosarcoma show any different susceptibility than normal human lines, which are very easy to grow?

STRANDER

No, I think that osteosarcomas would come in the same class as myeloma and also mammary carcinoma. On the other hand, the melanomas tested so far have been resistant.

TERRY

But how about normal cells?

STRANDER

Normal cells are not as sensitive as osteosarcoma cells, but if you add more interferon you can inhibit these also.

WESTPHAL

I wonder whether you know anything about long-term application of exogenous interferon? Would there be any consequence for the endogenous interferon production — in other words, if you test the patients before and after long-term treatment, do they react normally to interferon inducers?

STRANDER

This has not been tested on these patients, and I do not know of anybody who has done it, in the virus studies either. This is very important, of course. It is very difficult to do such tests, though.

DE MARSILLAC

Knowing as I know the difficulties of treating osteosarcoma clinically, I would like to make a suggestion. Because we know that there is a special kind of osteosarcoma, which is much more favorable concerning dissemination and prognosis, which is the so-called paraosteal or juxtacortical osteosarcoma, I would like to suggest to put this in a kind of trial. I think it changes very much the prognosis.

STRANDER

All the paraosteal or juxtacortical osteosarcomas are excluded from this study. We do not have a single one.

EDMUND KLEIN

I would like to ask Dr. Strander if, knowing what he does now, if he started to study other tumors would he randomize?

STRANDER

Well, the oat cell carcinomas will be randomized and also the larynx papillomas when we know the dose required.

EDMUND KLEIN

What about the osteosarcoma?

STRANDER

The osteosarcomas cannot be randomized. At the hospital in Stockholm, with the people that we have there — staff, relatives and so on — it is impossible.

EDMUND KLEIN

But if you had the doctors and the personnel, would you randomize on the basis of the interferon stock you have available?

[17] *Strander* - p. 22

STRANDER

I would, since we could then randomize all patients in Sweden and still treat the same number of patients totally with the interferon stock we have available.

LEVI-MONTALCINI

I would just like to know how you obtain the large amount of interferon needed for the treatment.

STRANDER

It is made by Prof. Kari Cantell's group in Helsinki — I worked there for five years on the production system — we have continued our close collaboration. This is the reason why we receive it. But now there is also a large production going on at the Red Cross Transfusion Service in Helsinki. Blood bags from about 400 leukocyte donors a day are used for interferon production. The reason why Finland has been so excellent in production is that they have a centralized blood transfusion service that can get all the local "buffy coats" for this production.

OETTGEN

As to the toxicity of interferon, there was one patient, I believe, who experienced visual disturbances — what was their nature?

STRANDER

It was very difficult to get this information — he had some problems when he looked at television. When the ophthalmologist investigated him he could not verify any visual disturbance.

OETTGEN

Are the cell lines that produce interferon themselves inhibited by interferon, or are they more resistant than non-producer cell lines?

STRANDER

There is a slight correlation between production and resistance, so very good interferon producer lines tend to be interferon resistant. So you can mix, for example, a cell line like Namalva, which produces interferon spontaneously and is resistant, with Daudi, which is very sensitive and does not produce. The Namalva will then completely wipe out Daudi. The lines sensitive to leukocyte interferon have also, to a variable extent, always been sensitive to other interferons.

SOME ASPECTS OF THE INTERACTIONS BETWEEN CANCER, DRUGS AND IMMUNITY

FEDERICO SPREAFICO and ENZO BONMASSAR

The Mario Negri Institute of Pharmacological Research
Milan, Italy

Department of Pharmacology, University of Perugia
Perugia, Italy

Introduction

Cancer immunotherapy, at least in the form at present more widely adopted in humans and based on the use of non specific immunomodulatory agents, is the object of active discussion among both experimental and clinical oncologists. Although it is widely accepted that host reactivity towards established tumors can be beneficial to the patient and that efforts are thus justified in attempting to increase and/or modulate this reactivity, disagreement exists regarding the ways and means of immunological manipulation having the greater therapeutic potential.

A number of possible answers can be found in this volume to the question: how can the effectiveness of immunological intervention in cancer treatment be improved? With the same general aim, this paper will examine two aspects of the complex web of interactions between the neoplasm, anticancer drugs and host reactivity which may both be of some relevance for the design of more effective approaches to the immunotherapy of malignancy.

Experiments on drug interactions in cancer chemoimmunotherapy

It is well known that in the majority of clinical conditions in which it is applied, immunotherapy is employed in combination with other treatment modalities. More specifically, treatment with non specific immunomodulators is most frequently preceded by chemotherapy. Although some findings may suggest that, at least in certain experimental conditions, the use of these agents before chemotherapy, or surgery, may also have a rationale [1], this type of treatment sequencing has not yet been systematically explored. Conversely, the injection of immunostimulants after chemotherapy is based on a now relatively large body of evidence [2] indicating that the immune system can be expected to effectively cope with relatively limited neoplastic burdens, hence the necessity of applying cytoreductive treatments before attempting immunological manipulations. A number of aspects with direct relevance to the design of the most effective chemoimmunotherapeutic protocols, e.g. timing between treatments, their frequency and duration, pairing of drugs, are however still to be more extensively analyzed.

It is widely known that at least the majority of cancer chemotherapeutic agents impair host defence mechanisms, a fact whose importance in the therapeutic efficacy of these drugs has recently been reemphasized [1]. However, evidence is accumulating that both quantitative and qualitative differences can be recognized between cytotoxic agents in their interaction with the various immunocyte subpopulations [3]. The antineoplastic mode of action of immunomodulators whether of bacterial origin such as BCG and *Corynebacterium parvum* (*C. parvum*) or of chemical nature (e.g. Levamisole or Pyran copolymer), is still not completely elucidated. However, sufficient evidence is already available to indicate that this class of agents is, to a certain extent, heterogenous in its effect on the various cells mediating the different antitumor immune effector mechanisms. For instance, the macrophage appears to play a major role in the mode of action of *C. parvum* [4] whereas T cells would seem to be a main target in the case of Levamisole (Leva) [5]. An example of the relative heterogeneity of nonspecific immunomodulators may be given by their effect on K cells, i.e. the elements mediating Antibody-dependent Cellular Cytotoxicity. BCG, *C. parvum* and Pyran copolymer stimulate these cells although the kinetics and the potency of the stimulatory effect are quite different, whereas Leva is inactive in this respect [6]. Differences between these agents on suppressor cell activity in the thymus have also been

[18] *Spreafico, Bonmassar* - p. 2

recently described [7]. Given this type of background, the hypothesis at the basis of the work discussed in this section was that a
better understanding, a more in depth analysis of the different interactions of cancer chemotherapeutic and immunostimulatory agents
with relevant host defence mechanisms could be of value in the
design of more effective chemoimmunotherapeutic protocols.

In the past few years we have been involved in investigating
Adriamycin (Adria) and Daunomycin (Dauno) (Fig. 1), two agents
on which much attention has recently been focused in view of their
high activity on a wide range of animal and human neoplasms [8].
More specifically, we have been interested in trying to understand
the possible bases on which Adria is a more effective antitumoral
than its earlier and structurally closely related analog. Although
differences in metabolism and pharmacokinetics have been recognized
for the two agents [9, 10], these have failed to provide a complete
explanation for the different antineoplastic effectiveness of the two
drugs seen in most *in vivo* conditions. *In vitro*, these analogs have

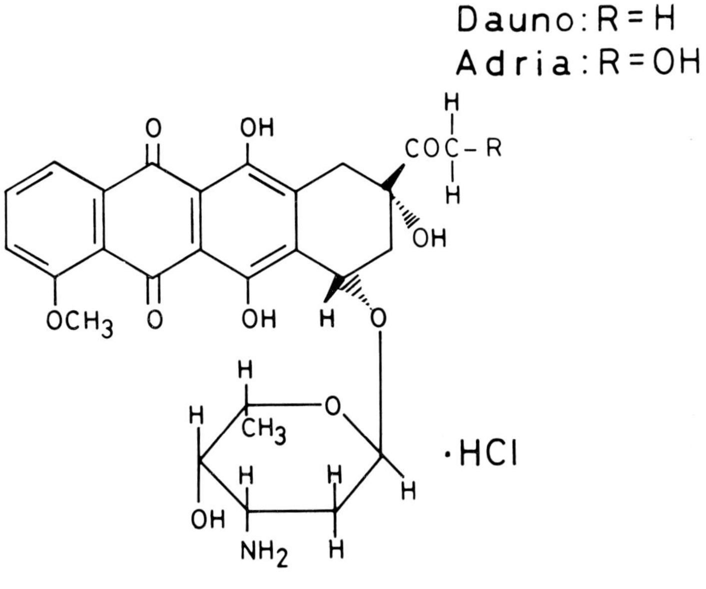

FIG. 1 — Chemical structure of Adriamycin and Daunomycin.

also been shown to be equally cytotoxic for tumor cells when prolonged exposure times are used as for instance shown by the data
of Table 1 employing two different lymphoma lines.   Moreover,
spontaneous lymphocyte DNA synthesis is equally inhibited by these
antibiotics and Concanavallin A and LPS-induced blastogenesis
in vitro are similarly depressed by Adria and Dauno.   In the course
of our investigations, a complex *in vivo* differential interaction of
the two drugs with immune reactivity was evidentiated [11-13];
the differences observed, although allowing us to advance the contention that this differential interaction could be an important determinant of the relative antineoplastic effectiveness of the two compounds,
still did not provide a completely satisfying explanatory picture.
To further elucidate this problem and considering also the important
role currently attributed to macrophages in the control of neoplastic
progression [14, 15], it was of interest to investigate the effect
of both agents on these elements.   It has been found that marked
differences in the sensitivity of macrophages to Adria and Dauno
exist.   Employing firstly peritoneal murine macrophages, Dauno was
markedly more toxic *in vitro* than Adria as judged by an assessment
of the number of surviving macrophages by the ^{89}Rb technique or
by microscopic examination of the cultures (table 1).   Although a
preferential accumulation of Dauno into lysosomes has been described
[16], the mechanism(s) responsible for the different sensitivity

TABLE 1 — In vitro *cytotoxic activity of Adriamycin and Daunomycin on different murine cells.*

Target cell	Assay	ED$_{50}$ (μg/ml)	
		Adria	Dauno
dSL 2 lymphoma	^{125}IUdR uptake	0.06	0.07
TLX9 lymphoma	^{125}IUdR uptake	0.05	0.04
Norm. splenocytes	^{125}IUdR uptake	0.15	0.12
Macrophages	^{89}Rb uptake	0.65 *	0.13

* = p < 0.01
exposure time was 24 hrs.

[18] *Spreafico, Bonmassar* - p. 4

of this cell type to these drugs, a differential which initial data indicate is present also for human macrophages, are still a matter of discussion. One subsequent step was to examine whether the functional capacity of these elements was also differentially affected by these drugs. To this end, mice were given *C. parvum* and injected 12 days later with graded doses of these antitumorals and the non specific cytotoxicity of activated phagocytes towards tumor cells evaluated. As shown in table 2, a marked, dose-dependent inhibition of macrophage cytotoxic capacity was found after injection of Dauno, whereas cells obtained from Adria-treated mice were not significantly different from controls in their damaging activity on tumor cells. This differential inhibitory capacity is observable employing a range of Attacker to Target cell (A:T) ratios and testing the cytotoxic activity at different times after drug injection [17]. It would thus appear that both *in vivo* and *in vitro* Adria is significantly less damaging for macrophages than Dauno: after injection of the former drug to mice lower numbers of these cells will be destroyed and the functional capacity of the surviving elements will be better preserved. More direct evidence for the importance of macrophages in the antitumoral activity of these drugs could be obtained when animals depleted in these cells by pretreatment with the selective macrophage toxins Silica and Carrageenan were investigated. Table 3 shows, for instance, that the injection of optimal

TABLE 2 — *Effect of Adriamycin and Daunomycin on spleen macrophage cytotoxic activity versus murine tumor target cells.*

Exp. group	% inhibit. ^{125}IUdR uptake on day		
	1	2	7
Control	60 ± 3	68 ± 4	61 ± 2
Adria	58 ± 4	52 ± 3	70 ± 3
Dauno	29 ± 4	19 ± 5	28 ± 2

CD2F$_1$ mice were injected with 0.7 mg i.v. *C. parvum* on day -12, drugs were given on day 0 at the dose of 10 mg/kg i.v.; target cells were TLX9 lymphoma cells and the A:T ratio 50:1.

TABLE 3 — *Effect of Silica and Carrageenan on the antitumoral activity of Adriamycin and Daunomycin in the SL2 lymphoma system.*

Adria 10 mg/kg i.v.	Dauno 15 mg/kg i.v.	Silica 5 mg i.v.	Carrag. 0.25 mg i.v.	M S T
—	—	—	—	13.8
+	—	—	—	24.0
+	—	0.2	—	15.6 *
+	—	5.7	—	18.6 *
+	—	—	0.2	18.4 *
—	+	—	—	22.3
—	+	0.2	—	20.9
—	+	—	0.2	21.5

* = p < 0.05

10^5 SL2 lymphoma cells i.p. on day 0; Adria or Dauno on day 1.

Adria doses to $CD2F_1$ mice bearing the compatible SL2 lymphoma is followed by a clear increase in survival time; however, when the same drug dose is administered to Silica or Carrageenan-pretreated animals, a marked reduction in lifespan or indeed the disappearance of chemotherapeutic effect is observed. On the other hand, no significant changes in the therapeutic activity were found when Dauno was employed in the same or other tumor systems. Since the treatments employed with these macrophage toxins did not influence the pharmacokinetics of Adria, these data are compatible with the hypothesis that a sparing of macrophages is an important factor of the higher antitumoral efficacy of Adria over Dauno.

These results suggested the possibility that the two analogs might differ in their capacity to synergize with a well known macrophage activator as *C. parvum*; therapeutic synergism could in fact have been expected in the case of the Adria-*C. parvum* combination and not with Dauno-*C. parvum*. This prediction appeared to be borne out in reality. Fig. 2 shows, for instance, that in the L 1210 Ha lymphoma system, the combination Adria-*C. parvum* was clearly superior in terms of increase in survival as well as of percentages

[18] *Spreafico, Bonmassar - p. 6*

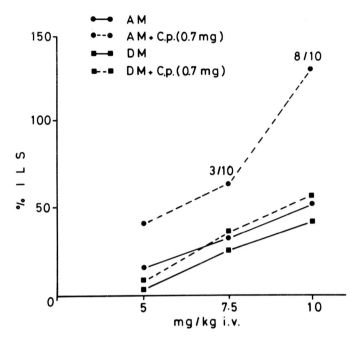

Fig. 2 — Antitumoral effectiveness of Adriamycin and Daunomycin when combined with *C. parvum* in CD2F₁ mice transplanted with 10^5 L 1210 Ha leukemia. Drugs were given on day 1 and *C. parvum* on day 6.

of cures than the Dauno-*C. parvum* combination, which showed at best only borderline therapeutic advantage over chemotherapy per se. A similar superiority of Adria over Dauno in chemoimmunotherapy with *C. parvum* has been confirmed in a number of other experimental neoplastic models including solid tumors.

In another series of experiments, the capacity of Adria to synergize with other immunomodulators known to be effective in influencing tumor progression in various experimental conditions, was evaluated in the L 1210 Ha leukemia model. It was found (table 4) that although increases in the therapeutic efficacy of Adria could be obtained with BCG and Leva, employing the optimal doses and schedules the results with these drug combinations were inferior to those observable with Adria-*C. parvum* [18]. In parallel, the effect of the latter immunomodulator when combined with other

[18] *Spreafico, Bonmassar* - p. 7

TABLE 4 — *Antitumoral effect of Adriamycin when combined with different immunomodulators in the L 1210 Ha leukemia system.*

Adria	C. parvum	BCG	Leva	% T/C	% cures
+1	—	—	—	162	0
—	+6	—	—	102	0
—	—	+6	—	98	0
—	—	—	3-6	104	0
+1	+6	—	—	200	90
+1	—	+6	—	184	60
+1	—	—	3-6	210	10

10^5 leukemia cells were transplanted i.p. on day 0; *C. parvum*: 0.7 mg i.v.; BCG: 1 mg i.v.; Leva: 3 mg/kg i.p.; Adria: 10 mg/kg i.v.

antitumorals was explored, employing doses of these drugs producing comparable increases in lifespan in these experimental conditions. As a further indication of the possible importance of an appropriate choice of agents in combination chemoimmunotherapy, table 5 shows that the 5-Fu-*C. parvum* combination was not therapeutically better

TABLE 5 — *Antitumoral effect of different chemotherapeutic agents when combined with C.* parvum *in the L 1210 Ha leukemia system.*

Day 1	Day 6	% ILS	% cures
Adria	—	70	0
Cy	—	83	0
5-Fu	—	75	0
Adria	C. parvum	120	80
Cy	C. parvum	140	45
5-Fu	C. parvum	145	0

10^5 leukemia cells i.p. on day 0; Adria: 10 mg/kg; Cy: 55 mg/kg; 5-Fu: 200 mg/kg; *C. parvum*: 0.7 mg

[18] *Spreafico, Bonmassar* - p. 8

than chemotherapy alone, whereas Cyclophosphamide (Cy) showed synergistic antitumoral activity when followed by C. parvum but the percentage of cures given by this combination was significantly lower than that seen with Adria-C. parvum.

As frequently observed in chemoimmunotherapy [19] the timing of administration of the two agents is critical in controlling the therapeutic efficacy of the Adria-C. parvum combination. This is for instance shown in table 6 for the L 1210 Ha leukemia system in which, as true also for other tumor models, optimal therapeutic activity was found either when C. parvum preceded Adria by 8 days or when Adria was injected 5 days prior to the immunostimulants. In an effort to explain the basis for this type of finding and to obtain indications as to the possible mechanisms sustaining the Adria-C. parvum synergism, the effect of Adria on the induction and expression of C. parvum-induced macrophage cytotoxicity were investigated. As presented in table 7, treatment with Adria 2 days after or up to 3 days prior to the injection of the immunostimulant (i.e. employing non synergistic in vivo schedules) resulted in marked impairments of spleen macrophage-mediated cytotoxic activity assessed in terms of inhibition of ^{125}IUdR uptake in SL2 lymphoma target cells. This dose-dependent inhibitory effect of Adria given shortly before C. parvum (24 hrs before) on the induction of macrophage

TABLE 6 — Antitumoral effect of different schedules of Adria - C. parvum treatment in the SL2 lymphoma system.

Adria on day	C. parvum on day	M S T	% cures
—	—	13	0
+1	—	22	0
+1	+6	35	40
+1	+3	25	0
+1	+1	19	0
+1	−1	20	0
+1	−7	33	40

10^5 SL2 cells i.p. on day 0; Adria: 10 mg/kg i.v.; C. parvum: 0.7 mg i.v.

[18] Spreafico, Bonmassar - p. 9

TABLE 7 — *Effect of Adriamycin on the induction and expression of* C. parvum-*induced macrophage cytotoxicity on tumor target cells.*

Day of Adria inject	% Inhibition ^{125}IUdR uptake
—	83 ± 2
− 5	85 ± 1
− 3	72 ± 1 *
− 1	55 ± 2 *
+ 2	50 ± 2 *
+11	84 ± 1

* = p < 0.05

C. parvum (0.7 mg i.v.) was given on day 0 and tests were performed on day 12; A:T ratio was 50:1 and SL2 lymphoma cells were used as targets.

cytotoxicity, was detectable even using quite high Attacker to Target cell ratios (table 8). Conversely, when *in vivo* synergistic schedules were used (e.g. Adria preceding *C. parvum* by 5 days), the cytotoxicity values observed were similar to those found in Adria-untreated, *C. parvum*-injected controls. Similarly, when Adria was administered after the induction of macrophage cytotoxicity by *C. parvum* (day 11) no reductions in the expression of phagocyte-mediated cytotoxicity were seen. Table 9 shows the time course of the Adria effect when a non-synergistic (1 day interval between treatments) and a synergistic (5 days interval) schedule were employed; it is apparent the prolonged inhibition of cytotoxic capacity in the first case and the fact that in the second case, actual increases in cytotoxicity could also be obtained at certain times. Thus it would appear that maximal therapeutic synergism was seen when Adria was combined with *C. parvum* according to schedules which did not interfere with the induction or expression of the cytotoxic activity of macrophages [20]. While these data support our contention that this cell type plays an important role in this chemo-immunotherapy protocol, it is possible that a complementarity of the two agents at the level of other immune effector mechanisms

[18] *Spreafico, Bonmassar* - p. 10

TABLE 8 — *Effect of Adriamycin on* C. parvum-*induced macrophage cytotoxicity.*

Day of Adria injec.	A : T	% Inhibition ^{125}IUdR uptake
—	75 : 1	89 ± 2
	50 : 1	94 ± 1
	25 : 1	78 ± 1
− 5	75 : 1	85 ± 1
	50 : 1	88 ± 3
	25 : 1	72 ± 1
− 1	75 : 1	82 ± 3
	50 : 1	45 ± 1 *
	25 : 1	15 ± 1 *

* = $p < 0.01$

C. parvum (0.7 mg i.v.) was given on day 0 and tests performed on day 12 using SL2 lymphoma cells as targets.

TABLE 9 — *Macrophage cytotoxicity at various times after different* Adria-C. parvum *treatments.*

Day of Adria inject.	% inhibition ^{125}IUdR uptake on day			
	6	7	12	19
—	55	77	91	58
−1	12 *	52 *	69 *	65
−5	85 *	83	88	52

* = $p < 0.05$

Spleen macrophage cytotoxicity was assessed against SL2 lymphoma target cells at an A:T ratio of 50:1; Adria: 10 mg/kg i.v.; *C. parvum*: 0.7 mg i.v. on day 0.

[18] *Spreafico, Bonmassar* - p. 11

27

may also be of some relevance. This possibility could be hypothesized considering that *C. parvum* activates the cellular arm of ADCC [21] and Adria has been found to relatively spare K cells whereas treatment with Dauno results in marked depressions in this activity [13]. Preliminary results indicate that no reduction in ADCC activity in respect to *C. parvum* alone is seen when the Adria-*C. parvum* combination is given in a synergistic schedule.

In conclusion cancer chemotherapeutic agents even when closely related structurally as Adria and Dauno, can markedly differ in their interactions with host defence mechanisms. Since also currently available immunomodulators appear to be heterogeneous in their influence on different immunocyte subpopulations, it may be expected that the pairing of agents in combination chemoimmunotherapy could critically affect the therapeutic outcome of these approaches. The findings presented suggest that a better understanding of the effect of chemoimmunotherapeutic combinations with relevant antitumor effector mechanisms can be instrumental to the design of more effective therapeutic protocols.

Cancer chemotherapeutic agents and tumor cell immunogenicity

Among the various and not mutually exclusive mechanisms which have been advanced to account for the inability of the host to successfully control tumors, the low immunogenicity of neoplastic cells is generally considered to play an important role, especially in the case of the so-called spontaneous malignancies [22]. Various approaches aimed at increasing this immunogenicity and/or at conferring new antigenic specificities to tumor cells have accordingly been proposed [23-26], although the majority of the procedures described would appear to have experimental rather than clinical interest because of practical difficulties of exploitation and/or theoretical limitations.

In view of the fact that cancer chemotherapeutic agents exhibit *in vivo* a degree of selectivity for neoplastic elements and that the majority of these compounds are known to directly or indirectly affect nucleic acid synthesis and/or function, the hypothesis could have been advanced that drug-induced disruption of cellular metabol-

[18] *Spreafico, Bonmassar* · p. 12

ic machinery could also have resulted in modifications of the cell antigenic profile. In other words, the hypothesis was conceivable that exposure of neoplastic cells to not immediately lethal concentrations of anticancer agents could lead, through a variety of possible mechanisms (drug-induced mutations, changes in codon recognition at ribosomal level, etc.), to modifications in membrane composition and/or architecture resulting ultimately in modified immunogenicity-antigenicity.

The studies hereafter summarized provide evidence that *in vivo* treatments with cancer chemotherapeutic drugs can modify tumor cell immunogenicity-antigenicity, a fact which should be considered not only for a better understanding of the mode of action of these agents but which could also be of relevance in the planning of more effective chemoimmunotherapeutic approaches. Although this discussion will be centered on one antineoplastic drug, i.e. 5-(3,3-dimethyl-1-triazeno-imidazole)-4-carboxamide (DTIC) in view of its higher capacity to influence tumor cell immunogenicity, it should be emphasized that a similar capacity has been demonstrated for a large number of chemotherapeutic compounds possessing different mechanisms of cytotoxic action [27].

A typical experiment [28] showing DTIC-mediated antigenic transformation of tumors is presented in fig. 3. When Balb/c mice transplanted i.p. with 10^6 cells of the compatible Moloney virus-induced LSTRA lymphoma are treated with DTIC (100 mg/kg i.p. for 8 days), it can be seen that drug-treated animals survive longer than untreated controls because of the modest but significant antineoplastic activity of DTIC on this tumor, although eventually all animals succumb with generalized lymphoma. When ascitic growth is detected in DTIC-injected mice, tumor cells are collected from the peritoneal cavity of 1 or 2 donors and 10^6 cells transplanted i.p. into two groups of Balb/c hosts which are given the same DTIC treatment or left untreated. It can be observed that at this transplant generation 1 (TG1) the difference in survival between drug-treated and untreated mice is reduced, disappearing at TG2 as would be expected from the progressive emergence of DTIC-resistant cells. However, after TG2 an apparently paradoxical phenomenon can be observed since the untreated recipients of lymphoma cells obtained

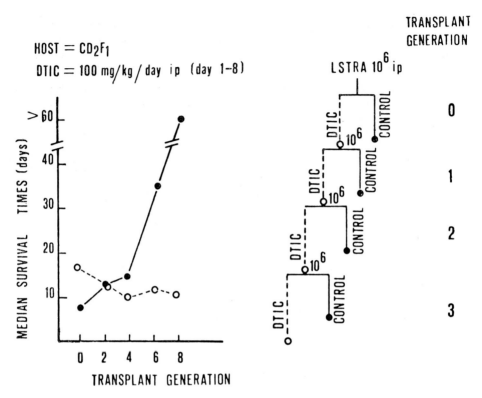

FIG. 3 — DTIC-mediated antigenic transformation of LSTRA lymphoma.

from DTIC-treated donors survive longer than similar mice sub-jected to further drug injections or control animals inoculated with the same number of parental line leukemia cells. Indeed, at TG8 the majority of the recipients of DTIC-cells survive beyond the 60 days observation period and these long-term survivors are resistant to subsequent transplants with either the parental leukemia or the DTIC-subline. If, however, the untreated recipients of TG8 LSTRA-DTIC cells are immunodepressed prior to tumor transplant, i.e. given 400R x-rays, antilymphocytic serum or Cyclophosphamide (Cy, 200 mg/kg i.p.), no long-term survivors are seen and these animals show median survival times (MST) similar to those of mice treated again with DTIC or syngeneic hosts transplanted with pa-

[18] *Spreafico, Bonmassar* - p. 14

rental lymphoma cells.   On the basis of similar findings obtained initially with the L 1210 leukemia [29], the following interpretation for the paradox phenomenon was advanced.   DTIC treatment *in vivo* leads to an increase in tumor cell immunogenicity capable of inducing a strong antitumor response resulting ultimately in the rejection of the tumor.   This response is absent in the recipients of DTIC-cells which are further treated with the drug because of the high immunodepressive activity of DTIC in rodents [30] which permits the progressive growth of the DTIC-cells chemoresistant to this agent.   A number of data are now available which not only support this interpretation but have also provided insights on the biological and immunological properties of DTIC-treated tumor sublines (DTTS) and on the mechanism(s) which might be at their origin.   This topic has recently been presented in detail [31], thus only an abbreviated review of available evidence will here be made.

DTIC-induced increases in tumor cell immunogenicity (and/or changes in antigenicity) have been observed for a large number of experimental tumors (table 10); it is evident that a variety of leukemia-lymphomas of chemical, viral and spontaneous origin and of different *H-2* haplotype and different sensitivity to the chemotherapeutic activity of DTIC are susceptible to DTIC-mediated immunogenicity modification.   For its possible practical and mechanistic implications, it is worth noting that the emergence of drug resistance does not appear to be a necessary prerequisite for the appearance of modified immunogenicity after DTIC treatment.   Tumors naturally resistant to DTIC (e.g. L 1210 Ha) can in fact be easily modified by the drug.   It should additionally be mentioned that indications exist that also solid neoplasms can be modified in their immunogenicity-antigenicity by antitumorals [32, 33] although this has not yet been sufficiently investigated with DTIC and that human cells can also undergo immunogenicity increases after exposure to cytotoxic compounds [34].   The range of susceptible tumors and of agents capable of inducing immunogenicity modifications would thus appear sufficiently wide to support the conclusion that the phenomenon described is not a curiosity of selected experimental conditions but may have broader biological and possibly therapeutic implications.

[18] *Spreafico, Bonmassar* · p. 15

TABLE 10 — *Murine tumors modified in their immunogenicity by antitumor drugs.*

Tumor	Host of origin		Degree of immunogenicity	
	strain	H-2	one cycle	multiple cycles
L 1210 Ha	DBA/2	d	+ +	+ + + +
L 1210 Cr	DBA/2	d	±	+ + +
L 5178 Y	DBA/2	d	±	+ + +
LPC-1	DBA/2	d	+ +	±
LSTRA	Balb/c	d	+	+ + +
EL-4	C57Bl/6	b	—	+
RBL-5	C57Bl/6	b	+	+ + +
S-1033	C57Bl/10	b	—	+ +
LSBM-1	C57Bl/10	b	—	+ + +
L5MF-22	B10.129 (5M)	b	—	—
K 36	AKR	k	—	+
GL	C3H	k	—	+
LAF-17	B10.A	a	—	—

The capacity of DTIC-transformed cells to growth in immunodepressed syngeneic recipients [29, 35] as well as the ability of DTIC-sublines of different lymphomas to give lethal takes in athymic nude mice [36] permit us to exclude drug-dependence of the DTIC-cells as a basis for the paradox phenomenon. The same finding rules out a decrease in oncogenic potential of DTTS as a major mechanism responsible for the longer or indefinite survival of animals transplanted with DTIC-cells. Two types of information have, however, prompted us to reexamine this possibility in more detail. Although in certain systems (e.g. L 5178Y leukemia) [29, 35] the MST of immunodepressed recipients of DTIC-cells was similar to that of untreated hosts challenged with the parental line (see table 11), in other systems (e.g. LSTRA and LSMB-1 lymphomas) it was appreciably longer [36]. In addition, a decrease in the growth potential of tumor cells treated with triazenes has been reported [37]. However, detailed cytokinetic analysis of different DTIC-sublines

TABLE 11 — *Survival of CD2F$_1$ mice inoculated with L5178 Y leukemia cells at different transplant generations of DTIC treatments.*

Transplant generation	Treated with DTIC		Untreated		BCNU-treated		Immunodepressed		Immunodepressed and BCNU-treated	
	MST	D/T	MST	D/T	MST	D/T	MST	D/T	MST	D/T
0	20	10/10	15	10/10	19	10/10	16	10/10	21	10/10
1	18	10/10	14	10/10	19	10/10	17	10/10	21	10/10
2	16	10/10	21	10/10	90	5/10	16	10/10	22	10/10
3	15	10/10	26	10/10	90	2/10	19	10/10	24	10/10
4	16	10/10	40	10/10	90	0/10	18	10/10	20	10/10
5	17	10/10	90	0/10	90	0/8	17	10/10	22	10/10
6	15	10/10	90	0/10	NT	NT	18	10/10	23	10/10
20	17	10/10	90	0/10	NT	NT	18	10/10	24	10/10
100	16	10/10	90	0/10	90	0/8	15	10/10	21	10/10

10^5 leukemia cells transplanted i.p. on day 0; DTIC treatment was 100 mg/kg i.p. for 10 days from day 1; BCNU dose was 10 mg/kg i.p. on day 4; immunodepression was given by 400 R x-rays on day −1. Transplant generation 0 is the untreated parental L5178 Y leukemia; TG 100 was obtained from DTIC-treated donors at the 6th transplant generation and passaged in CD2F$_1$ mice immunodepressed with Cyclophosphamide (200 mg/kg i.p. on day −1) until the 100th transplant generation. D/T: dead with tumor/total transplanted; MST: median survival time in days.

have failed to evidentiate significant differences with the appropriate parental, non drug-modified leukemias [38]. More directly, the data of fig. 4, which closely mimick what is seen when lymphomas are transplanted into allogeneic recipients [18], clearly indicate that the long-term survival of mice challenged with DTIC-cells results from a true rejection process rather than from a no-growth phenomenon. Therefore, even if in some cases a decrease in the growth capacity of drug-modified cells may occur, this factor does not appear to play a major role. It may further be noted that early in the course of these studies, evidence was obtained to the effect that

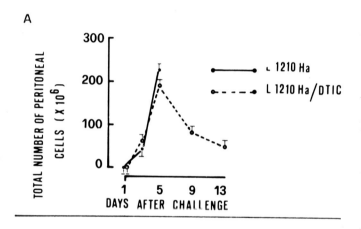

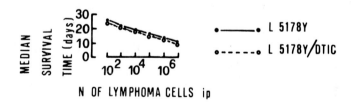

Fɪɢ. 4 — (A) Growth and rejection kinetics of L 1210 Ha/DTIC subline in CD2F₁ mice. (B) Survival of irradiated (400 R) CD2F₁ mice inoculated with L 5178 Y or L 5178 Y/DTIC lymphoma.

[18] *Spreafico, Bonmassar* - p. 18

the higher immunogenicity of Drug-treated tumor sublines (DTTS) is not sustained by a DTIC-haptenization process. Not only in fact can even single drug injections give tumor sublines which will not progress or give much longer MST in compatible hosts [39], but DTIC-sublines passaged (up to 100 passages, see table 11) in immunodepressed syngeneic hosts not subjected to drug treatment will still be rejected by normal compatible recipients while killing immunodepressed hosts [35]. These changes in tumor cell characteristics induced by DTIC or other drugs are thus inheritable, a point of relevance in understanding the mechanism(s) at their basis.

The data of fig. 3 showing the obtainment of long-term survivors after inocula of high numbers of DTIC-cells and the finding that these hosts are resistant to subsequent challenges with such cells even after a prolonged period (over 6 months in the L 1210 Ha or LSTRA systems) [28], suggest that the increase in immunogenicity induced by DTIC can be very marked. A measure of the immunogenic strength of DTTS can be obtained by comparing it with that of alloantigens associated with the entire H-2 complex, with different regions of the complex or with minor histocompatibility loci (MIHL). By this approach it was found that, in general, the immunogenic strength of early transplant generations (TG1-TG3) is comparable to that of MIHL [28], as indicated by the finding that mice inoculated with $10^5 - 10^6$ cells of DTTS-TG1 or of MIHL-incompatible lymphomas do not survive longer than immunodepressed or histocompatible recipients. It should be emphasized however that, as in the case of MIHL-incompatible tumors [40], strong synergistic effects with clear increases in survival and/or proportion of cures can be observed when chemotherapy is combined with these seemingly minor increases in immunogenicity. Also in view of its possible therapeutical relevance, the synergism between chemotherapy and early DTTS is illustrated by the representative data of table 11 for the L 5178Y leukemia system. It may be seen that when mice transplanted with DTIC-cells are also given a very limited course of BCNU chemotherapy, significant increases in lifespan are seen already at TG2 and 80% long-term survivors are observable already at TG3 whereas full survival in the absence of chemotherapy is seen only at TG5 - 6. The chemotherapeutic effect of BCNU alone in these conditions can be evaluated by the differences in MST between similar mice which before receiving the DTIC-cells and chemotherapy, had been immunodepressed. If thus the immunogenic strength of early TG of DTTS is operationally comparable to that of MIHL, when a full increase in immunogenicity is attained upon continuation of DTIC treatment, i.e. when compatible immunocompetent hosts resist challenges of up to 10^7 DTIC-cells even without BCNU chemotherapy, the change in immunogenicity is comparable to that of H-2 alloantigens. In our hands in fact the TD_{50} for L 1210, LSTRA or L 5178Y cells in H-2 incompatible C3H or C57Bl/6 hosts is of the order of $5.10^6 - 2.10^7$ cells. Whether the increased immunizing capacity of early TG of DTTS is the result of the appearance of novel antigenic specificities (see below) at low density or of an increased expression of tumor-associated transplantation antigens (TATA) already present in the parental line, is still undetermined.

The question should now be approached as to which is the basis for the higher immunizing ability of DTTS. More specifically, the question concerns the problem of whether the *in vivo* exposure of tumor cells to DTIC leads to the appearance of novel antigenic specificities or whether DTIC-cells are only quantitatively, but not qualitatively, modified in respect to the parental line.

A number of data [31] are available to indicate that DTIC-cells retain, at least in part, TATA associated with the parental line, a fact of clear relevance for the possible immunotherapeutical exploitation of DTTS. The first evidence in support of this conclusion was represented by the finding that animals which survived challenges with DTIC-cells were resistant also to high inocula of the parental leukemia [29]. More recently, the sharing of common TATA between DTTS and the parental tumor was confirmed by the observation of the absence of transplantation resistance towards the parental LSTRA lymphoma in mice rendered tolerant to LSTRA/DTIC cells [28]. This result is, in addition, not in support of the possibility that an increase in TATA density is at the basis of the rejection of DTTS. The conclusions that can be advanced from these *in vivo* studies are reinforced by *in vitro* findings. The cytolytic capacity of spenocytes sensitized *in vitro* to LSTRA cells was more pronounced against LSTRA targets than against LSTRA/DTIC cells [28]. In parallel, in both the L1210 Ha [41] and

LSTRA lymphoma systems [31], splenocytes from mice sensitized with DTTS were cytotoxic for both the specific DTIC-cells used for immunization as well as for the parental cells, although the degree of cytolysis, as measured by the extent of ^{51}Cr release, was significantly lower with the latter elements. It should be noted that at variance with the *in vivo* protection given by challenges with DTTS against parental cells, when relatively weak TATA are associated with the parental tumor (e.g. L 1210 Cr, L5178Y or LSBM-1 lymphomas) no cross-reactivity between parental and DTIC-cells can usually be detected in *in vitro* cytotoxicity assays. A number of findings are on the other hand, available to indicate the existence of cellular antigens associated with DTTS and not detectable in the parental tumor as reviewed more extensively elsewhere [31]. In support of this conclusion are for instance the results of transplantation resistance studies in which the capacity of limited doses of radiation (400 R) to inhibit primary immune responsiveness to drug-mediated specificities without impairing anamnestic responses [42], was exploited. Thus, when CD2F$_1$ mice presensitized with L 5178Y/DTIC or inactivated L5178Y cells were given 400 R x-rays and subsequently transplanted with parental or DTIC-cells, it was found that specific protection against the DTTS was given only by pre-immunization with the L5178Y/DTIC cells but not with the parental tumor [35]. Another, possibly more cogent, type of evidence in support of the conclusion that DTIC induces novel antigenic specificities is given by the data of table 12. It can be seen that CD2F$_1$ mice previously rendered tolerant to the TATA of the compatible LSTRA leukemia are still capable of rejecting LSTRA/DTIC cells whereas mice tolerant to the LSTRA/DTIC subline do not exhibit transplantation resistance to either the parental or the drug-modified tumor. It would thus appear that LSTRA/DTIC and LSTRA cells share common antigens but the DTTS carries specificities (drug-mediated tumor antigens, DMTA) not detectable in the parental tumor. Although the generation of highly immunogenic sublines in systems where the parental cells show little or no immunogenicity (e.g. the EL-4 and S-1033 lymphomas) does not provide direct support for the existence of DMTA, this finding is at least suggestive for such a conclusion. Thus, for instance, all attempts at showing sensitization of mice after challenges with the

TABLE 12 — *Presence of novel DMTA in LSTRA/DTIC as evidenced in CD2F₁ mice tolerant to the parental LSTRA lymphoma.*

Host tolerant to:	Transplantation Resistance against			
	10^7 LSTRA/DTIC		17^7 LSTRA	
	MST	D/T	MST	D/T
None	—	0/8	9	8/8
LSTRA	—	0/7	10	7/7
LSTRA/DTIC	18	6/7	10	7/7

Tolerance was induced with 5×10^7 irradiated lymphoma cells followed by Cy (250 mg/kg) 24 hrs later.

radiation-induced LSBM-1 (H-2^b) lymphoma have been unsuccessful, indicating that possible TATA associated with this tumor are at least not easily detectable. Yet, at TG16 the LSBM-1/DTIC subline is capable of inducing a strong transplantation resistance (fig. 5) so that syngeneic C57Bl/10 hosts will survive inocula of up to 10^7 DTIC-modified cells, a type of finding which may have important implications in the therapeutic exploitation of DTTS.

Another aspect of both practical and theoretical interest regards the possible cross-reactivity among various DTTS of the same or different tumors. Results so far available are relatively scarce and limited exclusively to DTIC-modified cells. With this proviso, when the cytotoxic capacity of splenocytes collected from mice sensitized to a given DTTS was tested *in vitro* against other DTTS in a number of combinations, in the majority of the experiments no significant cross-reactivity was seen [31]. Although the evidence is admittedly still inconclusive, it would at present appear that not only cells of different tumors modified by the same drug but also different DTTS of the same lymphoma possess unique DMTA(s).*

---

* Whether DMTA recognized by *in vivo* transplantation-protection assays are distinct from those detectable by *in vitro* tests is, at this time, purely a matter of speculation.

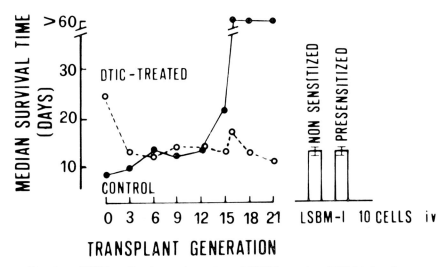

FIG. 5 — DTIC-mediated transformation of TATA-negative LSBM-1 lymphoma.

Related to this point is the question of whether the expression of normal histocompatibility antigens on DTTS is altered. The data of both *in vivo* and *in vitro* studies appear to lead to the conclusion that DTTS retain at least in part, a large amount of normal histocompatibility alloantigens associated with the parental line. For instance, B10.A (5R) and B10.A (2R) mice incompatible with B10 donors for the *S-D* and *K-1A-1B* regions of *H-2* respectively, normally succumb to i.v. inocula of the LSBM-1 lymphoma of B10 origin. If recipients are presensitized with LSBM-1/DTIC or parental cells, both the *S-D* and the *K-1A-1B*-incompatible hosts are capable of rejecting the LSBM-1 cells [43], suggesting that the LSBM-1/DTIC subline retained a significant complement of alloantigens associated with either the *S-D* or *K-1A-1B* regions of the *H-2* complex. In the same direction, when the susceptibility of DTTS to cell-mediated cytolysis by allogeneic and xenogeneic (rat) lymphocytes preimmunized to normal mouse tissue was evaluated *in vitro*, no differences in ^{51}Cr release could be found between parental and DTIC-cells of the L 1210 Cr and L5178Y lymphomas of DBA/2 origin [44]. Similar results were obtained with anti-DBA/2 sera raised in allogeneic mice or in rabbits and tested against parental and DTTS cells. In addition, both the cytotoxicity-inhibition assay with unlabelled cells as well as the absorption of the antisera with parental or DTIC-cells confirmed that comparable amounts of DBA/2 antigens were detectable in the parental and DTTS of these tumors. On the other hand, the loss of the Thy 1.2 antigen by DTIC/EL4 and DTIC/GL lymphoma cells has been described [31].

In this connection, an aspect not yet discussed and of some importance for a better understanding of the biology of drug-induced antigenic modification of tumor cells concerns the immunosensitivity of DTTS. In principle, an increased immunosensitivity of DTIC-cells could have been advanced as explanation for the increased or indefinite survival of DTTS-recipient animals. Against this hypothesis are however the data of table 13; it can be seen that parental and DTIC-cells were equally susceptible to cytolysis by lymphoid cells immune against histocompatibility antigens associated with the parental cells. That DTTS are not more susceptible *in vivo* to anti-TATA responses is further indicated, for instance, by the observation that the growth of L5178Y/DTIC cells is not inhibited by adoptive transfer of lymphoid cells immune against the parental leukemia [35].

Since this topic has recently been reviewed [31], only a limited discussion will be devoted to the types of immune reactivities elicited

TABLE 13 — *Cytotoxic effect of C3H or C57Bl/10 mouse or rat spleen cells against normal DBA/2 tissues or original parental lymphoma cells.*

Effector splenocytes		Target cells (% ^{51}Cr release)			
Strain	immune to	L 1210	L 1210/DTIC	L5178Y	L5178Y/DTIC
C3H	DBA/2	18±0.5	16±0.5	14±0.2	13±0.2
	L 1210	52±1.7	56±0.4	34±0.4	31±2.2
	L 5178 Y	55±0.6	54±0.5	45±1.2	43±0.9
C57Bl/10	DBA/2	12±0.6	12±0.4	14±0.7	13±0.3
	L 1210	60±1.9	57±1.3	NT	NT
Rat	DBA/2	34±1.5	37±1	33±0.9	32±0.4

[18] *Spreafico, Bonmassar* - p. 24

by DTTS. The resistance of compatible hosts to DTIC-cells appears to be essentially sustained by cell-mediated reactivities rather than by humoral mechanisms. Little or no cytotoxic antibodies have in fact been detected in mice challenged with fully immunogenic DTTS whereas cytotoxic cells are easily recognizable in such animals and specific protection can readily be transferred with such cell preparations [35]. T-dependent reactivity appears to be clearly involved as for instance indicated by the lethal growths of DTTS in nude mice [36] and by the loss of cytotoxic effects against DTTS if attacker lymphocytes sensitized *in vivo* or *in vitro* (by coculturing with DTTS) are preincubated with anti-Thy 1.2 serum [45]. Recent data have also been obtained supporting the possibility that T-independent, radioresistant responses of the type at play in the case of bone marrow incompatibility at the Hh locus [46] and which can also be operative in the rejection of lymphomas in certain conditions [47] could also be elicited by DTTS [31]. However, suggestive evidence against a major contribution of this type of reactivity (a mechanism whose cellular basis is still not completely characterized and which could be related to Natural Cytotoxicity) [48, 49], in the rejection of DTTS by compatible, immunocompetent mice is given by the fact that DTIC-cells progress in nude recipients which are strong responders for T-independent, radioresistant responsiveness [50]. Similarly, lethal growths of DTTS occur in lethally irradiated compatible recipients.

The finding that highly immunogenic tumor cells carrying novel specificities can be generated after *in vivo* treatment with antineoplastic agents raises obvious questions on the possible mechanism(s) underlying this phenomenon. Several important points are still obscure in this regard; however, available evidence permits at least the exclusion of a number of possible explanatory mechanisms. The experimental bases for rejecting a decrease in oncogenic potential, an increase in immunosensitivity, a DTIC-haptenization mechanism and an increase in TATA density as playing major roles in the long-term survival of DTTS recipients have already been discussed. Considering that DTIC is a potent immunodepressant [30], the appearance of DTTS could in principle have been explained by the progressive emergence in the immunodepressed hosts of preexisting cell clones possessing spontaneously a higher immunogenicity [51]. Such cells would in normal hosts be subjected to negative selection being easier targets for host immunity. Disregarding the fact that this hypothesis would additionally require that a growth advantage exists for tumor cells with higher immunogenicity, against this hypothesis it may just be cited that the passage for a number of TG of the L 1210 Ha or LSTRA leukemias in nude mice did not result in tumors of higher immunogenicity. On the contrary (table 14) strong immunogenicity was detectable only when these T-deficient hosts were also subjected to DTIC treatment.

As discussed above, data have been obtained supporting the conclusion that DTTS carry novel DMTA; on this basis two additional hypotheses could be advanced for the generation of these cells, i.e. viral activation and drug-induced somatic mutation. In addition to the fact that the biologic and immunologic properties of DTIC-cells cannot be transferred by cell-free filtrates of DTTS, the limited or no cross-reactivity among different DTTS of the same tumor would not seem to militate in favour of a viral activation mechanism. On the other hand, no arguments are presently available against the hypothesis that DTIC could induce somatic mutations in the neoplastic cells resulting in the appearance of novel antigenic specificities. The antineoplastic mode of action of DTIC is believed to be that of an alkylating agent and the drug has been reported to be mutagenic and cancerogenic [38]. In this respect, it is tempting to draw an analogy between the non cross-reactivity among DTTS

TABLE 14 — *DTIC-induced transformation of L 1210 Ha and LSTRA lymphomas in nude Balb/c mice.*

Tumor	Treatment in nude mice	Transplant generation	N. cells injected i.p.	Recipient mice			
				nude		CD2F$_1$	
				MST	D/T	MST	D/T
L 1210 Ha	none	7	10^5	9	7/7	10.5	6/6
L 1210 Ha	DTIC	5	10^5	14	4/4	—	0/6
LSTRA	none	15	10^6	8.5	8/8	10	6/6
LSTRA	DTIC	9	10^6	6	8/8	—	0/6

[18] *Spreafico, Bonmassar* - p. 26

and the unique antigenic specificities generally attributed to chemically-induced neoplasms [52].

Whatever its mechanism, the fact that antineoplastic agents can induce *in vivo* modifications in cancer cells antigenic structure could have a series of consequences for the more rational use of these agents and in immunochemotherapeutic approaches. For instance, the design of chemotherapeutic combinations could also take into account the efficiency of the drugs in inducing antigenicity changes or "good" transforming agents could be added to the combination. As mentioned above, also cells resistant to DTIC can be "modified" by the drug and the data of table 11 indicate that marked increases in antigenicity would not be necessarily required for obtaining strong therapeutic synergism between chemotherapy and host antitumoral reactivity. Table 15 shows that not only limited treatments with DTIC but even single injections can produce increases in immunogenicity sufficient to give a majority of long-term survivors when combined with BCNU chemotherapy [53]. On the other hand, although a variety of antitumorals have been found to induce DTTS their efficiency in so doing has varied considerably [27]. It should be noted however that detailed investigations on the most effective conditions for obtaining strongly immunogenic DTTS with agents other than DTIC have not yet been conducted, although clear indications exist in the case of DTIC that treatment conditions (e.g. dose and drug schedule) can markedly influence the rate of appearance of DTTS [53]. For its practical implications it should be mentioned that DTIC treatments capable of inducing strong DTTS have been found not to alter the antigenic profile of normal tissues. Skin from mice treated with schedules of the drug capable of inducing marked immunogenicity increases in various leukemias, was ineffective in sensitizing syngeneic hosts or in cross-reacting with DTIC-induced antigens on leukemia cells. Moreover, splenocytes from DTIC-treated mice failed to stimulate syngeneic lymphocytes in a mixed lymphocyte reaction [54]. On this basis, the possibility that treatment with DTIC may cause the appearance of new specificities in normal tissues with the risk of the induction of autoimmunity, does not seem to be supported.

The potential of DTTS for immunotherapeutic purposes has so far been explored only to a very limited extent. The possibility

TABLE 15 — *DTIC transformation of L 1210 Ha leukemia in CD2F$_1$ mice : effect of limited DTIC treatments.*

Donors		Recipients							
DTIC mg/kg i.p.	days of treatment	Untreated		BCNU		Immunodepr.		Immunodepr. + BCNU	
		MST	D/T	MST	D/T	MST	D/T	MST	D/T
150	1-5	25	8/8	—	0/8	13	8/8	15	8/8
150	1-5	13	8/8	—	0/8	12	6/6	16	8/8
50	1-5	11	8/8	—	0/8	10	8/8	15	8/8
150	1-3	12	6/6	22	3/8	9	8/8	12	8/8
400	1	10	8/8	13	6/8	9	8/8	10	8/8
400	3	14	8/8	—	0/8	10	8/8	15	8/8
400	6	10	8/8	20	6/8	9	8/8	12	8/8

10^5 L 1210 Ha (MST: 9 days) or L 1210 Ha/DTIC cells transplanted i.p. on day 0; BCNU: 10 mg/kg i.p. on day 6; immunodepression: 400 R x-rays on day −1.

[18] *Spreafico, Bonmassar* - p. 28

is currently being investigated of employing adoptively transferred DTTS-sensitized lymphocytes for instance in these conditions in which the "transforming" agent (e.g. DTIC) is strongly immuno-depressant thus preventing effective host reactivity against the DTTS. Similarly, a still restricted number of data are available on the use of DTTS, which still carry parental line antigens, for inducing strong anti-TATA responses in hosts bearing the parental tumor. In comparison with other procedures aimed at increasing tumor cell immunogenicity-antigenicity and relying on *in vitro*-processed, inactivated cells, the advantages of DTTS would essentially consist in the use of living elements undergoing proliferation in the host before rejection (see fig. 4) thus resulting in more efficient sensitization. The markedly better protection given by preimmunization with DTIC- L 1210 Ha cells in comparison to x-irradiated leukemia cells against subsequent challenges of the parental tumor is exemplified by the data of table 16. Fig. 6 on the other hand shows representative results in the LSTRA system of a therapeutic approach in which DTTS, in conjunction or not with chemotherapy, were given after tumor transplantation. While immunotherapy alone in this system (but not in others) was ineffective, clear therapeutic synergism could be obtained when DTIC-cells were associated with BCNU chemotherapy; no synergism occurred when allogeneic L5MF-22 lymphoma was used [28].

TABLE 16 — *Protective effect of L 1210 Ha/DTIC and L 1210 Ha-irradiated cells.*

Immunization			Challenge		
Tumor	No. cells	Day	Day 0	MST	D/T
—	—	—	10^6 L 1210 Ha	8	8/8
L 1210 HaRx[a]	10^7	−14	10^6 L 1210 Ha	10	8/8
L 1210 Ha/DTIC	10^5	−14	10^6 L 1210 Ha	—	0/8
L 1210 Ha/DTIC	10^5	−33	10^6 L 1210 Ha	—	0/8
L 1210 Ha/DTIC	10^5	−54	10^6 L 1210 Ha	—	1/8
L 1210 Ha/DTIC	10^5	−70	10^6 L 1210 Ha	22	3/8

[a] = 5,000 R x rays *in vitro*

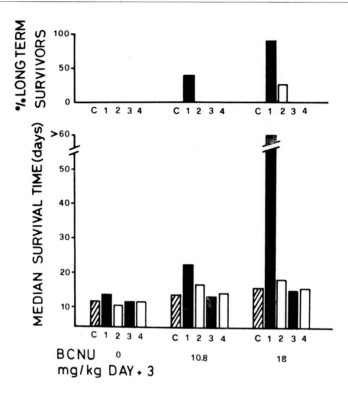

Fig. 6 — Immunochemotherapy of LSTRA lymphoma with a DTIC-subline and BCNU. Balb/c mice were transplanted with 10^3 LSTRA cells on day 0. C: controls not receiving treatment; 1 and 2: mice transplanted with 10^6 LSTRA/DTIC cells 1 or 7 days after LSTRA, respectively; 3 and 4: mice transplanted with 10^6 cells of the unrelated, allogeneic L5MF-22 lymphoma 1 or 7 days after LSTRA, respectively.

In connection with possible practical exploitation of this approach, it seems worth noting that DTTS of murine lymphomas can be produced in nude mice and that such DTTS retain the TATA detectable in the parental lines [36]. Since it is well known that nude mice can sustain the growth of a variety of human tumors, this finding could in principle be exploited for obtaining human DTTS for immunotherapeutic purposes. Further studies are however required to show whether human tumors are consistently susceptible to DTIC-mediated antigenic alteration without loss of the TATA possibly present on the neoplastic cell.

[18] *Spreafico, Bonmassar* - p. 30

REFERENCES

[1] MATHÉ G., « Cancer Immunol. Immunother. », 2, 81 (1977).

[2] MATHÉ G., in: *Cancer Active Immunotherapy: Immunoprophylaxis and Immunorestoration. An introduction.* Springer Verlag, Berlin (1976).

[3] SPREAFICO F. and ANACLERIO A., in: *Immunopharmacology*, Hadden J. W., Coffey R. G., Spreafico F. (Eds.), Plenum Press, New York (1977).

[4] SCOTT M. T., « Sem. Oncol. », 1, 367 (1974).

[5] SPREAFICO F., MANTOVANI A., VECCHI A., POGGI A., TAGLIABUE A. and GARATTINI S., in: *Modulation of Host Immune Resistance in the Prevention or Treatment of Induced Neoplasias*, Chirigos M. A. (Ed.), Fogarty Inter. Ctr. Proc., No. 28 (1976).

[6] TAGLIABUE A., MANTOVANI A., POLENTARUTTI N., VECCHI A. and SPREAFICO F., « J. Natl. Cancer Inst. », 59, 1019 (1977).

[7] ANACLERIO A., MORAS M. L. and SPREAFICO F., « Eur. J. Cancer », in press

[8] CARTER S. K., « J. Natl. Cancer Inst. », 55, 1265 (1975).

[9] DI FRONZO G., GAMBETTA R. A. and LENAZ L., « Rev. Eur. Etud. Clin. Biol. », 16, 572 (1971).

[10] YESAIR D. W., SCHWARTZBACH E., SCHUCK D., DEVINE E. P. and ASBELL M., « Cancer Res. », 32, 1177 (1972).

[11] VECCHI A., MANTOVANI A., TAGLIABUE A. and SPREAFICO F., « Cancer Res. », 36, 1222 (1976).

[12] MANTOVANI A., TAGLIABUE A., VECCHI A. and SPREAFICO F., « Eur. J. Cancer », 12, 381 (1976).

[13] MANTOVANI A., VECCHI A., TAGLIABUE A. and SPREAFICO F., « Eur. J. Cancer », 12, 371 (1976).

[14] EVANS R. A. and ALEXANDER P., in: *Immunobiology of the Macrophage*, Nelson D. S. (Ed.), Academic Press, New York (1976).

[15] ALEXANDER P., ECCLES S. and GAUCI C. L. L., « Ann. N. Y. Acad. Sci. », 276, 124 (1976).

[16] NOEL G., TROUET A., ZENERBERGH A. and TULKENS P., in: *Proc. Second Int. Symp. on Adriamycin*, European Press, Medikon (1975).

[17] MANTOVANI A., « Cancer Res. », 37, 815 (1977).

[18] TAGLIABUE A., POLENTARUTTI N., VECCHI A., MANTOVANI A. and SPREAFICO F., « Eur. J. Cancer », 13, 657 (1977).

[19] CURRIE G. A. and BAGSHAWE K. D., « Br. Med. J. », 1, 541 (1970).

[20] MANTOVANI A., TAGLIABUE A. and SPREAFICO F., « Proc. Am. Ass. Cancer Res. », *18*, 34 (1977).

[21] MANTOVANI A., TAGLIABUE A., VECCHI A. and SPREAFICO F., « Eur. J. Cancer », *12*, 113 (1976).

[22] PREHN R. T., « J. Natl. Cancer Inst. », *59*, 1043 (1977).

[23] RIOS A. and SIMMONS R. L., « J. Natl. Cancer Inst. », *51*, 637 (1973)

[24] BEKESI J. G., ROBOZ J. P. and HOLLAND J. F., « Ann. N. Y. Acad. Sci. », *277*, 313 (1976).

[25] GREEN A. A., PRATT C., WEBSTER R. G. and SMITH K., « Ann. N. Y. Acad. Sci. », *277*, 396 (1976).

[26] PRAEGER M. D. and BAETCHEL F. S., « Methods Cancer Res. », *9*, 339 (1973).

[27] NICOLIN A., VADLAMUDI S. and GOLDIN A., « Cancer Res. », *32*, 653 (1972).

[28] HOUCHENS D., BONMASSAR E., GASTON M., KENDE M. and GOLDIN A., « Cancer Res. », *36*, 1347 (1976).

[29] BONMASSAR E., BONMASSAR A., VADLAMUDI S. and GOLDIN A., « Proc. Natl. Acad. Sci. », *66*, 1089 (1970).

[30] VECCHI A., FIORETTI M. C., MANTOVANI A., BARZI A. and SPREAFICO F., « Transplantation », *22*, 619 (1976).

[31] BONMASSAR E., NICOLIN A. and SPREAFICO F., in: *Tumor-Associated Antigens and their Specific Immune Response*, Spreafico F., Arnon R. (Eds.), Academic Press, New York, in publication.

[32] ASAKUMA R. and YOKOBAMA I., « Arch. Jap. Chir. », *34*, 1413 (1965).

[33] BOON T. and KELLERMANN O., « Proc. Natl. Acad. Sci. », *74*, 272 (1977).

[34] PIOUS D., SODERLAND C. and GLADSTONE P., « Immunogenetics », *4*, 437 (1977).

[35] NICOLIN A., SPREAFICO F., BONMASSAR E. and GOLDIN A., « J. Natl. Cancer Inst. », *56*, 89 (1976).

[36] CAMPANILE F., HOUCHENS D., GASTON M., GOLDIN A. and BONMASSAR E., « J. Natl. Cancer Inst. », *55*, 207 (1975).

[37] SCHMID F. A. and HUTCHISON D. J., « Cancer Res. », *34*, 1671 (1974).

[38] SILVESTRINI R., TESTORELLI C., GOLDIN A. and NICOLIN A., « Int. J. Cancer », *19*, 664 (1977).

[39] SPREAFICO F., MANTOVANI A. and BONMASSAR E., in preparation.

[40] BONMASSAR E., CUDKOWICZ G., VADLAMUDI S. and GOLDIN A., « Cancer Res. », *30*, 2538 (1970).

[41] NICOLIN A., BINI A., FRANCO P. and GOLDIN A., « Cancer Chemother. Rep. », *58*, 325 (1974).

[42] MAKINODAN T., SANTOS G. W. and QUINN R. P., « Pharmacol. Rev. », *22*, 189 (1970).

[43] FIORETTI M. C., in preparation.

[44] NICOLIN A., TESTORELLI F., FRANCO P. and GOLDIN A., « Cancer Res. », *36*, 222 (1976).

[45] NICOLIN A., BINI A. and CORONETTI E., « Nature », *251*, 654 (1974).

[46] CUDKOWICZ G. and LOTZOVÀ E., « Transplant. Proc. », 5, 1339 (1973).

[47] BONMASSAR E. and CUDKOWICZ G., « J. Immunol. », 117, 697 (1976).

[48] HERBERMAN R. B., NUNN M. E. and LAVRIN D. H., « Int. J. Cancer », 16, 230 (1975).

[49] KIESSLING R., KLEIN E., PROSS H. and WIGZELL H., « Eur. J. Immunol. » 5, 117 (1975).

[50] CUDKOWICZ G., « Proc. Am. Ass. Cancer Res. », 16, 170 (1975).

[51] KITANO M., MIHICH E. and PRESSMAN D., « Cancer Res. », 32, 181 (1972).

[52] BALDWIN R. W. and PRICE M. R., « Ann. N. Y. Acad. Sci. », 276, 3 (1976).

[53] SPREAFICO F., MANTOVANI A. and BONMASSAR E., in preparation.

[54] TESTORELLI F. and NICOLIN A., in preparation.

DISCUSSION

MATHÉ

You have briefly mentioned in your talk that differences in therapeutic effect were seen when you employed methyl-CCNU or RFCNU
in chemoimmunotherapeutic treatments in mice. I would like to point
out that RFCNU is a sugar derivative of nitrosourea, which is not immunosuppressive at the minimal dose of the maximally efficient dose interval,
when applied after the antigen in the Jerne test and in an allogeneic skin
graft assay. At higher doses, it is. My question is: when you combine
two adjuvants which are *C. parvum* and BCG, and you get an increased
effect, do you get potentiation or only addition? And is this at the
maximally efficient dose or at the low dose?

SPREAFICO

As regards RFCNU, we have seen immunodepressive effects with
this compound at doses having a relatively low antileukemic activity.
However, I quite agree with you on the main point, since our data show
that this nitrosourea is clearly less immunodepressive than other nitrosoureas. We can obtain better results when we use RFCNU in combination with *C. parvum* than when we use for instance methyl-CCNU.
As regards the dosages of BCG and *C. parvum* when used in combination,
I will say that with this specific combination we have investigated only
the doses giving maximal antitumoral effect when injected singly. In
these conditions, our experience has not been very suggestive for better
therapeutical results employing the combination in comparison to the use
of the single agents and we have seen cases of paradoxical effects. I would
emphasize, however, that with this specific combination we have only
limited experience. We are working on it. On the other hand, as men-

tioned previously, with other combinations of immunostimulants we have obtained synergistic antitumoral effects employing optimal doses of each compound when used singly.

MATHÉ

When you gave them in combination, was it at high doses?

SPREAFICO

Yes — and in most of our experience we have never seen a potentiation between *C. parvum* and BCG, and occasionally we have seen better tumor growth.

NOSSAL

I would like to ask a general question, about the effects of these anti-cancer drugs on the immune response in man. My question relates to the gathering of data rather than listing of preconceptions. We were quite interested some time ago to look at the human immune response in patients with auto-immune diseases, patients who have been treated for long periods with corticosteroid drugs and immunosuppression. The surprising thing that came out was that in fact their response to test antigens was surprisingly good. In fact, we did not show evidence of B cell immunodepression despite the long period of time for which these patients had been receiving drugs. That left us of course wondering why the auto immune state was kept under such excellent control and why their auto immune disease frequently recurred if you removed the drugs; the drugs were doing something but they were not doing something we could measure very readily when test antigens were given. That led us to look at the group of renal transplant recipients, who of course get the same drugs but in higher dosage, particularly as our renal transplants are all cadaver transplants. And here, surprisingly enough, what turned out was that there were pretty good B cell responses in these patients and a moderate reduction of T cell responses. So I like the drift of what you are trying to do but I would like to know whether these anti-cancer drugs are as immunodepressive as we think they should be.

[18] *Spreafico, Bonmassar* - p. 36

SPREAFICO

To your comments I would like to offer firstly one general answer. It is my belief that many of the existing studies on the immunodepressive capacity of drugs in man are quite bad: the number of patients is often limited, study design questionable and analysis of results often wanting. My impression is that a true pharmacology of immunodepression is almost nonexistent even at the experimental level. With regard to the second part of your comment, one may answer that since your patients were indeed immunodepressed and yet you could not see laboratory indications of such a depression, then it was possibly the choice of the parameters of immune reactivity which was not the most representative.

WEISS

I should like to refer briefly to a clinical observation in support of Dr. Spreafico's remarks. In the trial of MER conducted in acute myelocytic leukemia patients by the Cancer and Acute Leukemia Group B cooperative trials body, it appears that addition of MER to the chemotherapy regimen prolongs remission and survival duration only when the chemotherapy arm includes vincristine and dexamethasone. Addition of these two drugs to the standard chemotherapy without MER does not improve the results over standard chemotherapy only. It is the combination of MER with vincristine and dexamethasone which seems to be required for remission and survival prolongation. This may be a positive effect, additive or synergistic between the immunological intervention and the activities of these drugs; or, it may be a therapeutic effect arising from the circumstance that patients given vincristine and dexamethasone receive that standard chemotherapy by a somewhat different schedule.

I also point out that in mouse experiments with several different solid tumors, challenge being with syngeneic implants, the combination of radiation therapy and MER is often, under the appropriate conditions, significantly more efficacious in slowing tumor growth and in prolonging animal survival than either modality alone; our findings have already appeared in the literature. Thus, both radio-immunotherapy and chemoimmunotherapy may be the means of accomplishing maximum therapeutic effects.

Westphal

I would like to remind us that, already a long time ago, the combination of non-specific agents with chemo or antibiotic therapy, for example against bacterial infection, was found to be much more efficient in many instances than chemo or antibiotic treatment alone. The late pharmacologist Rolf Meier did a series of investigations when there was the first concern about the development of resistance of microorganisms against antibiotics. In animal experiments they found that resistant strains responded when the, otherwise non-effective, antibactericidal agent was given together with adjuvants, like endotoxin etc. (1).

Rapp

Several years ago Dr. Eichwald under contract to the National Cancer Institute tried to determine whether mice, when given drugs under conditions similar to those used in humans to promote allografts, would be more susceptible to carcinogenesis during the time they were receiving these drugs, and he never got past the first part of the experiment because, to his great surprise, no matter what the relationship between the donor and recipient mice was in terms of their histocompatibility antigens or the dose of the drug, or the kind of the drug, he could never get prolongation of skin graft survival in the mouse. I would like to ask you what you really mean by a "more rational approach" because what I see here is more empirical studies where you are by intuition combining different doses of drugs and agents and seeing what comes out at the other end.

Spreafico

I may mention that the experience you mentioned has not been shared by other authors; there are in fact a number of reports in the literature on the possibility of obtaining prolongation of skin allografts in mice, employing chemicals. As concerns the second part of your remarks

---

(1) Neipp L., Kunz W. and Meier R.: *Selektive Erhöhung der « natürlichen » Resistenz gegenüber bakterieller Infektion durch Polysaccharide und andere Pharmaka.* « Schweiz. Med. Wschr. », *89,* 532-36 (1959).

[18] *Spreafico, Bonmassar - p. 38*

which refers to chemoimmunotherapy work described, I may point out that the synergism of the combination Adriamycin-*C. parvum* and non synergism between Daunomycin-*C. parvum* had been hypothesized on the basis of data previously obtained by us on the effects of these agents on the immunocyte subpopulations. Synergism and absence of synergism, respectively, were then experimentally confirmed and experiments conducted to examine whether our original hypothesis for expecting synergism was tenable. The evidence so far gathered seems in support of our concept, so it was not really only mixing agents blindly and hoping for the best.

CLERICI

I was quite interested in the timing of administration of Adriamycin and *Corynebacterium Parvum* and I am not able to figure out why, if you administer Adriamycin on day one and *Corynebacterium parvum* on day six you get a 100% cure, while if you administer *Corynebacterium parvum* on day four or five the percentage of cures is greatly reduced. Can you suggest a reason why such timing is so important?

SPREAFICO

As detailed in the text, available evidence indicates that *in vivo* synergistic schedules of Adriamycin-*C. parvum* are those which did not impair the induction and expression of macrophage cytotoxicity.

TERRY

It is extraordinarily difficult to properly design experiments that would allow one to determine the effects of chemotherapeutic agents on the immune systems of cancer patients. There are such a large number of variables that coming up with any kind of a reasonable answer is very difficult. For example, one could attempt to evaluate the immunosuppression induced by a drug. Such a study would have to take into account the immunosuppression that is induced by some tumors. The degree of immunosuppression varies from patient to patient and may depend upon the bulk of tumor.   If the drug is effective, tumor bulk will decrease and tumor induced immunosuppression will decrease, at a time when drug induced suppression is increasing.   While many of us believe it is important to try to understand what effects drugs have on the immune system, despite considerable effort we have very little information.

LYSOSOMOTROPIC CHEMOTHERAPY

CHRISTIAN DE DUVE and ANDRÉ TROUET

International Institute of Cellular and Molecular Pathology
B-1200 Brussels, Belgium

The Need for Chemotherapy

Cancer, it is often claimed, could be largely eradicated by preventive measures. Remove carcinogens from the diet, clean up the environment, stop cigarette smoking; and the incidence of cancer may drop to as low as one-tenth of what it is today. This figure could possibly be reduced even further by immunization.

Nobody can quarrel with the desirability of prevention. One ounce of it is still worth a pound of cure, as the old saying goes; probably much more today, with the rising cost of medical care. But whatever advances are made in prophylaxis, the need for an effective therapy will remain. The experience with infectious diseases is very eloquent in this respect. In spite of all the progresses that were achieved through sanitation, vaccination, vector control and other public health measures, the discovery of sulphonamides, and later of mold antibiotics, still played a decisive role in our conquest of microbial infections. With cancer, the need for therapy is likely to be even greater, in view of the complex etiology, insidious nature and long incubation of the disease.

Of the various forms of therapy available, chemotherapy is undoubtedly a choice one, at least in principle, since chemicals can seek cancer cells wherever they are, in contrast to the surgeon's knife or radiation. Immunotherapy has the same theoretical advantage, and appropriately has evoked increasing interest in recent years. But unless new breakthroughs are made in the future, it is likely to serve in most cases as an adjunct to, rather than as a complete replacement for, other forms of therapy.

These considerations are not restricted to cancer. They apply also to the many communicable diseases that still confront us today, in particular the tropical parasitic diseases which afflict two-thirds of the world population. Whatever advances are made in prophylaxis, the need for better drugs is urgent and undeniable.

The Problem of Selective Cell Killing

The aim of chemotherapy is to kill undesirable cells selectively. The problem lies, of course, in the requirement for selectivity. Cell killing, in itself, hardly raises any difficulty.

In principle, selectivity can be achieved on the basis of either accessibility or vulnerability of the target-cells. One can either use a drug that kills all cells, and see to it that it goes preferentially to the target-cells; or use a drug that goes to all cells but kills target-cells preferentially. In practice, the "magic bullet" of the first kind has remained largely a dream. Until now, selective cell killing has relied almost exclusively on differential sensitivity.

With bacteria this has proved relatively easy. A number of important enzyme systems of prokaryotes do not exist in the human hosts, and are susceptible to inhibition by compounds that are harmless to human cells. It is of some historical interest that most of these compounds were discovered by accident or by conventional screening procedures, often before much was known of their biochemical point of attack. In fact, several of them have played a major role in the elucidation of the metabolic pathways on which they act. It is also interesting that most of the failures of antibacterial chemotherapy, when they are not due to drug resistance, arise from problems of accessibility. They concern bacteria that entrench themselves in tissular or cellular sites that are not easily reached by the appropriate antibiotics.

Selective killing of eukaryotic pathogens — fungi, protozoa and other parasites — has been distinctly less successful so far. The reasons for this are not clear. Perhaps we have just been unlucky, and tomorrow will witness the chance discovery of a fungicide or schistocide comparable to prontosil or penicillin. It is more likely, however, that the odds of hitting upon such a wonder drug, even by the most educated form of screening, are distinctly poorer than they were in the case of anti-bacterial agents. Since the metabolic gap between attacker and victim is narrower, the number of possible biochemical targets for a selective action is also smaller. Furthermore, active compounds may be less likely to occur in nature, due to weaker selective pressures favoring their development. Finally, as with certain bacterial infections, problems of accessibility of the pathogen often complicate chemotherapy against eukaryotic invaders.

Viruses and cancer cells offer the greatest obstacles to successful chemotherapy, the former because they have almost no metabolism of their own and simply use the biochemical machinery of their host-cells, the latter because they are nearly identical to normal cells, both genetically and metabolically. In searching for selective anti-cancer agents, investigators have aimed almost exclusively at the property of cancer cells most obviously related to their ability to cause disease, namely unbridled growth. This effort has produced the anti-mitotic agents, a highly heteroclite group of compounds having in common the ability to interfere at some stage with cell division. In this way post-mitotic cells tend to be spared, although protection is rarely perfect due to side-effects of the drugs. But stem-cells in the bone marrow and elsewhere perforce share with cancer cells their ability to divide and their sensitivity to anti-mitotic agents. This functional kinship opposes an almost insurmountable barrier to the selective eradication of cancer by pervasive chemical means. Fortunately, considerable gains can already be achieved by simply slowing down the pathological process, and chemotherapy has become increasingly useful in this connection, as more drugs have become available and clinicians have learned to use them more efficiently. But the fact remains that complete cure is still a very rare outcome of chemotherapy.

Choice of a Strategy

The decision as to how to set about developing new chemotherapeutic agents depends largely on whether one views past achieve-

[19] De Duve, Trouet - p. 3

ments optimistically or pessimistically, as half-successes or half-failures. The optimist will be tempted to ask for more of the same, the pessimist for something new. The realist should ask for both.

One must keep in mind the simple historical fact that enlightened empiricism, if not sheer luck, certainly not rational design, has given us most of our active chemotherapeutic drugs. And this is so not simply because no other approach has been tried. The lure of fitting a key to a lock has attracted many a chemist, though rarely led him to success. It is understandable, therefore, that those who are closest to the problem, the investigators and managers of the pharmaceutical industry, should be reluctant to abandon the strategy that has given them most of their victories and on which their whole organization has long been geared.

At the same time, it must be realized that two important changes have taken place in the last few years. On one hand, the cost-effectiveness of empirical screening procedures has risen sharply. In some cases huge sums have been invested, as in the search for better anti-malarials, with negligible returns. Perhaps there are not so many wonder drugs left to be discovered empirically or accidentally. On the other hand, there has been a similarly sharp rise in the store of fundamental knowledge on which drug design can be based, as well as in the technology for acquiring more. The latter point is of importance. The pillars of modern biology have been bacteriophage, *E. coli*, rat liver and guinea-pig pancreas, which for a variety of reasons, some of them accidental, turned out to be convenient objects for the elucidation of a number of basic biological processes, but have hardly any bearing on pathology. However, the knowledge that has been gained and the techniques and approaches that have been worked out in the course of these developments can now profitably be exploited for studies of diseased cells and of pathogenic organisms.

Leaving out the important approach which consists in the strengthening of the host's natural defenses and forms the main object of this symposium, two main lines of research may be considered. One is to look for new drugs, trying to achieve better selectivity by zeroing in on whatever biochemical differences can be uncovered between target-cells and host-cells. Fungi and parasites,

[19] *De Duve, Trouet* · p. 4

which are separated from us by about a billion years evolutionary divergence, are most likely to yield to such an approach. It is certainly remarkable how little is known of the metabolic peculiarities of most pathogens. One of the reasons for this lies in the difficulties that attend mass cultivation of many of the organisms. But another is that this kind of study simply has not attracted much interest so far. The situation is different for cancer cells, which have been the object of many detailed biochemical studies. But here the early hopes evoked by the work of Warburg and later of Greenstein have not been fulfilled. The likelihood of finding a cancer-specific reaction or property against which chemotherapy can be directed, or even of the existence of such a potential target, seems slim.

The other line of research that can be envisaged is to try and achieve selectivity by means of differential uptake of a drug rather than by differential sensitivity to it. Ideally one could think of taking a completely unspecific cytotoxic agent, and equipping it with a homing device that will cause it to be taken up exclusively by the target-cells. Obviously, the approach need not yield such a dramatic result to be useful. Even a small gain in target-specific delivery of an agent already endowed with a certain degree of biochemical selectivity may provide the edge that is needed for successful therapy. The lysosomotropic approach developed in our laboratories over the last few years falls in this category.

The Lysosomotropic Approach

The principle of this approach is illustrated schematically in Fig. 1. The drug is linked to a carrier in such a way as to form a complex that is stable in the extracellular fluids, unable to permeate across membranes and essentially inert pharmacologically, but susceptible to pinocytic uptake and to subsequent lysosomal breakdown with concomitant release of the drug.

The main basis of selectivity in this approach is represented by differences in the rates at which different cell types capture the drug-carrier complex by endocytosis. This process, in turn, depends on two factors, one quantitative, the other qualitative.

[19] *De Duve, Trouet* - p. 5

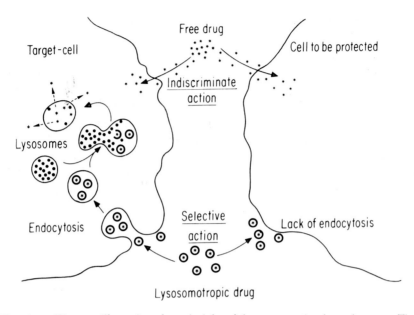

FIG. 1 — Diagram illustrating the principle of lysosomotropic chemotherapy. The drug (star) is bound to a carrier (circle) to form a stable, inert, nonpermeant complex that is taken up by endocytosis, and processed in lysosomes with release of the drug in free and active form. Selectivity depends on rate of endocytic uptake and lysosomal processing.

The quantitative factor may be expressed in terms either of the volume of extracellular fluid, or of the surface area of plasma membrane, interiorized per unit of time. These two measurements are related to each other by a factor equal to one-third the average radius of the endocytic vesicles. SILVERSTEIN, STEINMAN and COHN [1] have recently reviewed our knowledge of the endocytic activity of cells. Although very few accurate data are available, it is already clear that large differences in endocytic rate may exist between different cell types. For instance, macrophages interiorize every hour a volume equal to 26% of their own volume, together with 190% of their surface area, whereas L-cells take in only 3% of their volume and 48% of their surface area per hour [2]. There are also indications that the endocytic activity of a given cell type may itself be influenced by certain internal and external factors.

[19] *De Duve, Trouet* - p. 6

One such factor is the cell cycle.   In our Brussels institute, QUIN-
TART, BARTHOLEYNS and BAUDHUIN [3] have found on HTC
hepatoma cells that the endocytic rate is minimal during the M phase
and goes through a maximum at the end of the G_1 or the beginning
of the S phase.   The difference between the two extrema may be
as much as 5- to 10- fold.

The qualitative differences in endocytic uptake are mediated
by specific binding sites (pinocytic receptors) present on the plasma
membrane.   Molecules attached to these binding sites are carried
inward by the portions of plasma membrane that invaginate in the
course of endocytosis (Fig. 2).   Only a few such receptors have
been investigated so far, but there is already good evidence that
some of them at least are cell-specific as well as ligand-specific.
Furthermore, their affinity for their ligand is such that they may
bring about a highly selective uptake of certain molecules present at
low concentration in the medium.   Under favorable circumstances,
a cell equipped with the appropriate receptor may pinocytize several
hundred times more of a given molecular species than a cell having
the same endocytic activity but no receptor.

Expressed in simple terms, what these findings tell us is:
1) that some cells are constitutionally "greedier" than others; 2) that
the cellular "appetite" varies according to circumstances, including
the phases of the cell cycle; and 3) that different cells have different
"tastes".   Due to these three factors, different cells exposed to the
same medium may each selectively extract from it a very different
"meal".   This is the basis of the lysosomotropic approach.   Instead
of poisoning the whole environment indiscriminately as is done in
the ordinary form of chemotherapy, we poison only a certain kind
of food that we have reasons to believe will be eaten preferentially
by our target-cells (see: Fig. 1).

To be effective, the poisoned food must not only be eaten;
it must reach the stomach and be digested there, releasing the poison.
Which means, at the cellular level, that the endocytic vacuole containing the drug-carrier complex must fuse with a lysosome and that
the complex must be broken down in the resulting phagolysosome,
with release of the drug in free and active form.   Molecules bound
to the membrane of an endocytic vacuole may fail to undergo this
fate, either because they inhibit phagosome-lysosome fusion, or be-

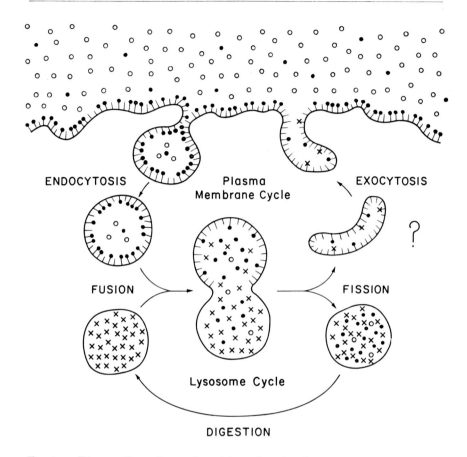

FIG. 2 — Diagram illustrating preferential uptake of molecules (black circles) bound by membrane receptor, delivery into lysosomes following phagosome-lysosome fusion, and hypothetical mechanism of recycling of plasma membrane. Open circles are molecules taken in non-selectively (fluid endocytosis). Crosses are lysosomal hydrolases.

cause they are recycled back to the cell surface. The former phenomenon was found to occur with concanavalin A by EDELSON and COHN [4]. The latter was first observed in our laboratory by SCHNEIDER, TULKENS and TROUET [5] with anti-plasma membrane antibodies which they found to remain attached almost indefinitely to the cell surface. At first, they thought this to be so because of lack of interiorization of the membrane patches to which the antibodies were bound.   But subsequent experiments disproved this interpretation and led instead to the conclusion that the membrane of endocytic vacuoles does not remain as part of the lysosomal membrane after phagosome-lysosome fusion, but rather separates from it again and returns to the plasma membrane, carrying back with it any ligand that has not become detached during contact with the lysosomal milieu, and eventually also some intralysosomal materials capable of binding to it.   The existence of such a membrane shuttle had been previously predicted by STEINMAN, BRODIE and COHN [2] on kinetic grounds.   How it takes place is not known. A likely possibility is that the membrane detaches from the phagolysosome in the form of flattened sacs or vesicles and fuses with the plasma membrane as in the exocytic discharge of secretory granules (Fig. 2).   This finding carries a number of important implications which will cause us to revise several of our ideas concerning the functioning of the lysosome system.   It may also be important for the design of lysosomotropic drugs.

After delivery to the lysosomes, the drug-carrier complex must still be broken down, usually as a result of enzymic attack, but possibly also under the influence of the prevailing acidity, and this process must take place in such a way as to release the drug in free and active form.   The drug itself must resist inactivation in the lysosomes and it must be able to travel from the lysosomes to its final target, which in most cases will be extra-lysosomal.

The rate and efficiency of these successive steps in the processing of the endocytized complex may play an important role in determining how much of the drug taken up in the form of a lysosomotropic complex actually ends up on its biochemical target. Differences in these factors may have a bearing on cellular selectivity, but in what way is difficult to predict.

Many other factors may be expected to change when a drug is given in lysosomotropic form, including its rate of clearance from the blood, access to other humoral compartments, renal excretion, distribution between tissues, metabolism, etc.   It is obvious that the whole pharmaco-toxicology of a drug-carrier complex is bound to be very different from that of the free drug.   Some of these differences may be favorable to our ends; others may not.   For instance, to the extent that fairly complex molecules have to be used as carriers to provide the necessary specificity, we run the risk that the complexes may be prevented from reaching their target-cells by capillary or other structural barriers, or that their prolonged administration may elicit immune reactions.

There is thus a considerable margin of uncertainty surrounding the design of a lysosomotropic drug, with plenty of room for unforeseen complications, but also for serendipitous benefits. At least the main cellular parameters of a rational design are amenable to direct experimentation. Techniques exist for the accurate assessment of pinocytic kinetics and of lysosomal processing. From such measurements, the molecular characteristics of the appropriate homing device and of its connecting link can be derived. To translate this information into a real drug-carrier complex may pose some technical difficulties, but not insoluble ones. The guidelines to be followed have been discussed in detail elsewhere [6, 7, 8].

Indications of Lysosomotropic Therapy

There are three groups of diseases in which a lysosomotropic approach may prove beneficial, namely cancer, parasitic diseases and intracellular infections.

Cancer. As pointed out above, selective eradication of cancer cells has proved very difficult to achieve on the sole basis of differential drug-sensitivity. This in itself would be a good enough reason for trying to improve selectivity by means of a lysosomotropic approach. But there are other, more positive reasons for doing so. The cell surface is known to be a major site of expression of the malignant transformation, and there is thus a real possibility that new pinocytic receptors may appear on the plasma membrane of cancer cells. Another favorable factor is provided by the observation, alluded to above, that cells are at their greediest just about when they are getting ready to duplicate their DNA [3]. Finally there is the possibility that cancer cells may be more accessible than their normal counterparts, due to the poor tissular organization of many tumors.

These, however, are all theoretical or conjectural arguments. So far, except for a few hints that certain cancer cells may have a

[19] *De Duve, Trouet* - p. 10

high endocytic activity [see ref. 6], essentially no hard facts are available concerning the feeding habits of human tumor cells. Clearly needed is some sort of primary screening test applicable to clinical specimens, which could provide some orienting guidelines for a more systematic search for appropriate carriers.

Parasitic diseases. The feeding mechanisms of protozoa, although often more elaborate than those of mammalian cells, rely on the same basic cellular processes of endocytic ingestion and lysosomal digestion. Thus pathogenic protozoa should be susceptible to a lysosomotropic therapy, especially if they occur freely in blood or other extracellular fluids. The problem of intracellular parasites will be considered below.

As an extension of the lysosomotropic approach, one might consider also the selective poisoning of parasitic worms by means of drugs linked to preferred nutrients. Uptake and digestion of such complexes might not take place by the cellular mechanisms of Fig. 1. But the principle would be the same, except for the drug being "enterotropic" rather than lysosomotropic. Such an approach merits some consideration, since parasitic worms have notoriously impermeable cuticles and probably take in drugs mostly by the oral route in any event.

Intracellular infections. This is a particularly interesting application of the lysosomotropic approach since intracellular infections are among the most resistant to chemotherapy due to the poor accessibility of the pathogen. It differs from the two previous applications by the fact that the drug-carrier complex is not taken up and processed by the target-cells themselves, as illustrated in Fig. 1, but by host cells that harbor the pathogens. This means, among other advantages, that the lysosomotropic approach can be extended in this case to microorganisms lacking a vacuolar feeding mechanism, in particular bacteria. We take advantage of the feeding habits of their host-cells to concentrate drugs selectively at the sites of infection. This will be done most efficiently in those cases where the pathogens actually reside in the lysosomes of the host-cells, as in leprosy. But such pin-pointing is not essential. There is, however, an advantage in knowing where in the cell the pathogens are located, since we will want to use a drug that tends to remain within the lysosomes, or on the contrary is capable of readily diffusing out of them, depending on whether the pathogen is intra- or extra-lyso-somal [7].

Another favorable feature of this kind of application is that the host-cells of intracellular parasites are often active phagocytes related to macrophages. Thus they are among the "greediest" cells known, richly fitted with endocytic receptors. One major exception is represented by malaria, although even here one should not give up all hope. Malaria has an early hepatic stage involving a host-cell with highly selective endocytic properties. As to the erythro-cytic stage, even though red blood-cells are generally not considered as carrying out pinocytosis, they can be induced to do something closely similar to it, as demonstrated by their engulfment of the malarial plasmodium itself. Where the latter can get in, presumably we should be able to follow. Release of the drug from its carrier might, however, still pose a problem.

DNA as Lysosomotropic Carrier

The first attempt to apply the lysosomotropic approach was made some seven years ago, when DNA was introduced as carrier for such intercalating drugs as daunorubicin [6] and adriamycin [9]. Initially these experiments were started with little hope or intention of developing a clinically usable drug-carrier complex. The main purpose of the exercise was to test the lysosomotropic concept which, until then, existed simply as a logical inference from our know-ledge of lysosomes [10], but lacking experimental validation. It was felt that if the concept could be verified on a simple experimen-tal model, this might provide enough incentive for the more so-phisticated, but also considerably more laborious, type of search that might lead to clinical application.

For such a purpose, DNA appeared as a particularly convenient carrier, since in addition to being a good inducer of pinocytosis [11] and substrate of lysosomal digestion [12], it was known to bind daunorubicin so tightly that a covalent linkage might possibly be dispensed with [13]. This was an immense practical advantage to the amateur-chemists that we were, since the main difficulty in the construction of a lysosomotropic complex lies in the attachment of

[19] *De Duve, Trouet* - p. 12

the drug to the carrier. The linkage must be stable in all extra-cellular fluids, and at the same time it must readily be broken down in the lysosomes in a way that releases the drug in free and active form. With DNA there was the possibility that a linkage satis-fying these conditions might form simply upon mixing of the drug with the carrier.

This prediction was verified and the DNA complexes were found to behave in various "in vitro" systems essentially as expected on the basis of the lysosomotropic model of Fig. 1. Given to ani-mals, either intra-peritoneally or intra-venously, they were found to be less toxic than the same amount of drug given in free form, to reach higher plasma levels and to be cleared more slowly from the blood. When administered to DBA/2 mice inoculated with L1210 leukemia cells, they consistently gave better therapeutic results than the same dosage of free drug. Since DNA binding allowed the dosage itself to be increased appreciably over what would normally be tolerated, some dramatic results could be obtained, with long-term survivals of as much as 80% or more [6-9].

Since these first results were published, a number of other workers have performed similar experiments with the DNA com-plexes of daunorubicin [14-17] and adriamycin [15, 16, 18-20a], as well as of other intercalating agents such as actinomycin D [15, 16], ethidium bromide [21] and ellipticin [17]. In our own laboratory, a considerable amount of work, much of it unpublished, has been carried out on the comparative cytopharmacology [22, 23] of daunorubicin, adriamycin and their DNA complexes and on their toxicological and histopathological properties [23]. In addition, another successful application of the use of DNA as carrier has been carried out in a completely different kind of disease, namely ex-perimental infection with *Trypanosoma cruzi*, the agent of CHAGAS disease [24]. This corresponds to the third type of application en-visaged above, where the "greediness" of host-macrophages is ex-ploited to selectively concentrate a chemotherapeutic agent at the sites occupied by intracellular parasites. The agent in this case is ethidium bromide.

In general, all these investigations have tended to confirm the original findings, as well as their interpretation. There have been minor discrepancies and disagreements, mostly explainable by the

[19] *De Duve, Trouet* - p. 15

choice of inappropriate experimental conditions. The molecular properties of the DNA used, and the mode of preparation of the complexes have proved to be the most sensitive variables, capable in some cases of seriously altering the therapeutic efficiency [25, 26].

Leaving a detailed discussion of these points to a more technical publication, we may summarize as follows the present state of our knowledge concerning the behavior of DNA complexes in experimental systems:

1) The complexes are less toxic than the free drugs, with LD_{50} values increased by a factor of 2 on an average. Since their plasma concentrations are much higher and decrease more slowly, this fact indicates a considerably enhanced tolerance by certain tissues. Prominent among these are liver, kidney and digestive mucosae. Heart is also spared [27, 28], a point of considerable importance from the point of view of clinical application. On the other hand, stem-cells in the bone-marrow and in lymphoid tissues are poorly protected.

2) Therapeutic effects vary with a number of factors, including the type of tumor cell, the strain of animals, the site and mode of inoculation, the size of the inoculum, the dosage and route of administration of the complexes, and, as already mentioned, the manner in which the latter are prepared. Even so, there is practically no case on record where the DNA complex of an intercalating drug has given distinctly poorer results than the same amount of free drug administered in the same way. In most cases, the complexes are at least as good as the free drugs, and often better than them. The significance of this point has not always been properly appreciated. Since animals will tolerate higher doses of complexes than of free drugs, even equal efficiency can be turned to advantage. Higher efficiency, combined with higher dosage, may give striking therapeutic successes, as has been found in our laboratory both in experimental leukemia [6-9] and in acute experimental CHAGAS disease [24].

3) The exact mode of action of the complexes is not entirely clear. When added to cultured cells "in vitro", there can be little doubt that they enter cells and act on them in the way predicted by the lysosomotropic model. Presumably this behavior extends

[19] *De Duve, Trouet* - p. 14

to the "in vivo" situation. But other factors come into account in the intact animal. One concerns the manner in which the complexes leave the blood, cross barriers and reach different cell types. The other concerns the ability of the complexes to dissociate and release free drug molecules when in contact with plasma. The level of plasma DNase activity is of course very important in this respect and has been found to account for certain strain differences. But, in addition, we have indications, especially with daunorubicin, that the drug may detach significantly from its complex in circulating blood. On the whole, however, available data show that the results tend to be better in terms of lowered toxicity and increased thera-peutic efficiency, the tighter the complex. This is consistent with the lysosomotropic mechanism being largely responsible for the fa-vorable properties of the complexes.

As mentioned above, when these experiments were initiated, the possibility of a clinical application was hardly envisaged. But the animal results appeared so encouraging as to justify a trial in human leukemia patients. These tests were started some six years ago in collaboration with Professor GÉRARD SOKAL and his asso-ciates. They were run with utmost caution on terminal patients who had become resistant to other forms of therapy [29]. When the complexes were found to be well tolerated, as well as therapeu-tically effective, the trials were progressively extended. To date, hundreds of patients have been treated, or are being treated, with daunorubicin-DNA or adriamycin-DNA, administered alone or in combination with other drugs, in a number of clinical centers in Belgium and elsewhere. Some of the results obtained have been published [26, 29-34]. Others are still in the process of being evaluated. Although no large-scale rigorously controlled testing of the kind that would be required for unequivocal appreciation of the new therapy has yet been performed, some preliminary conclu-sions may already be formulated.

Firstly, there can be no doubt that the complexes are active in a number of human neoplastic diseases, including various forms of lymphoblastic and nonlymphoblastic leukemia [29-32], metastatic breast cancer [33], bronchogenic carcinoma [34], and a number of other solid tumors [31, 32]. Whether they are superior, equivalent or inferior to the free drugs or to other medications is an unanswerable question at the present time. The only available hint is provided by the experience with nonlymphoblastic leukemia, for which the percentage of complete and partial remissions registered so far with DNA-daunorubicin [29, 30] and with DNA-adriamycin [31, 32] is considered to be comparable to the best published statistics for this disease.

Secondly, it is already clear that the DNA complexes are not miracle drugs. A number of cases have been reported where they evoked little or no response. And they tend to lose their efficiency in time as do other chemotherapeutic agents. On the other hand, it is probable that they are not yet used optimally. Their pharmacokinetic properties are very different from those of other drugs and they obviously present the clinician with novel problems which only large-scale empirical trials will allow to solve.

Finally, all the results obtained so far indicate that patients can tolerate considerably larger doses of daunorubicin and of adriamycin without showing signs of cardiotoxicity, when the drugs are administered as their DNA complexes than when they are given in free form. This is in contrast to certain other toxic signs such as alopecia, thrombopenia or leucopenia, where little advantage of the DNA complexes over the free drugs has been recorded [26].

On the basis of these indications, it would appear that more extensive trials with the DNA complexes are justified. If these complexes should turn out to be equally effective therapeutically as the free drugs and to be less toxic than the latter, especially on heart, this would already be a considerable advantage. Unfortunately, large-scale use of DNA as drug carrier meets with certain practical difficulties. DNA is expensive, and it is difficult to purify, characterize and standardize in a manner that will at the same time ensure a reproducible product and satisfy regulating agencies. Objections of an ethical nature have also sometimes been formulated against the administration of animal DNA to human patients, though on what rational basis is difficult to understand. The possibility of causing some freaky transformation of somatic cells, or genetic change of germ-cells, is clearly too farfetched to be entertained seriously. A more realistic potential hazard is the development of

[19] *De Duve, Trouet* - p. 16

immune reactions, although DNA has proved essentially non-immunogenic, outside of the spontaneous pathological situation of lupus
erythematosus. So far, no antibodies against DNA have been detected in the blood of patients treated with DNA-drug complexes,
despite routine testing.

Whatever the future of the DNA complexes, they are very
unlikely to represent the ultimate in lysosomotropic therapy. As
mentioned above, DNA was chosen as carrier more for reasons of
expediency than because it was expected to have specially favorable
homing properties. The difficulties of having to depend on a dis-
sociable linkage of variable strength have already been commented
upon. Clearly, the future of lysosomotropic therapy lies in the use
of more rationally developed carriers binding the drugs covalently.

In a way, the unexpected successes obtained with DNA complexes have, paradoxically, slowed down new developments in this
direction. One of their consequences has been a regrettable shift
in emphasis from the theoretical and general to the practical and
particular. Ensuing debates have focused primarily on the use of
DNA as carrier, rather than on the lysosomotropic approach which
it was meant to illustrate. Conceptual misunderstandings have
arisen, to the point that the possible use of DNA as carrier for
drugs that do not form tight complexes with it has come under
discussion.

The Future of Lysosomotropic Chemotherapy

All drugs that are not inactivated in lysosomes are potential
candidates for guidance by means of a lysosomotropic carrier, provided their properties allow them to move easily from their site of
liberation in the lysosomes to their final intra-cellular target. Interestingly, even drugs that have been rejected on account of ex-
cessive toxicity may come under consideration, since reduced toxicity
is one of the major benefits to be expected from a good lysosomotropic drug-carrier complex. The DNA-complexes of daunorubicin
and adriamycin illustrate this point. According to present experience, they are distinctly less toxic on heart muscle than the free
drugs, and as a consequence may continue to be used clinically far

beyond the customary dosage threshold of appearance of severe cardiotoxicity.

Binding the drug to its carrier by an appropriate linkage may require some chemical legerdemain, though hardly ever to the point of overtaxing the resources of modern technology. We are after all sending the drug-carrier complex into an environment where very few hydrolyzable bonds can survive.

The main problem, therefore, lies in the selection of the carrier. Here is where groundwork is needed for optimal design. We must explore the pinocytic preferences of the target-cells (or of the host-cells in the case of intra-cellular infections) so as to find out which type of chemical specificity the carrier should have. Any promising substance must be investigated further with respect to its ability to reach the lysosomes. As mentioned above, binding to the membrane and pinocytic interiorization do not necessarily suffice for efficient discharge into the lysosomes. Final selection will have to include also consideration of the relative accessibility of the target-cells in the organism. If they are reached easily, as for instance in leukemia, one would be inclined to choose a carrier of restricted distribution range. If the target-cells are shielded by barriers, a carrier capable of crossing these barriers will obviously be required. Or some other means must be found to take it across.

Under present research priorities, such custom-tailoring is beyond our reach. But there is no reason why it should remain so. There is certainly no compelling reason why the methods presently used for the measurement of pinocytic kinetics in the few laboratories that are interested in the problem could not be converted into a battery of routine tests suitable for the screening of cells isolated from surgical specimens. No major breakthrough is required. Only a modicum of imagination and organization, and a great deal of labor.

What we want to present to the cells in such a screening test is a sufficiently large selection of potential carrier molecules. If you are going to investigate the tastes of your customers measuring consumption, you must of course give them a sufficiently varied menu to choose from. This could comprise a variety of carbo-hydrates, including glycoproteins or glycopeptides, hormones or parts of them, antibodies (or their fragments) against certain target-

[19] *De Duve, Trouet* - p. 18

specific antigens, possibly other proteins or peptides, liposomes, nucleic acid derivatives, certain synthetic macromolecules, etc.... Within each of these groups there is already evidence of preferential uptake of certain compounds by certain cells. All that is needed is a more systematic inventory, and streamlining of the assay procedures.

Compared to some of the other screening programs that have been implemented before, this would be a small price to pay for an effective guided missile, especially since the information required for the design of the homing device will at the same time enrich considerably our basic knowledge of an important cell function, as it is carried out by different cells, both normal and transformed.

[19] *De Duve, Trouet* - p. 19

REFERENCES

[1] SILVERSTEIN S. C., STEINMAN R. M. and COHN Z. A., « Ann. Rev. Biochem. », *46*, 669 (1977).

[2] STEINMAN R. M., BRODIE S. E. and COHN Z. A., « J. Cell Biol. », *68*, 665 (1976).

[3] QUINTART J., BARTHOLEYNS J. and BAUDHUIN P., « J. Cell Biol. », *70*, 134a (1976).

[4] EDELSON P. J. and COHN Z. A., « J. Exp. Med. », *140*, 1364 (1974).

[5] SCHNEIDER Y.-J., TULKENS P. and TROUET A., « Biochem. Soc. Trans. », *5*, 1164 (1977).

[6] TROUET A., DEPREZ-DE CAMPENEERE D. and DE DUVE C., « Nature New Biology », *239*, 110 (1972).

[7] DE DUVE C. and TROUET A., in: *Non-specific Factors Influencing Host Resistance*, W. Braun and J. Ungar, editors, Karger, Basel, p. 153 (1973).

[8] DE DUVE C., DE BARSY T., POOLE B., TROUET A., TULKENS P. and VAN HOOF F., « Biochem. Pharmacol. », *23*, 2495 (1974).

[9] TROUET A., DEPREZ-DE CAMPENEERE D., DE SMEDT-MALENGREAUX M. and ATASSI G., « Europ. J. Cancer », *10*, 405 (1974).

[10] DE DUVE C., in: *Biological Approaches to Chemotherapy*, R. J. C. Harris, editor, Academic Press, London-New York, p. 101 (1961).

[11] COHN Z. A. and PARKS E., « J. Exp. Med. », *125*, 213 (1967).

[12] DE DUVE C., PRESSMAN B. C., GIANETTO R., WATTIAUX R. and APPELMANS F., « Biochem. J. », *60*, 604 (1955).

[13] CALENDI E., DI MARCO A., REGGIANI M., SCARPINATO B. and VALENTINI L., « Biochim. Biophys. Acta », *103*, 25 (1965).

[14] OHNUMA T., HOLLAND J. F. and CHEN J.-H., « Cancer Res. », *35*, 1767 (1975).

[15] SEEBER S., BRUCKSCH K. P., SEEBER B. and SCHMIDT C. G., « Z. Krebsforsch. », *89*, 75 (1977).

[16] MARKS T. A. and VENDITTI J. M., « Cancer Res. », *36*, 496 (1976).

[17] SORACE R. A. and SHEID B., « Fed. Proceed. », *36*, 335 (1977).

[18] ATASSI G., TAGNON H. J. and TROUET A., « Europ. J. Cancer », *10*, 399 (1974).

[19] ATASSI G., DUARTE-KARIM M. and TAGNON H. J., « Europ. J. Cancer », *11*, 309 (1975).

[20] DECKERS C., MACE F., DECKERS-PASSAU L. and TROUET A., in: *Adriamycin Review*, European Press Medikon, Ghent, p. 79 (1975).

[20ª] BROWN I. and WARD H. W. C., « Cancer Letters », *2*, 227 (1977).

[21] Heinen E., Bassleer R., Calbert-Bacq C. M., Desaive Cl. and Lepoint A., « Biochem. Pharmacol. », *23*, 1549 (1974).

[22] Noel G., Peterson C., Trouet A. and Tulkens P., « Europ. J. Cancer », in press (1978).

[23] Trouet A., Deprez-De Campeneere D., Maldague P., Jadin J.-M. and Van Hoof F., in: *Drug Design and Adverse Reactions*, Alfred Benson Symposium, *10*, 77 (1977).

[24] Trouet A., Jadin J.-M. and Van Hoof F., in: *Biochemistry of Parasites and Host-Parasite Relationships*, H. Van den Bossche, editor, North-Holland, Amsterdam, p. 519 (1976).

[25] Trouet A. and de Duve C., « Cancer Chemother. Rep., Part 1 », *59*, 260 (1975).

[26] Rozencweig M., Kenis Y., Atassi G., Staquet M. and Duarte-Karim M., « Cancer Chemother. Rep., Part 3 », *6*, 131 (1975).

[27] Langslet A., Oye I. and Lie S., « Acta Pharmacol. Toxicol. », *35*, 379 (1974).

[28] Henry D. W., « Cancer Chemother. Rep., Part 2 », *4*, 5 (1974).

[29] Sokal G., Trouet A., Michaux J. L. and Cornu G., « Europ. J. Cancer », *9*, 391 (1973).

[30] Cornu G., Michaux J. L., Sokal G. and Trouet A., « Europ. J. Cancer », *10*, 695 (1974).

[31] Michaux J. L., Cornu G., Sokal G. and Trouet A., in: *Adriamycin Review*, European Press Medikon, Ghent, p. 216 (1975).

[32] Lie S. O., Lie K. K. and Langslet A., in: *Adriamycin Review*, European Press Medikon, Ghent, p. 226 (1975).

[33] Longueville J. and Maisin H., in: *Adriamycin Review*, European Press Medikon, Ghent, p. 260 (1975).

[34] Bosly A., Prignot J., Ledent C., Sokal G. and Trouet A., « Europ. J. Cancer », in press (1978).

DISCUSSION

RAPP

We tend to think of leukemia as a disease of the blood, but it starts in blood forming organs. Everyone does not agree with your statement that tumor cells divide more rapidly than normal cells. I think there is evidence that cells in carcinomas divide slowly — and it is also possible that leukemia cells in blood forming organs also divide slowly.

DE DUVE

I mentioned leukemia because it turns out that this is the disease in which we made our first clinical application, but in fact we worked on a number of solid tumors also. As to whether cancer cells divide rapidly or slowly I think this is irrelevant. The main point is that what makes a cancer a cancer is that the cells divide. If they did not divide, they would not bother us. And I think that you will agree that most chemotherapeutic drugs are aimed against some metabolic step concerned with cell division.

RAPP

But if normal cells divide more rapidly than carcinoma cells, drugs on carriers may accumulate more readily in normal cells than in cancer cells.

DE DUVE

Well, that would be true of any of the anti-mitotic agents that are used now. Our approach aims precisely at obviating this drawback. We take the common drugs and try to send them more selectively to the target cells by binding them to an appropriate carrier.

RAPP

Why not introduce them directly into the area that you are interested in?

DE DUVE

But that is what we are doing.

RAPP

No, no — by just taking a needle with your material and putting it
into the tumor.

DE DUVE

Well, I have nothing against it, but if it were so simple why has it
not been done before?

RAPP

It *is* being done.

BALDWIN

Dr. De Duve, there are a number of principles that I think we ought
to discuss. If you compare your model here, are you implying that there
is a quantitative difference in the endocytosis of the malignant cell versus
the normal cell? or are there qualitative differences? or are you suggesting
that you can now take recognition of substances on the cell surface such
as you mentioned — fetal antigens — and use those as receptors for the
drug, and so by binding the drug to the surface, then inducing the endocytosis? The question that I would like to ask is: whether this is a
quantitative difference to the normal and the malignant, or whether you
try to select qualitatively the cell surface components if you can then
induce endocytosis.

[19] *De Duve, Trouet* - p. 24

DE DUVE

The final aim is to take advantage of qualitative differences, that is, using the receptors that are present only on the cancer cell membrane if they exist. So far we have taken advantage only of quantitative differences. At least that is what we suspect. And we have also protected the cells that have little endocytic activity.

BALDWIN

In quantitative terms, can you give us an example of, say, a normal and a malignant cell where the endocytosis rate is quantitatively different?

DE DUVE

I cannot give you an example because the measurements are still to be made.

MATHÉ

There are tumor cells which are very rich in lysosomes, such as monocytic and granulocytic tumors, and others which are much poorer, like lymphocytic tumors. Have you seen any difference in your preliminary test between both?

DE DUVE

No. All cells have lysosomes, even lymphocytes have lysosomes.

MATHÉ

Yes, but much less than monocytes or granulocytes.

DE DUVE

Yes, but that may not be true of lymphoblasts. They are large cells and they have a big cytoplasm with many organelles. Certainly in experimental leukemia, such as the L-1210 mouse leukemia, and also in human leukemia, we obtain very good results with our approach.

[19] *De Duve, Trouet* - p. 25

MATHÉ

But your results may not be related to your hypothesis. There may be several mechanisms, such as an " effet retard".

DE DUVE

That would be fine as long as it works. Serendipity is something that I would always welcome with great pleasure.

MATHÉ

My other question is: what about Kupffer cells? What is the proportion of your complex which is taken up by Kupffer cells?

DE DUVE

Well, it all depends on the complex. It is certainly possible to use carriers that will not go to Kupffer cells, because the appropriate receptor is missing in these cells.

TERRY

There are several ways of taking materials across the cell membrane and internalizing them. The mechanism of capping seen in lymphoid cells leads to some internalization of the cell surface material. Does that material fuse with lysosomes as well, or is it handled in a different manner?

DE DUVE

According to all the evidence in the literature, it fuses with lysosomes and is degraded in lysosomes.

ROSENBERG

The problem with the principle that you have mentioned would be that of destruction not only of the carrier but of the drug itself, by contact with lysosomal enzymes. Now is that a problem for most drugs? Can

[19] *De Duve, Trouet* - p. 26

most drugs be inactivated by contact with this wide variety of lytic enzymes?

De Duve

Obviously this approach is restricted to drugs that are not destroyed in lysosome. You could not do this with insulin for instance.

Oettgen

Some of the drugs that are used at present are highly reactive agents. It is probably too simplistic to assume that they will get into the cell as they are injected into the blood. Do you think that the principle that you have outlined here may already be applied to some extent in that drugs bind to macromolecules before getting into the cell, in the way that you described, without being artificially attached to carriers?

De Duve

This is certainly not excluded. In the particular case of adriamycin and daunorubicin, which have been studied in great detail in our laboratory, all our results indicate that the drugs cross by diffusion across the cell membrane.

Weiss

There is a climate of opinion that "fetal" antigens on the surface of tumor cells do not constitute effective transplantation antigens, i.e. antigens which evoke, and which are the targets of, protective immunological responses. Whether this is true in general, or only in some instances, is still open to question, I believe. Even if fetal antigens do not serve as TATA, however, they may still bestow on neoplastic cells antigenic qualities of sufficient distinction from analogous normal cells to act as targets for antibodies carrying cytotoxic drugs; even if incapable of inciting protective reactions in their own right, they might make the target cell susceptible to drugs coupled to antibodies directed against them.

[19] *De Duve, Trouet* - p. 27

DE DUVE

Yes, I think we will come to this when Michael Sela gives his presentation; I think our two presentations sort of overlap and there will be some very exciting and interesting discussion. But obviously there may be receptors on the cell surface that, as you mention yourself, will not evoke an immune response but may nevertheless act as binding sites for materials that are taken up by pinocytosis.

CLERICI

If I am not wrong, when you calculate the phagocytosis rate according to the K and corrected α indexes there is no difference among tissues. In other words, the phagocytosis exerted by the spleen, which is rich in macrophages, is apparently greater than that exerted, for instance, by the lungs, which have a minor concentration of phagocytes; such difference disappears if the phagocytosis rate is calculated according to the K and corrected α indexes. So, I am wondering from what causes the selectivity of the lysomonotropic chemotherapy, since it is likely that tumors phagocytize to the same extent as normal tissues do.

DE DUVE

Dr. Clerici, you are thinking in terms of the classical concept of reticulo-endothelial system, which is the system of fixed phagocytes or histiocytes, that are present all over the body and characteristically take up carbon black and other such inert particles that are injected. But you have to realize that every cell type in the body has the ability to ingest selectively certain macromolecules. Here there are marked differences in specificity between cells. For instance, glycoproteins with sialyl endgroups are taken up avidly by macrophages and poorly by hepatocytes. Remove the sialic acid to expose a β-galactosyl residue and the relationship is reversed.

TERRY

A few brief questions. In the L-1210 study that you reported, when was the drug given relative to the implantation of the tumor?

[19] *De Duve, Trouet* - p. 28

DE DUVE

One, 2, 3, 4, 5 days after implantation.

TERRY

And it was given intraperitoneally?

DE DUVE

It was given intraperitoneally in the case where the inoculation was done intraperitoneally; it was given intravenously in the adriamycin experiment, where the cells were also inoculated intravenously.

TERRY

Has the experiment been done, in such a way that cells are given intravenously and drugs intraperitoneally?

DE DUVE

No, but the reverse experiment has been done, giving the cells intraperitoneally either as such or in diffusion chambers, and the drug intravenously. In general, the DNA complexes gave better results than did the free drugs, especially with adriamycin and, strangely enough, more so when the cells were in diffusion chambers.

TERRY

And have you used this with spontaneous AKR leukemia or any other tumor models other than L-1210?

DE DUVE

Yes. Other models on which tests have been made include (see reference list of my paper), in the mouse: P-388 leukemia and Madison carcinoma 109 [16], B-16 melanoma and Lewis lung carcinoma [19], Ehrlich ascites [15] and mammary adenocarcinoma [20a]; in the rat:

[19] *De Duve, Trouet* - p. 29

L-311 leukemia, S-250 sarcoma and immunocytomas [20]. The DNA complexes were active in all these systems, sometimes more so than the free drugs, being at the same time less toxic than the latter.

TERRY

If you mix a given amount of adriamycin with a given amount of DNA, is the binding complete?

DE DUVE

Yes.

ROSENBERG

Is it possible that the reason there is less cardiotoxicity — if there is less cardiotoxicity — is that part of the drug is just inactivated when attached to the DNA and therefore you are really giving less active drug?

DE DUVE

It may be, but how do you explain the therapeutic activity?

ROSENBERG

Well, in the human situation you really have not shown that it is active. What I think we would need to see would be equivalent activity with less toxicity and you have not shown us that data. You have shown us some activity in the mouse system; you claim that there was less toxicity in the human system, but I think it would be very important in the same system to show that one is getting these effects.

DE DUVE

I have not mentioned the clinical results for lack of time. Appropriate references are listed in my written paper [26, 29-34]. They indicate that so far the DNA complexes have given encouraging results, comparable to, or better than, those obtained with the free drugs, in a number of

[19] De Duve, Trouet - p. 30

conditions including various types of leukemia, metastatic breast cancer and lung carcinoma.   These are the patients who so far have shown no sign of cardiotoxicity.   Results on animals confirm this conclusion [see: references 27 and 28, and JAENKE R.S., CRADOCK J.C. and RAHMAN A., 1978, manuscript submitted to Cancer Research].

WOLFF

A few brief questions.   1. The source of DNA for the human studies. 2. Have you seen any antibodies develop in the humans that you have given DNA to?   3. Have these patients that you say were drug-resistant already received either of these drugs without DNA before and are now responsive to it with DNA?

DE DUVE

1) The DNA is Type VII, highly polymerized, from Sigma.   It was first extracted from calf thymus; now it comes from herring sperm. 2) Our patients are systematically tested for anti-DNA antibodies.   Results are uniformly negative so far.   3) It has happened that patients who become resistant to one of the free drugs have responded to the same drug given as the DNA complex.   Others, however, have not.

MATHÉ

I think I read a paper from Staquet and Kenis showing that the life span of your complex in the serum is longer than that of adriamycin. Do you confirm that?

DE DUVE

Definitely.

MATHÉ

This might be a very interesting mechanism in my opinion, in complement of your first hypothesis.   So there is a new series of drugs which we have been working on, the ellipticins, which are intercalating agents, which work very well on experimental leukemia and work very poorly in human beings; the reason may be that they disappear very quickly. So would you be ready to work on them, to give them a chance?

DE DUVE

Richard Storace and Bertrum Sheid, at the New York Downstate Medical Center in Brooklyn, have recently found that the DNA-complex of ellipticin may advantageously replace free ellipticin in certain *in vitro* tests. They have obtained particularly good results with a mixture of daunorubicin and ellipticin bound to DNA. So far they have not tested these complexes *in vivo*.

SPREAFICO

Two short questions and a comment. I may have missed in your slides the data of the control group treated with DNA and Daunomycin given simultaneously but not bound together. Has this been done?

DE DUVE

Yes, this has been done and the results are very interesting (ATASSI G., TAGNON H.G. and STAQUET M., in: *Adriamycin Review*, European Press Medikon, Ghent, p. 70, 1975). If the DNA is injected a few minutes before the drug, the results are comparable to those obtained after injection of the complex. But this is not true if the reverse is done. This is understandable in view of the rapid rate of clearance of the free drugs from plasma.

SPREAFICO

Secondly, have you checked the comparative immunodepressive activity of the complex and Daunomycin per se? The comment regards the possibility that you may have different levels of cardiotoxicity because, with the complex, you have changed the pharmacokinetics of the drugs in respect to free Adriamycin or Daunomycin. Indeed, one can markedly reduce the concentration of Adriamycin in the heart of mice, without loss

[19] *De Duve, Trouet* - p. 32

of antitumoral effect if instead of using single high dosages as is done in the clinic, one divides the same dosage in a number of injections.

DE DUVE

Yes.

SPREAFICO

Further, have you checked the immunosuppressive activity of the complexes?

DE DUVE

Not directly, but a lot of work has been done on the comparative toxicology of the free drugs and their DNA complexes. This work indicates that the lymphoid tissues are equally affected by the free and by the DNA-bound drugs. The bone-marrow appears less damaged histologically when the drugs are given as their DNA complexes. However, when the bone-marrow stem-cells were assessed by their ability to form colonies, it was found that they were partly protected against adriamycin by giving this drug as the DNA complex, but not against daunorubicin which appeared even more toxic when bound to DNA than in free form. This is explained, we believe, by the fact that daunorubicin is released more easily from its DNA-complex than is adriamycin under *in vivo* conditions. The greatest protection against either drug was observed on liver and kidney which were almost unharmed by the DNA complexes. Digestive mucosa were partly protected (see: reference 23, and HUYBRECHTS M., SYMANN M. and TROUET A., 1978, manuscript submitted to Cancer Chemother. Rep. and unpublished results).

NOSSAL

My comment is a more cell biological one, and I think it could be a useful link to Michael Sela's talk. I do not think the audience should allow to slip by the extremely important new concept in cell biology that Christan de Duve revealed to us, namely, this idea of a membrane shuttle. The point that he told us was that there were agents that attach to a cell membrane — in this particular case antibodies to cell surface constituents which were endocytosed but were actually never subjected to enzymic degradation because some membrane component was reshuttled back to the surface. Scott Linthicum had independently made a parallel observation, suggesting that this may not be a unique or unusual situation relating to antibodies attaching to the cell membrane but may be illustrating a general principle. In his case, PHA was attached to the surface of T lymphocytes, and the observation made was that this material was rapidly endocytosed and after a longish — in this particular case I must say a longish — interval, 24 to 36 hours, there was clearcut indication of the reappearance of the material on the surface of the cell. So I think that does open a new dimension as to how we should look at the whole question of guided missiles, of magic bullets, and I am very happy to have this fascinating aspect read into the record and, if you want, in a very small way confirmed.

[19] *De Duve, Trouet* - p. 34

USE OF ANTIBODIES FOR DELIVERY
OF CHEMOTHERAPEUTIC DRUGS (*)

MICHAEL SELA (**), ESTHER HURWITZ and RUTH MARON
The Weizmann Institute of Science
Rehovot, Israel

INTRODUCTION

Chemotherapy constitutes a major therapeutic approach for the treatment of cancer, alongside with surgery, radiotherapy and, to a lesser extent, immunotherapy, non-specific or specific. It is used effectively for disseminated as well as localized cancer. Its major drawback, however, is that agents effective in killing neoplastic cells usually also have detrimental effects on normal cells, particularly the rapidly proliferating ones of the gastrointestinal tract and bone marrow. This toxicity often puts limitations on their effective employment in cancer chemotherapy.

One possible approach aimed at overcoming these limitations is by attaching the chemotherapeutic drugs to high molecular weight carriers. Macromolecular conjugates of anti-tumor drugs could affect their distribution in the body and facilitate slow and continuous release, while exerting better stability of the active substances. This attachment could thus decrease the overall toxic effects of these compounds without reducing their profitable activity. This approach

(*) Studies from our laboratory reported here were partially supported by the National Cancer Institute, National Institutes of Health, Public Health Service, USA.
(**) M.S. is an Established Investigator of the Chief Scientist's Bureau, Ministry of Health, Israel.

[20] *Sela, Hurwitz, Maron* - p. 1

was demonstrated for various biologically active substances (MOL-
TENI and SCROLLINI, 1974) and also with some anti-cancer drugs:
(SZEKERKE *et al.*, 1967, 1972; CHU and WHITELEY, 1977).

The ideal carrier, however, would be one that could recognize
the target cell so as to selectively increase the local concentration of
drug, thus performing site-directed killing of the tumor cell. The
specific targeting of the cytotoxic agent could allow for the use of
non-toxic drug doses which would by themselves be ineffective.

PAUL EHRLICH (1906) was the first to suggest that molecules
with an affinity for certain tissues might be able to serve as carriers
of cytotoxic agents, to concentrate them on the appropriate target
cells *in vivo*. Various macromolecules have been shown to localize
in tumor cells *in vivo* and were suggested as possible carriers for
cytotoxic drugs (ISLIKER *et al.*, 1969). With the development of
tumor immunology, many investigators have sought to use antibodies
to antigenic determinants expressed preferentially on tumor cells as
carriers of cytotoxic agents. The question whether genuinely tumor-
specific antigens exist is still open. However, without going too
deeply into this controversy it is clear that antibodies can be prepared which can recognize tumor cells from normal ones in a selective
fashion, and may thus be adequate by virtue of their selectivity. For
this approach to succeed, both the antibody and the toxic agent must
retain their activity when the two are linked together or, alternatively, as discussed by ISLIKER *et al.* (1969), they might be linked
in a manner allowing the release of the active agent after reaching
the target cell.

Complexes and covalent conjugates of drugs with immunoglobulins and other tumor recognizing macromolecules have also been
studied in treatment of tumors (GHOSE *et al.*, 1972a, 1972b;
DAVIES and O'NEIL, 1973a, b; FLECHNER, 1973; RUBENS and
DULBECCO, 1974; LINFORD *et al.*, 1974; MOOLTEN *et al.*, 1970,
1972; PHILPOTT *et al.*, 1973; ROWLAND *et al.*, 1975; ROWLAND,
1977; VARGA *et al.*, 1977; KITAO and HATTORI, 1977). The resulting conjugates and complexes were shown to have selective toxicity
towards cells bearing on their surface the determinants to which the
antibodies or other biological compounds such as lectins or melano-
tropin were specific. In two of these studies, (DAVIES and O'NEIL,
1973a, b; and RUBENS and DULBECCO, 1974) it was shown that

similar effects could be obtained by administration of the free drug and antibody separately, so it is possible that when the drug is administered as a noncovalent complex with antibody it dissociates *in vivo* and acts separately and synergistically with the antibody, as suggested also by SEGERLING *et al.* (1974).

In the present study it was attempted to use conjugates in which the drug is chemically bound to the carrier. Cytotoxic drugs of low molecular weight may retain their activity after covalent linkage to macromolecules. Thus, methotrexate bound *via* azo bond to hamster immunoglobulin (MATHÉ *et al.*, 1958) as well as to fibrinogen and human serum albumin (MAGNENAT *et al.*, 1969) retained significant activity. Likewise did conjugates of a methyl hydrazide derivative with fibrinogen and albumin (MAGNENAT *et al.*, 1969), or conjugates of several nitrogen mustards with proteins and synthetic polypeptides (SZEKERKE *et al.*, 1967).

The drugs we have used (HURWITZ *et al.*, 1975; LEVY *et al.*, 1975) are the anti-tumor antibiotics daunomycin and adriamycin, two of the most useful cancer chemotherapeutic agents presently available (FREI, 1972; O'BRYAN *et al.*, 1973). They have been linked either to a model system of antibodies (anti-BSA) or to antibodies reactive with several experimental murine tumor cells. The resultant conjugates have been investigated for their properties, and in particular their selective cytotoxic activity both *in vitro* and *in vivo*. The results obtained so far are summarized in the following.

BINDING OF DAUNOMYCIN AND ADRIAMYCIN TO ANTIBODIES

Binding Procedures

The drugs daunomycin and adriamycin were covalently linked to the immunoglobulin fraction (prepared by precipitation with ammonium sulfate at 33% saturation), of the following antisera: *a*) Rabbit antiserum to bovine serum albumin (BSA); *b*) Rabbit antiserum against B leukemia cells (a dimethylbenzanthracene-induced leukemia in SJL/J mice [HARAN-GHERA and PELED, 1973]); *c*) Rabbit antiserum against a plasmacytoma (PC5) induced in BALB/c

[20] *Sela, Hurwitz, Maron* - p. 3

mice (POTTER and ROBERTSON, 1960); *d*) Rabbit antiserum against a Moloney virus induced lymphoma (YAC) in A/J mice (KLEIN and KLEIN, 1964). In the YAC system purified antibodies were used as well, as will be described later; *e*) Fab dimers prepared from the anti BSA, anti-PC5 and anti-YAC immunoglobulins.

Three different methods of binding were used, in two of which binding was covalent taking advantage of the amino sugar moiety of the drugs, whereas the third made use of the property of the drugs to intercalate with nucleic acids.

1. *The direct binding procedure.* Periodate oxidation of the drugs was performed to cleave the bond between C_3 and C_4 of the amino sugar. This produced carbonyl groups capable of reacting with free amino groups on the protein, and the resulting Schiff base linkages were subsequently reduced with sodium borohydride.

2. *Linking of daunomycin or adriamycin to immunoglobulins via a dextran bridge.* Dextran was oxidized by periodate (FOSTER, 1975). The polyaldehyde dextran was reacted first for 20 hours with daunomycin at room temperature and then for 20 hours with the antibody at 4°C. The Schiff bases thus formed were reduced by sodium borohydride at a slight excess over the total oxidized groups of the polyaldehyde dextran. The antibody-dextran-daunomycin conjugate was separated from the free drug by gel filtration on Biogel P-60 or on Sephadex G-100 (Fig. 1). Apparently not all the formed Schiff bases were reduced under these conditions. Dialysis of the conjugates against 0.1 M acetate buffer at pH 4.2 released about 30% of the drug. However, too rigorous reducing conditions had dismal effects both on the drug and on the conjugate.

3. *Complexing daunomycin onto t-RNA covalently bound to the immunoglobulin.* Commercial *E. coli* t-RNA was oxidized by 0.05 M $NaIO_4$ for 1 hr at room temperature. Antibodies to YAC cells were incubated with the oxidized t-RNA at pH 9.5 overnight at 4°C. Reduction by sodium borohydride for 1 hr at 37°C followed. The drug was then allowed to react with the t-RNA-antibody compound by incubation for 2 hrs at 37°C. The final conjugate was separated from unbound drug, drug-t-RNA, and reagents, on a Biogel P-60 column.

[20] *Sela, Hurwitz, Maron* · p. 4

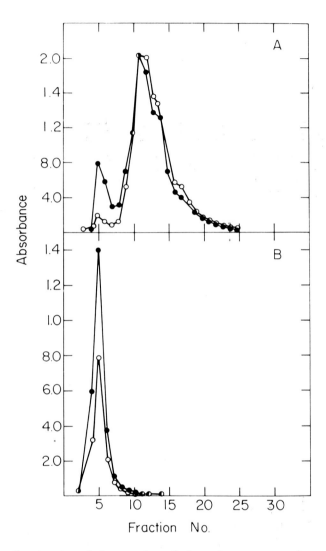

FIG. 1 — *Fractionation of daunomycin-antibody conjugates on a column of Bio-gel P-60.* A comparison between the two binding techniques: The direct binding of the antibody to the drug and the binding *via* a dextran bridge.

(A) Direct binding procedure, 5 moles drug per mole antibody.

(B) Binding through a dextran bridge. 25 moles drug per mole antibody. Absorbance at 280 (●), at 495 (O). (From HURWITZ *et al.*, 1978b).

ACTIVITY OF THE CONJUGATES

One of the prerequisites of the approach used in this study is that both the activity of the drug, namely its cytotoxicity, and the activity of the antibody, namely the capacity to recognize the tumor cell, will be retained.

The drug activity of the conjugates was measured by their inhibition of cellular RNA synthesis, as quantitated by the inhibition of [³H]uridine incorporation into test cells (ROSENBERG *et al.*, 1972). Fig. 2 depicts the activity of free daunomycin, and the two preparations of daunomycin bound to the immunoglobulin of anti-BSA or anti-B-leukemia by the periodate-borohydride method.

Binding of daunomycin *via* a dextran bridge caused a more drastic reduction in its activity, but this effect could be compensated by increase of concentration or prolongation of incubation, by which

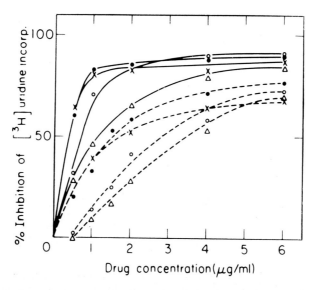

FIG. 2 — Inhibition of [³H]uridine incorporation (*incorp.*) by daunomycin and by daunomycin bound to immunoglobulin (coupled by the periodate-borohydrate method). B leukemia test cells. - - - -, 2 hr incubation; ———, 4 hr incubation; ●, free daunomycin; X, free daunomycin treated with periodate and sodium borohydride; Δ, daunomycin bound to anti-BSA, 6 moles/mole; O, daunomycin bound to anti-B leukemia. (From HURWITZ *et al.*, 1975).

90-95% cytotoxicity was eventually achieved (BERNSTEIN *et al.*, in press).

Binding by complexing the drug to the antibody via t-RNA did not affect appreciably the drug activity. A comparison between the activity of the various conjugates and the free drug is summarized in Table 1.

Another assay of drug effect, namely direct cell killing (non-complement dependent) as estimated by trypan blue uptake, confirmed the results of the [^{3}H]-uridine incorporation assay, again demonstrating the activity of protein-bound drug.

Antibodies to tumor cells

Xenogeneic antibodies to tumor cells were prepared by injecting whole tumor cells into rabbits or goats. The antisera thus obtained were repeatedly absorbed on cells from normal lymphoid tissues from their respective mice strains, until they no longer reacted with those normal cells in a cytolysis assay. In the YAC tumor system immunization was carried out not with the intact cells but rather with a soluble fraction of its membranes obtained by papain proteolysis. Immunization of a goat or rabbits with this fraction yielded an antiserum, which in the unadsorbed form exhibited selectivity towards the YAC cells, as compared to normal spleen and thymus cells of A/J mice (Fig. 3). Although it was not monospecific, this serum reacted with YAC cells more strongly than with normal spleen or thymus cells: at 50% lysis the effect was 3-4 times stronger against YAC cells than against normal cells, while at a 1 : 100 dilution it was cytotoxic only towards the YAC cells. The IgG fraction of this antiserum exhibited the same selective cytotoxicity, but still consisted of a large excess of irrelevant immunoglobulins over the specific antibodies.

Purified antibodies were prepared from this antiserum by adsorption on, and elution from, an immunoadsorbent consisting of gluteraldehyde fixed YAC cells. These purified antibodies, although not exhibiting more specificity than the total IgG fraction, were five fold more effective in their cytotoxic activity.

[20] *Sela, Hurwitz, Maron* - p. 7

TABLE 1 - *In vitro activity of daunomycin and daunomycin-conjugates.*

Yac cells (10^6) were incubated for 2 hrs at 37°C in the presence of daunomycin or daunomycin-conjugates. Incorporation of [³H]-uridine into cellular material precipitable by trichloroacetic acid was measured and expressed as percent inhibition (100% of control culture containing no drug).

Dau conc. µg/ml	Dau	Dau-dex	% inhibition of ³H-uridine incorporation					
			Dau-dex-anti-Yac	Dau-dex-NIg	Dau-anti-Yac	Dau-NIg	Dau t-RNA	Dau t-RNA-anti-Yac
.25	11	0	—	—	—	—	—	—
.50	42	2	8	4	22	39	21	12
1.00	60	50	9	17	44	62	39	34
5.00	90	80	44	48	86	90	74	76
15.00	—	—	63	58	—	—	—	—
50.00	—	—	90	92	—	—	—	—

[20] *Sela, Hurwitz, Maron* - p. 8

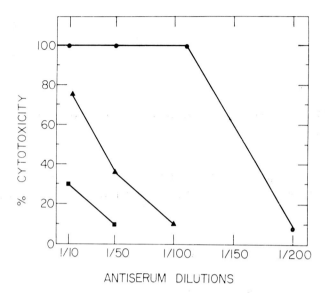

FIG. 3 — *The anti-tumor activity of a goat antiserum prepared against a papain digest of the YAC cell membrane.* The antiserum activity was assessed by C'- mediated cytotoxicity and the % of dead cell determined by trypan blue exclusion. Target cells: YAC (●), normal spleen (▲), normal thymus (■). (From HURWITZ *et al.*, 1978b).

Fab dimers of anti-tumor immunoglobulins as carriers of daunomycin

In all the systems described above, which involved experimental murine tumors, xenogeneic antibodies have been employed. A similar situation will probably exist if the approach will ever be applied to patients. In such case, the removal of the Fc portion of the immunoglobulins that are to be administered might be advantageous for several reasons:

1) Anti-tumor antibodies may still be toxic to normal cells. This toxicity — which is either residual or due to a shift of specificity (DRAKE and MARDINEY, 1975) — is most probably complement-mediated. Thus the removal of the Fc portion should prevent any toxic effects induced by complement.

2) The purpose of the drug-antibody conjugate is to reach the tumor target cell and react with it. It would be most desirable

that fragments not attached to the cellular antigen, should be removed from the circulation as quickly as possible. Thus the (Fab') dimer, with a shorter half life *in vivo* should be superior to the intact antibody molecule (SPIEGELBERG and WEIGLE, 1968; WOCHNER *et al.*, 1967).

3) The lower immunogenicity of the Fab dimer should reduce the antibody response against it in the host.

Fab dimers from the anti-tumor IgG fractions were prepared by pepsin (NISONOFF *et al.*, 1960) cleavage and separated from digested Fc fractions and intact IgG by gel filtration (HURWITZ *et al.*, 1975).

Antibody activity of sera, IgG fractions and antibodies against tumor cell were assayed by C' mediated cytotoxicity and evaluated by trypan blue exclusion or ^{51}Cr release. The antibody activity of Fab dimers was determined by a double binding technique with iodinated goat anti-rabbit (Fab')$_2$.

Antibody activity in the drug-antibody conjugates

The activity of daunomycin-anti-BSA conjugates, whole IgG and Fab dimers were measured by BSA-T4 bacteriophage inactivation (HAIMOVICH *et al.*, 1970). Approximately 55% of the IgG activity (Fig. 4), and 70% of the (Fab')$_2$ activity were retained (HURWITZ *et al.*, 1975).

The antibody activities of the conjugates with antitumor Ig and with purified antibodies were measured by complement-dependent cytotoxicity of the conjugates on the respective tumor cells (Fig. 5). In most cases the cytotoxic activity decreased in relation to the extent of drug substitution, with the residual antibody activity in the conjugates ranging between 25% and 64% of the unmodified antibodies. The antibody activity of Fab dimers prepared from anti-tumor antibodies was likewise maintained. This was established for daunomycin linked anti-BSA (Fab')$_2$ by the modified bacteriophage technique (HAIMOVICH *et al.*, 1970). The anti-YAC (Fab')$_2$ activity was measured by its binding to YAC tumor cells.

[20] *Sela, Hurwitz, Maron* - p. 10

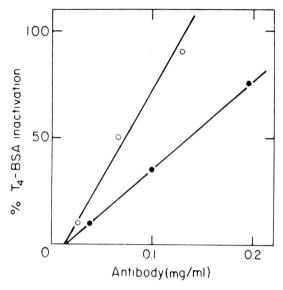

FIG. 4 — The effect of drug binding by the direct method on anti-BSA antibody activity as measured by BSA-T4 bacteriophage inactivation. (○), anti-BSA; (●) daunomycin-anti-BSA. (From HURWITZ et al., 1975).

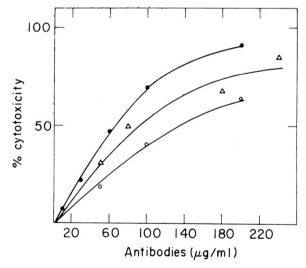

FIG. 5 — *The antibody activity of the daunomycin-anti-YAC conjugates.* The antibody activity was determined by C'-mediated cytolysis of YAC cells. The percent cytolysis was assessed by ^{51}Cr-release. Anti-YAC antibodies (●), dau-anti-YAC antibodies (direct binding procedure) (▲), dau-dextran-anti-YAC antibodies (○). (From HURWITZ et al., 1978b).

From these studies it is apparent that it is feasible to bind covalently both daunomycin and adriamycin to antibodies, with sufficient retention of both drug and antibody activity to be potentially useful.

THE SPECIFIC CYTOTOXIC EFFECTS «IN VITRO» OF THE CONJUGATES

The next step was to determine whether daunomycin bound to antibodies directed against individual tumors showed preferential cytotoxicity against their specific target cells. For that purpose experiments were carried out with a concentration of daunomycin-immunoglobulin conjugate which gave 40-60% inhibition of ^{3}H-uridine incorporation in test cells when it was left in contact with the target cells for the entire period of the incubation. To reveal the specificity of the conjugates, the test cells were exposed to them for only 5 minutes, to allow attachment of specific antibody, then washed to remove non-specific immunoglobulins. The toxicity of the daunomycin remaining in contact with the cells was assessed either by in vitro experiments, namely inhibition of uridine incorporation, or by interference with the transplantability of the tumor cells and their capacity to develop into established tumors in recipient animals.

The results of the in vitro experiments demonstrate that the specific antibody drug conjugate showed toxicity against the homologous PC5 target cell and against a cross-reacting rat lymphoma cell, but much less against the non cross-reacting YAC cells. Drug bound to non-relevant antibodies such as anti-BSA or antibodies directed against a different tumor cell, B leukemia, exhibited only very low toxicity levels. 7% and 16% respectively. The daunomycin bound to the anti-tumor Ig, was twice as efficient as the free daunomycin in spite of its rapid penetrability into mammalian cells (Table 2, Fig. 6). Similar results were obtained showing the specific cytotoxicity of daunomycin anti-YAC Fab dimers (HURWITZ et al., 1975).

The next step in testing the specific cytotoxicity of the drug-antibody conjugate was performed by treatment of the cells in vitro and testing its effect on the tumor growth in vivo. Indeed, as demonstrated in Fig. 7, the growth of the tumor cells subsequent

[20] Sela, Hurwitz, Maron - p. 12

TABLE 2 - *Specific cytotoxicity of daunomycin linked to anti-PC 5 immunoglobulin. Drug (1.5 µg) was incubated with 10^6 cells in a total volume of 100 µl. After 5 min incubation at 37° cells were washed and resuspended in fresh medium for 2 hrs.*

Incubated with	% inhibition of [³H]-uridine incorporation		
	PC5	Rat lymphoma	YAC
Daunomycin-anti-PC5	60 [a]	63 [a]	20 [b]
Daunomycin-anti-BSA	7 [b]	14 [b]	ND [d]
Daunomycin-anti B leukemia	16 [b]	14 [b]	62 [a]
Free daunomycin	32 [c]	53	67

[a, b, c] All *a* values different from all *b* values by $p < 0.001$ (Student's *t* test), *a* values different from *c* values by $p < 0.001$.
[d] ND, not done.

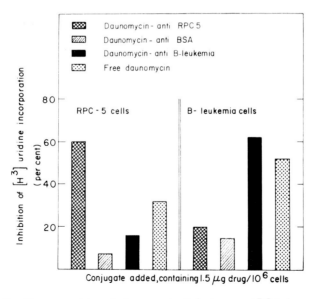

FIG. 6 — Specific cytotoxicity of daunomycin linked to anti-PC-5 immunoglobulin. (Details in table 2).

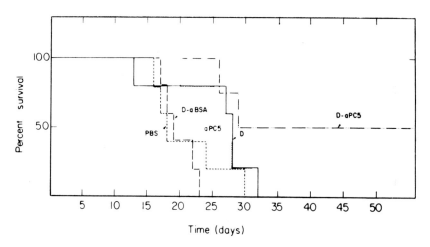

FIG. 7 — PC-5 cells were exposed for 5 min *in vitro* to 0.15 M NaCl:0.01 M phosphate (pH 7.2) (PBS), daunomycin-anti-BSA (D-aBSA), anti-PC-5 (a-PC 5), free daunomycin (D), or daunomycin-anti-PC-5 (D-aPC 5). Cells were then washed and transplanted into syngeneic BALB/c mice. 10^7 cells/animal. Drug, 1.5 µg were added per 10^6 tumor cells. (From LEVY *et al.*, 1975).

to their *in vitro* treatment was retarded and sometimes prevented entirely. The effect was due to the binding of antibodies to their specific target cells, since exposure to drug conjugated to unrelated immunoglobulins caused no delay of tumor growth.

EXPERIMENTS DESIGNED TO ELUCIDATE THE MODE OF ACTION OF THE CONJUGATES

The chemotherapeutic activity of daunomycin attached to antibody or other specific and non specific macromolecules demands the ability of the conjugates either to release the drug upon contact with the cell, or to penetrate the cell and release the drug intracellularily, or — alternatively — to penetrate the cell and the nucleus and possibly perform its activity in the macromolecular form. We have performed some experiments designed to elucidate the mechanism of action of the conjugates.

In order to test the ability of daunomycin, bound covalently to

[20] *Sela, Hurwitz, Maron* - p. 14

immunoglobulins, as compared to free daunomycin, to penetrate into the cell and to reach the nucleus, we have measured the uptake of labeled materials by the YAC cells (HURWITZ *et al.*, 1978a). The labeling was performed by using tritiated $NaBH_4$ for the reduction step in the conjugation procedure, so that the label was at the conjugation point or, alternatively, the antibody was labeled by iodination with [125]I.

The uptake of daunomycin and its conjugates by YAC cells or by normal cells (rat splenocytes) is depicted in Fig. 8. It is expressed as percentage of uptake of the total radioactivity added to a fixed number of cells. The distribution of daunomycin or daunomycin-conjugates in the membranes or the cytoplasm, and its possible attachment to the nucleus, were measured as a function of time of incubation. As can be seen, the free drug penetrated the cells very

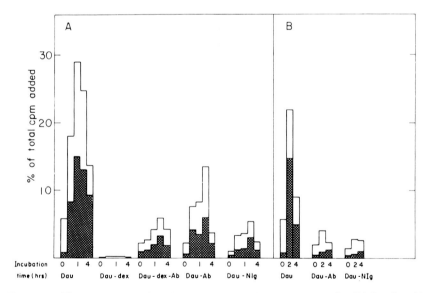

FIG. 8 — The *in vitro* uptake of daunomycin and its conjugates by YAC cells (A) and normal rat lymphocytes (B), measured as a function of time. Measurements of uptake were made at zero time and after 0.5, 1, 2, 3 and 4 hrs following the addition of drug. The total drug accumulation in the cells is denoted by the open bars, whereas the nuclear incorporation by the shaded areas. (From HURWITZ *et al.*, 1978a).

rapidly. The uptake of the free drug reached high levels already at zero point (at which the test was performed by centrifugation and washing at 0°C, immediately after the addition of the drug), reached a peak at 1 hr incubation, and declined after 3 hrs. The accumulation of the drug in or on the nuclei (shaded areas in the chart) paralleled its uptake by the intact cell and amounted roughly to two thirds of it.

Daunomycin-dextran was not readily taken up by the cells, either tumor or normal, although the compound retained drug activity. At the optimal uptake time (2 1/2 hrs) only 0.2% of the added radioactively labeled daunomycin-dextran was incorporated into the cells. Daunomycin-antibody conjugates, whether directly bound or *via* a dextran bridge, penetrated into the YAC cells and attached to their nuclei, although at a much lower rate than that of the free drug. Thus the results show that daunomycin bound directly to antibodies entered the cells at higher levels than when bound through dextran or when drug was bound to normal Ig. The optimal concentrations were similar to those obtained for free drug without a noted dependence on the amount of antibody in the preparation. The accumulation of drug on the nuclei was parallel at all times tested to the extent of uptake by the whole cells, amounting to half to two thirds of its value. We have not tested whether the conjugates have penetrated the nuclei or were just attached to them.

In normal unrelated cells (rat splenocytes) the uptake of free drug was lower than that by the tumor cells. The daunomycin conjugates with either anti-YAC antibodies or normal Ig (linked directly) were taken up at low rates and did not differ from each other. This was expected, since these cells do not bind goat anti-YAC. The uptake of daunomycin-dextran-anti-YAC, labeled both by ^{3}H at the linkage points and by ^{125}I on the antibody, similarly showed presence of both labels in or on the nucleus. Yet, it was not established whether the compound was the original one presented to the cell or whether breakdown products labeled by one or the other isotope simultaneously reach the nucleus.

It is possible that free drug released from the complexes *in situ* is the compound that performs the cytotoxic activity. Our results

[20] *Sela, Hurwitz, Maron* - p. 16

just demonstrate that immunoglobulin drug conjugates are capable of reaching the nucleus, particularly when bearing affinity to the cell surface.

« IN VIVO » STUDIES

The next step in the evaluation of these conjugates was to test their ability to prevent *in vivo* the development of tumors. We have tested the effect of daunomycin bound to anti-tumor antibodies, on two different murine tumors, namely the plasmacytoma PC-5, and the YAC Moloney virus induced lymphoma. The effect was assessed by the suppression of tumor growth, as indicated by prolongation of the life span of the mice, and by the prevalence of long term survivors.

In *the PC-5 system*, BALB/c mice, 2-3 months old, were implanted with 10^5 tumor cells, i.p., and the treatment by the drug or its conjugates was also given i.p. The conjugates tested in this system were only those prepared by the direct binding procedures. The control groups included treatments with free drug, a conjugate of drug and irrelevant antibodies, mixtures of the drug and antibodies, as well as antibodies alone. The *in vivo* experiments with the plasmacytoma system are summarized in Table 3. The results with all the groups treated with the drug and drug conjugates were variable from one experiment to the other and within the treated groups of each experiment, but they do allow some conclusions. The drug-anti-PC-5 conjugate was at least as effective as the free drug, and was more effective than a conjugate of daunomycin with the irrelevant anti-lysozyme.

The highest increase in the therapeutic value of daunomycin was observed when it was given in a mixture with the relevant antibodies, with median survival of 94 days (while the non-relevant anti-lysozyme did not increase the efficiency at all). Such synergistic effects of mixtures of antibodies to tumor cells and drugs were reported by several other groups in both *in vitro* and *in vivo* experiments (DAVIES, 1974; DAVIES and O'NEIL, 1973a, b; FERRONE *et al.*, 1974; RUBENS and DULBECCO, 1974; SEGERLING *et al.*, 1975; NEWMAN, 1977). The suggested explanation for this effect is that

[20] *Sela, Hurwitz, Maron* - p. 17

TABLE 3 - *The effect of daunomycin, daunomycin-Ig conjugates and a mixture of daunomycin and antibodies, on mice transplanted with a plasmacytoma (PC5).*[a]

Treatment	Total No. of exp.	Median[b] life span Days	Average[b] Survival %	Survival Day[c] Mean ±	S.E.
PBS	13	20	0	20.2 ±	3.7
Daunomycin	13	31	20	45.3 ±	25.4
Anti-PC5 + Dau	10	94.5	48	93.8 ±	20.9
Anti-PC5-Dau	9	41	26	54.7 ±	34.3
Anti-PC5	13	22	6	27.1 ±	6.3
Anti-Lysozyme + Dau	6	24	10	36.6 ±	15.6
Anti-Lyso-Dau	6	28.5	10	35.4 ±	14.4
Anti-Lysozyme	8	19	2.5	18.5 ±	2.3

[a] BALB/c mice at the ages of 2-3 months (with one exception where mice were 6 weeks old) were transplanted with 10^5 PC5 cells delivered i.p., received a total amount of 60 μg daunomycin/mouse. The drug was administered in 4 i.p. injections on two consecutive days, 6-8 hrs appart each day. The first portion was given at the time of the tumor transplantation.

[b] The median life span is calculated from the median of each of the experiments. The % survival is calculated from the number of mice which survived over 4 months, divided by the total number of mice tested in each group.

[c] The survival day is based on the analysis of variance assay.

the drug renders the cells more susceptible to the cytotoxic action of the antibodies.

Preliminary *in vivo* experiments using the $(Fab')_2$ derived from anti-PC5 as the drug carrier, similarly to the whole Ig fraction, demonstrated no loss in the original drug activity. However, mixtures of Fab' dimer and drug did not exhibit any advantage over the free drug, suggesting that the "mixture effect" is dependent on the Fc fragment of the antibody.

[20] *Sela, Hurwitz, Maron* - p. 18

In vivo studies with the YAC tumor system

In the *in vivo* experiments with the YAC system (HURWITZ *et al.*, submitted for publication [b]), groups of 5 to 10 mice were transplanted with 10^5 tumor cells and then treated with the drug conjugates, with either Ig fraction of the antiserum or purified antibodies, with control groups including free drug, conjugates of drug and normal Ig, mixtures of drug and antibodies, and antibodies alone.

In this system the tumor and the treatment were given by separate routes; whereas the tumor cells were transplanted i.p., the drug and drug-antibodies were injected i.v., usually 2 days and in some experiments 5 days following the implantation of tumor cells.

The daunomycin conjugates, either with the total IgG or with the purified antibodies, were prepared by linking *via* a dextran bridge. This enabled higher substitution of antibody by drug, from about 4-6 M/M, by the direct binding, to as much as 25 M/M, and thus it was possible to use the higher drug doses needed when the treatment was given systemically.

The effect *in vivo* of dau-dex-anti-YAC (Ig) as compared to daunomycin (Table 4) showed an advantage of the conjugate over the free drug at high doses ($p < 0.05$). A similar effect, however, was obtained by using drug conjugated to normal immunoglobulin or just to dextran. When purified antibodies were employed, again dau-dex-anti-YAC was more efficient in its chemotherapeutic effect than the free drug, but not significantly different from dau-dex or dau-dex-NIg. However, at the lower drug doses the results demonstrated an andvantage of the conjugate of the specific antibody over the preparation of daunomycin linked through dextran to normal immunoglobulin. The purified antibodies themselves had a small but reproducible effect in delaying the onset of the tumor.

Since the activity of the conjugated drug was reduced by the binding procedure by about 50-80% in different preparations, as determined in the *in vitro* assay (HURWITZ *et al.*, 1978a), an experiment was conducted in which the amounts of free drug were comparable, not by their actual concentration, but according to *in vitro* activity units, to the amounts present in the conjugates. In this experiment, 50 µg/mice of daunomycin were compared to 200 µg/mice dau-dex-antibody or dau-dex-Ig. Under

TABLE 4 - *The in vivo therapeutic effect of daunomycin bound through dextran, to anti-Yac (Ig), to anti-Yac (Ab) or to normal immunoglobulin.*

Treatment [a]	Drug dose: (µg/mouse)											
	50		100		150		200		250-300		350-450	
	M	% S [b]	M	% S	M	% S	M	% S	M	% S	M	% S
Daunomycin	23	0 (0/22)	53	40 (2/5)	27	26 (4/15)	120	46 (7/15)	93	44 (11/25)	20	3 (1/35)
Dau-anti-Yac (Ig)					25	10 (1/10)	34	0 (0/5)	120	80 (4/5)	120	60 (3/5)
Dau-anti-Yac (Ab)	20	0 (0/5)	40	40 (2/5)	35	30 (3/10)	45	44 (8/18)	27	40 (4/10)	120	80 (8/10)
Dau-NIg [c]			24	20 (1/5)	26	0 (0/11)	39	18 (4/22)	79	60 (6/10)	120	80 (12/15)
Dau + anti-Yac (Ig)					75	40 (2/5)						
Dau + anti-Yac (Ab)	35	0 (0/5)										
Dau + NIg					35	40 (2/5)	120	80 (8/10)				

Control groups	M	% S
PBS	18	0 (0/60)
anti-Yac (Ig)	20	0 (0/35)
anti-Yac (Ab)	24	4 (1/25)

[a] Treatment was given i.v. within 2 days after tumor transplantation. Tumor cells, 10^5/mice were transplanted i.p. The number of mice per group in each experiment was 5-10.
[b] The number of surviving mice out of total number of mice studied in one or more groups is given in parentheses.
[c] NIg: normal immunoglobulin.

such conditions the drug-dex-antibody showed advantage both over the free drug and over drug-dex-NIg (Fig. 3). These results, demonstrating a significant difference between the daunomycin-antibody conjugate and all the controls, encourage continued effort in this direction.

In the YAC system, like in the plasmacytoma (PC5) *in vivo* experiments, favorable synergism, between daunomycin and antibodies to YAC cells, was also observed. The amount of antibody necessary for a synergistic effect was usually higher than that needed for an efficient treatment with the daunomycin-dextran-antibody conjugate. The therapeutic effects with the mixture were more pronounced when the routes of tumor transplantation and treatment were the same, namely i.p. But an advantage over drug alone and antibody alone was also observed when the treatment was given i.v.

Drug-dextran

From the experiments with the drug-dextran-antibody conjugates, it appeared that the control drug-dextran, proved to be efficient

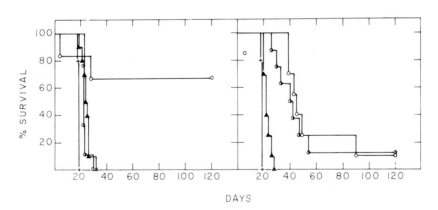

Fig. 9 — *The therapeutic effect of daunomycin bound to specific anti-tumor antibodies as compared to that of the drug bound to normal immunoglobulin.* Left figure: The treatment was given 2 days after the tumor transplantation. Right figure: The treatment was given 5 days after the tumor transplantation. Phosphate buffered saline (+), daunomycin, 50 ¡ɩg/mouse (▲) Daunomycin-dextran-anti-YAC(o), daunomycin-dextran-NIg (ᴑ). The amount of daunomycin delivered in the conjugates was 300 ¡ɩg/mouse. (From HURWITZ *et al.*, 1978b).

as the conjugate with the antibody at high drug doses. In view of
these results we have extended the experimentation with drug-dextran
conjugates (BERNSTEIN *et al.*, 1978). As can be seen in Fig. 10,
low doses, below 300 µg/mouse, are more effective when free daunomycin is given than when the treatment is with daunomycin-

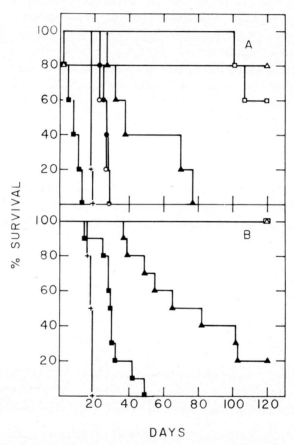

FIG. 10 — The therapeutic effect of daunomycin-dextran compared to that of the
free drug. A graphic representation of one experiment with 10 mice per group.
Mice were transplanted with 10^5 tumor cells, i.p. The therapeutic treatment was
given i.v. either 2 days after the tumor inoculation (A), or after 5 days (B). Daunomycin: 150 µg (●), 300 µg (▲), 450 µg (■) per mouse. Daunomycin-dextran:
150 µg (○), 400 µg (△), 500 µg (□) per mouse. PBS (+). (From BERNSTEIN
et al., 1978).

[20] *Sela, Hurwitz, Maron* - p. 22

dextran. This is probably a result of some loss in the drug activity upon binding which was also observed in the *in vitro* assay (Table 1). The free drug reaches its optimal activity at doses of 150-300 µg/mouse where the median survival day is day 78, and 40% of the mice are long-term survivors (do not die within 120 days). However, at concentrations above 300 µg/mouse the free drug has toxic effects, which are usually lethal at concentrations above 450 µg/mouse. Therefore, the concentration of 300 µg free daunomycin per mouse is optimal. The drug-dextran becomes effective at higher concentrations. Doses of 400 and 500 µg/mouse double the survival rate observed with the optimal dose of daunomycin. Thus, 80% of the mice are completely cured and the remaining 20% live longer than mice receiving unbound drug.

In an experiment in which the treatment with the drug or the drug-dextran conjugate was started at various intervals after the inoculation of the tumor cells, we observed that the daunomycin-dextran is effective up to about 6 days after the tumor transplantation, where it competed well with the free drug. When treatment was given after 12 days the free drug was somewhat more effective. This may be due to a quicker accessibility of free drug to higher tumor loads.

In another experiment, the treatment in all groups was given at day 2 after the tumor cell transplantation, but the load of inoculated tumor cells varied from 10^5 to 10^8/mouse. Here neither free drug nor drug-dextran cured effectively a tumor load of 10^8 cells, only a small delay in the median survival day was noted which was slightly longer with free drug. With a higher dose of daunomycin-dextran, 750 µg/mouse, using a conjugate of dextran T-40 with daunomycin substitution of 15 M/M, the effect was still only a small increase in life span. However, daunomycin-dextran was advantageous to the free drug at a lower tumor load, of 10^7 cells/mouse.

In the application of antibodies as carriers of the anti-cancer agent, two advantageous conditions could be operative: *a*) At low doses, too low for drug effectivity, selectively concentrating the drug at the site of the tumor. *b*) At high doses, when the free drug is toxic to normal tissues, by the lower toxicity of the conjugate.

[20] *Sela, Hurwitz, Maron* - p. 23

The results corroborate these conditions. The specific beneficial effect of the relevant conjugate using purified antibodies, as compared to all other drug conjugates, at low drug doses only, corresponds to the first extreme condition. The higher efficacy of all high molecular weight drug conjugates as compared to the free drug, at high drug doses, corresponds to the second extreme condition, and might be a direct result of lowering of the toxicity.

Homing and distribution of drug-antibody and drug-dextran conjugates

In preliminary studies we tested the *in vivo* homing of the anti-YAC antibodies and their drug conjugates. The experiments were performed by a double labeling technique. Antibodies were iodinated with ^{125}I, while the built-in control, NIg, with ^{131}I. Normal and tumoric mice at different stages of tumor development received a mixture of the two labeled immunoglobulins as such or in the drug conjugate form. Mice heavily infested by the tumor, indeed had accumulated specific antibodies in the ascitis as well as in several other tissues. However, mice at earlier stages of the tumor development could not localize these antibodies on the tumor cells.

The distribution *in vivo* of the free drug versus that of the conjugates was tested by injecting into normal and tumoric mice either tritiated or iodinated compounds. Results demonstrated a much slower clearing of drug conjugates, particularly with dextran-T-40 (M.W. = 40,000) than that of the free drug. This could indicate that the beneficial effects of the conjugates were the results of systemic persistance and slow release of the drug.

CONCLUDING REMARKS

The results reported in this article indicate that antibodies may serve as carriers for anti-cancer drugs to the tumor cells. It is still too early to decide whether this approach will develop into a therapeutic procedure for treatment of cancer. The main difficulty anti-

[20] *Sela, Hurwitz, Maron* - p. 24

cipated is the preparation of suitable antibodies which will be specific only for the tumor cells and thus will not interact at all with normal tissue. These antibodies should be immunospecifically purified so as to avoid the presence of high amounts of irrelevant immunoglobulins. With more information accumulated about "tumor associated" antigens it should become possible to prepare mono-specific antibodies. Alternatively, other compounds such as lectins or hormones shown recently to bind specifically to tumor could serve as the site directed carriers. With the introduction of highly specific carriers this approach might provide potential means for improvement of chemotherapy.

[20] *Sela, Hurwitz, Maron* - p. 25

REFERENCES

BERNSTEIN A., HURWITZ E., MARON R., ARNON R., SELA M. and WILCHEK M., « J. Nat. Cancer Inst. », in press (1978).

CHU B.C.F. and WHITELEY J.M., « Molecular Pharmacology », *13*, 80-88 (1977).

DAVIES D.A.L., « Cancer Res. », *34*, 3040-3043 (1974).

DAVIES D.A.L. and O'NEIL G.J., « Brit. J. Cancer », *28*, 285-298 (1973a).

DAVIES D.A.L. and O'NEIL G.J., « Brit. J. Cancer », *28*, Suppl. I, 285-298 (1973b).

DRAKE W.P. and MARDINEY M.R., « J. Immunol. », *114*, 1052-1057 (1975).

EHRLICH P., *Collected Studies on Immunity*. Vol. II, pp. 442-447. John Wiley & Sons, Inc., New York (1906).

FERRONE S., PELLEGRINO M.A., DIERICH M.P. and REISFELD R.A., « Tissue Antigens », *4*, 275-282 (1974).

FLECHNER I., « Eur. J. Cancer », *9*, 741-745 (1973).

FOSTER R.L., « Experientia », *31*, 773-774 (1975).

FREI E., « Cancer », *30*, 1656-1661 (1972).

GHOSE T. and NIGAM S.P., « Cancer », *29*, 1398-1400 (1972a).

GHOSE T., NORVELL S.T., GUCLU A., CAMERON D., BODURTHA A. and MacDONALD A.S., « Brit. Med. J. », *3*, 495-499 (1972b).

HAIMOVICH J., HURWITZ E., NOVIK N. and SELA M., « Biochim. Biophys. Acta », *207*, 115-124 (1970).

HARAN-GHERA N. and PELED A., « Nature », *241*, 396-398 (1973).

HURWITZ E., LEVY R., MARON R., WILCHEK M., ARNON R. and SELA M., « Cancer Res. », *35*, 1175-1181 (1975).

HURWITZ E., MARON R., ARNON R. and SELA M., « Cancer Biochem. Biophys », *1*, 197-202 (1976).

HURWITZ E., MARON R., ARNON R., WILCHEK M. and SELA M., « Eur. J. Cancer », in press (1978a).

HURWITZ E., MARON R., BERNSTEIN A., WILCHEK M., SELA M. and ARNON R., Submitted for publication (1978b).

ISLIKER H., CEROTTINI H.C., JATON J.-C. and MAGNENAT G., In: *Chemotherapy of Cancer*, pp. 278-288, Elsevier Publishing Co., Amsterdam (1969).

KITAO T. and HATTORI K., « Nature », *265*, 81-82 (1977).

KLEIN E. and KLEIN G., « J. Nat. Cancer Inst. », *32*, 547-568 (1964).

LEVY R., HURWITZ E., MARON R., ARNON R. and SELA M., « Cancer Res. », *35*, 1182-1186 (1975).

LINFORD J.H., FROESE G., BERCZI I. and ISRAELS L.G., « J. Nat. Cancer Inst. », *52*, 1665-1667 (1974).

MAGNENAT R., SCHINDLER R. and ISLIKER H., « Eur. J. Cancer », *5*, 33-40 (1969).

MATHÉ G., TRAN B.L. and BERNARD J., « Compt. Rend. », *246*, 1626-1628 (1958).

MOLTENI L. and SCROLLINI F., « Eur. J. Med. Chem. », *6*, 618-620 (1974).

MOOLTEN F.L. and COOPERBAND S.R., « Science », *169*, 68-70 (1970).

MOOLTEN F.L., CAPPARELL N.J. and COOPERBAND S.R., « J. Nat. Cancer Inst. », *49*, 1057-1062 (1972).

NEWMAN C.E., FORD C.H.J., DAVIES D.A.L., O'NEILL G.J., « Lancet », *2*, 163-166 (1977).

NISONOFF A., WISSLER F.C., LIPPMAN L.N. and WOERNLEY D.L., « Arch. Biochem. Biophys. », *89*, 230-244 (1960).

O'BRYAN R.M., LUCE J.K., TALKY R.W., GOTTLIEB J.K., BAKER L.H. and BONADONNA G., « Cancer », *32*, 1-8 (1973).

PHILPOTT G.W., SHEARER W.T., BOWER R.J. and PARKER C.W., « J. Immunol. », *111*, 921-929 (1973).

POTTER M. and ROBERTSON C.L., « J. Nat. Cancer Inst. », *25*, 847-861 (1960).

ROSENBERG S.A., LEVY R., SCHECHTER B., FICKER S. and TERRY W., « Transplantation », *13*, 541-545 (1972).

ROWLAND G.F., O'NEILL G.F. and DAVIES D.A.L., « Nature », *255*, 487-488 (1975).

ROWLAND G.F., « Eur. J. Cancer », *13*, 593-596 (1977).

RUBENS R.D. and DULBECCO R., « Nature », *248*, 81-82 (1974).

SEGERLING M., OHANIAN S.H. and BORSOS T., « J. Nat. Cancer Inst. », *53*, 1411-1413 (1974).

SEGERLING M., OHANIAN S.H. and BORSOS T., « Science », *188*, 55-57 (1975).

SPIEGELBERG H.L. and WEIGLE W.O., « J. Exp. Med. », *121*, 323-338 (1968).

SZEKERKE M., WADE R. and WHISSON M.E., « Nature », *215*, 1303-1304 (1967).

SZEKERKE M., WADE R. and WHISSON M.E., « Neoplasma », *19*, 211-215 (1972).

VARGA J.M., ASATO N., LANDE S., LERNER A.B., « Nature », *267*, 56-58 (1977).

WOCHNER R.D., STROBER W. and WALDMANN T.A., « J. Exp. Med. », *126*, 207-221 (1967).

DISCUSSION

CHEDID

Dr. Sela, I would like to ask you a question which is also directed to Dr. Rosenberg. Since fetal antigens are present *in vivo* on tumor cells, do they not therefore represent more helpful carriers than a specific antigen? Could you also tell us if the immunogenicity of daunomycin is increased by conjugating it to a carrier?

SELA

The first question was about the immunogenicity of daunomycin. Daunomycin is also, I believe, an immunosuppressive drug, and I do not think that daunomycin alone, unless it is attached to a macromolecule, leads to an important antibody formation. But it is possible to make antibodies to daunomycin by using for immunization conjugates of daunomycin with, in our case, serum albumin. Certainly daunomycin attached to a rabbit immunoglobulin is a good candidate when injected to form anti-daunomycin antibodies.

DAVIES

In connection with the last comment, we do have some data to suggest that carcinoembryonic antigen is *not* a candidate for drug-antibody synergism. I will mention it later. A comment I would like to make is this: in your experiment where you labelled the linkage to see where this complex was localizing in the cell, I thought that if you subtracted the localization index of your daunomycin-dextran-normal Ig from that of the daunomycin-dextran-immune Ig, there is really very little difference between those two.

SELA

I agree with you: this is not a very significant difference. I think the only thing that is very significant is the daunomycin-dextron, which is very effective *in vivo*.

MARINI-BETTÒLO

I think, Prof. Sela, that from the present discussion you have obtained a distribution pattern in the "target searching drugs". I believe that it would be most important at this point to learn something about the mode of action of the drug on the carrier, and about the type of binding between the drug and the carrier itself. Maybe the bond could be covalent, but in the case of the Schiff base we must consider that these substances are rather labile. Most probably the Schiff base could bind to the target and then, in the presence of particular enzymes, the drug could be liberated and in conditions to interact with the target. Have you any evidence about that?

SELA

Yes, I think so. First of all we make a Schiff base but we reduce it with sodium borohydride to make a very stable covalent linkage. The question is whether the reduction is totally quantitative. We have now some doubts about it but certainly at least 90% of the bonds are reduced.

MARINI-BETTÒLO

May I ask you — have you tried with other anti-tumor drugs like vinblastin or daunomycin?

SELA

No, all our work was at the beginning with adriamycin, which I did not discuss here.

MARINI-BETTÒLO

Being of different types maybe they can give some more information about the mode of action.

[20] *Sela, Hurwitz, Maron* - p. 30

SELA

This is correct, but I will confess that in this particular study I tried to be less curious than we would have wanted, because I thought that this is something which ultimately, at least for our purpose, is of an applied interest and I wanted first of all to spend enough effort to make sure that it is worth continuing. As to the mode of action, we went into that only several weeks ago after we had sufficient initial results to decide that it was worth probing into it. Now we are dealing with a lot of possible variations, we used half a dozen different techniques in binding the drug — we were using various handles, we were using various antibodies — I did not want to go into so many drugs (even though now we are starting some other drugs) so at this moment — for better or worse — we settled on daunomycin.

MARINI-BETTÒLO

Excuse me, one more question: Have you tried the dextrans bound with adriamycin? In this case it also reduced?

SELA   .

Yes, always reduced.

MARINI-BETTÒLO

In this case it is clear that it is not a question of releasing.

SELA

There has not been a question about it in my mind until a month ago, but some of our recent results suggest there is release. Daunomycin, attached to dextran, and with the bonds stabilized should not be at all released.

DE DUVE

There are obviously many questions one can ask because, as we have discussed many times before, we both start from different principles but may have reached more or less the same goal, perhaps by accident. Now, the only question that I would like to raise in connection with what Professor Marini-Bettòlo has asked is: how do these conjugates act? Especially how do they enter the cells? Because to my knowledge penetration of an intact macromolecule inside the cytoplasm to reach the nucleus is an extremely rare event. Certain viruses seem to be able to do this, but even they may enter by the normal mechanism of endocytosis and then somehow escape out of the vacuolar system. Some toxins seem to have solved the problem. I am thinking of substances such as abrin, ricin, diphtheria toxin, cholera toxin, etc. They are all made of two chains bound by disulphide bonds. One of these chains recognizes a receptor on the membrane and the other gets in, and inhibits an enzyme. How this happens is not known; it is a fascinating thing. But except for these highly specialized systems, I know of no example really authenticated of a macromolecule getting across the plasma membrane. Now you showed on your last slide that your conjugates had reached the nucleus: and I have to ask you again the question I asked you and Ruth Arnon six months ago: could the association with the nucleus be an adsorption artifact subsequent to disruption of the cytoplasm by detergent action?

SELA

Yes. We are at a stage where you ask us "how" and not "whether", because until a few months ago we did not know even whether anything of this goes on. Now, first of all, any criticism that was made here yesterday concerning radioactivity measurements is valid also here. We can only say that we have two different radioactivities which go on parallel — you might say that they were split and they are on small molecules and they happen to go at the same rate inside, because all we do at this stage is to see the radioactivity. Also I did not say that it is *in* the nucleus — I said in the nucleus or on the nucleus or going with the nucleus. But it is a fact that it is inside, so that the only thing which I would believe is that, considering the proportion of this drug conjugate that finds its way into the cytoplasm, I do not believe that it is totally digested. On the other hand, it is also clear that some of the daunomycin goes inside free — I do not think from this experiment but from others, including experiments with the drug-dextran conjugate.

[20] *Sela, Hurwitz, Maron* · p. 32

DE DUVE

I just want to make one point clear, because I think it is important for the general understanding of what you are doing. As I remember it, the cells are exposed to these conjugates. They are then lysed with a detergent — Triton if I remember rightly — and then the nucleus is that part that remains and is sedimented from the solubilized cytoplasm. Now such a treatment would release any material that is inside the lysosomes because lysosomes would be lysed by your detergent. If then the material released should secondarily adsorb to the nuclei, your results could be explained without the need of invoking an unorthodox route of entry. Of course, the mechanism of action of the conjugates would still have to be explained. That is a different problem.

MATHÉ

First I would like to answer the question which was asked you about other drugs: we did it in 1958 with methotrexate combined with heterospecific anti L1210 leukemia antibodies. The complex was more effective than methotrexate alone, but the complex methotrexate-albumin was also more effective than methotrexate. My first question is: have you studied the life span of the complex? My second one is: I know you have two lines of YAC: one which is very immunogenic and one which is less immunogenic. Do you have a better result with the more immunogenic one?

SELA

Of course the life span is longer. This is certainly not due to human complexes because these animals do not have any anti-daunomycin antibodies during the experiment. But the antibody as such has a much longer life span.

MATHÉ

What about toxicity?

[20] *Sela, Hurwitz, Maron* - p. 33

SELA

I do not know how much is known about cytotoxicity in mice.

MATHÉ

It is better in rabbits.

MATHÉ

We considered it but we have not studied it yet. Concerning the question about the two YAC lines, I think we worked only with one of them and I cannot tell you which one.

BALDWIN

I just wanted to make a comment about whether one can use specific antigens on the cell surface. I think that it is not advisable to do fetal antigens because they tend to shed very easily from the cell surface. In order to get tumor-specific antibodies, a very easy source that you might consider is to take immune-complexes from tumor-bearing mice and just by dissociating these immune complexes, you have a source of antigen which will produce tumor-specific antibody and that may be a simple way to produce an antibody for this particular approach.

CLERICI

Just a very short question. Daunomycin is linked at random to the antibody, including the Fab fragment. Is it possible to keep the Fab fragment free from Daunomycin? I feel it is quite important that the antibiotic be linked to the Fc rather than the Fab fragment, because, if the opposite takes place, the efficiency of the system would be definitely decreased.

SELA

That is very correct; we have used it in various situations in the past, and we would consider doing it if we do not find a way which is much simpler.

[20] *Sela, Hurwitz, Maron* - p. 34

OETTGEN

I have a question about the relevance of the animal model that you use to the clinical situation, if the mechanism is as you think it is. The mouse which you treat with your conjugated material has not yet had an opportunity to form antibody to the leukemia cells that were just inoculated into it. In human cancer patients there is already circulating antibody. Would additional treatment with small amounts of the antibody that is in the conjugate interfere with the effect in your mouse system?

SELA

You mean by previously immunizing the mouse or by giving it passively the antibody? That is a very good point.

CHAGAS

In your work you showed that daunomycin and dextran did not penetrate — you highlighted this point. But I would like to understand the mechanism by which dextran and daunomycin do not go into the cell and when you attach it to the immunoglobulin it goes in.

SELA

I will try to explain. What we labeled was not daunomycin and not dextran in this case but a link between them. If 10 or 15% of the daunomycin-dextran Schiff base was not reduced, it would not be labeled. The experiment of label would show that nothing penetrated, but the 10 or 15% of daunomycin could have been released.

RAPP

I would like to speculate on how these drugs are getting into cells and I think you have already alluded to the possibility that I want to raise but I just want to make sure. My speculation is based on your observation, Dr. Sela, that dextran-daunomycin conjugate gives you the best results so far. Is that correct?

[20] *Sela, Hurwitz, Maron* - p. 35

SELA

No, the daunomycin-dextran does not give the best results; it certainly is not as good as daunomycin-dextran-antibody. But this, of course, depends on the conditions. I would say that we have definitely conditions under which even daunomycin-dextran-normal immunoglobulin is at least as good as daunomycin-dextran or better. Daunomycin-dextran antibody is much better than either of them.

RAPP

If the daunomycin-dextran conjugate activates macrophages, and if you combine this with our findings and those of others that the most successful so-called immunotherapy has been that which activates the so-called nonspecific immune system, is it possible that what is happening is that the most phagocytic cell — the macrophage — takes up the complex first, goes through all the processes Dr. de Duve outlined, the cell dies and now you have the exposed, altered conjugate or what-have-you that can now be taken up in another form by the cell that you are interested in killing?

DAVIES

In connection with that point, we do have some evidence ourselves that macrophages are not involved. Also I would like to make a comment! You seem to be working very close to the toxic levels of your drug because in some treated groups you were losing mice earlier than in the controls, thus you would not have very much facility to maximize the effect. Is that right?

SELA

This was on purpose, and we have even much higher doses where we killed the animal much quicker, because I thought that this was the area in which we should concentrate. When we used a very high dose the animal died, of course, from the daunomycin much before it had any time to develop any tumor — it died on the average after 3 or 4 days. With the tumor it died in 8 or 10 days and when the same amount of

[20] *Sela, Hurwitz, Maron* - p. 36

drug was chemically bound to antibody, then 100 days later all the animals were still alive. This is not true for a mixture of daunomycin and drug because there the drug is still very toxic, and the animals also died within a few days.

DAVIES

I got the impression that using your complex in one test where you had some long-term survivors or one or two deaths early on, if you had lowered the dose a little you would not have had the toxic deaths and the result would have been better.

SELA

Yes.

WESTPHAL

For a chemist listening to all these challenging possibilities, it may be tempting to consider that dextran would not meet degrading enzymes in the lysosomes. Biologically, dextran is quite a stable compound. One may, thus, think of similar compounds and possible chemical derivatives which would be better substrates for lysosomal enzyme degradation: for example amylose. In the US they grow a certain mutant of corn which produces only amylose and no (branched) amylopectin. This amylose can be produced — and is in fact being purchased — in large quantities, which one can further chemically substitute in any wanted degree with acidic, basic or other groups, to make it slowly digestible by amylases and which, at the same time, allows its complexing with your active drug material. For the carbohydrate chemist there would be a wide field for playing around along these lines.

[20] *Sela, Hurwitz, Maron* - p. 37

APPROACHES TO SPECIFIC IMMUNOTHERAPY IN CLINICAL CANCER *

D. A. L. DAVIES and G. J. O'NEILL
Searle Research Laboratories
High Wycombe, England

For those who believe that all tumour cells have a specific antigen exposed on their surfaces, there is a ray of hope that this distinguishing feature can be put to use in therapy. No other characteristic consistently distinguishes cancer cells from normal cells, indeed, this is the crux of the problem posed by this disease. Tumour antigens have already been discussed this week and opinions do not wholly concur. However, a great deal of evidence indicates the existence of tumour associated antigens and also tumour specific membrane antigens but we are, in particular, unable to generalise for the latter. The history of the use of antibody in cancer, and that is mainly animal work, indicates lack of effectiveness. Risks of enhancement of tumour growth will be discussed later.

The idea that an antibody might be made effective by using it as a carrier for some lethal poison was distinctly hinted at by EHRLICH (1906) but it would seem to have been MATHÉ (1958) who first tried to use drug/antibody complex to treat cancer; he used an antibody directed against the L1210 mouse (DBA/2) lymphoma attached to methotrexate. Some years later claims were made (GHOSE, 1972) for successful treatment of a melanoma patient with a goat anti-melanoma immunoglobulin attached to Chlorambucil.

(*) Notes from lecture.

In studies of non-covalent Chlorambucil antibody complexes we were successful in showing an antibody directed drug toxicity for mouse thymocytes, using an anti-Thy.1 serum and including the appropriate controls (O'NEILL, 1975). With this encouragement we proceeded to test similar complexes in an *in vivo* situation using the EL4 lymphoma in C57BL mice, and rabbit anti-EL4 sera. The sera were absorbed with mouse spleens before use, such that all cytotoxicity for normal C57BL cells was removed. Such antisera were linked in the same way as for the Thy.1 tests, to Chlorambucil, and the progress of tumour growth could be retarded but the interpretation put on this was that the antibody and drug worked synergistically and that the effect seen was not due to a "guided missile". We concluded that the complex had fallen apart *in vivo* en route to the tumour. Hence there were two approaches which we have called ADC (Antibody-Drug-Complexes) and ADS (Antibody-Drug-Synergism).

ADC

It was apparent that some simple criteria could be set for ADC if any success were to come from this approach:

a) Antibody specificity must be retained.

b) Drug Activity must be retained.

c) The complex must remain stable up to the point of reaching its target.

d) The stability should be arranged to suit the events judged to take place at the target site, e.g. as follows:

If the drug is to be internalised, then it might be necessary for the drug to become detached intra cellularly; if the toxic agent acts from outside, (being e.g. an enzyme, such as a phospholipase) then internalisation and separation from the carrier might not be necessary etc. There is a very wide choice of toxic agents, chemical linkages, and specific carriers from which to choose. We have chosen particularly to study peptide linked nitrogen mustards. Linkage was made to immunoglobulin, separated by $AmSO_4$ fractionation of serum prepared in rabbits against mouse tumours, and, for clinical use, immunoglobulin made similarly but from goat antisera against human tumours. Absorption of antibody against normal tissue cells of the host has been checked by monitoring for complete removal of complement mediated lymphocytotoxicity (chromium release).

A pool of human spleen cells was used for absorbing the goat antisera because spleen had been successful in the mouse experiments. More recently we have done experiments which show the practicality of using placentas for absorption in mice, and in the human situation the logistics are thereby improved.

The compound phenylenediamine mustard (PDM) was synthesized and attached to Ig by water soluble carbodiimide and a similar complex could be made with Melphalan (phenylalanine mustard) but the reaction time is longer in the case. Melphalan has previously been used clinically, unlike PDM. These complexes favourably influence the lifespan of mice carrying transplanted tumours (especially EL4 in C57BL) but the interpretation is subject to reservations mentioned later (DAVIES and O'NEILL, 1974).

There are problems with direct linkages of this kind which can easily be visualised. One might wish to put on more drug molecules to provide greater toxicity, but this will result in increasing loss of antibody specificity, upon which the missile relies for correctly finding its target. In peptide links one is restricted to the use of carboxyl groups or amino groups on the Ig to link with either the carboxyl group or amino group on the chosen drug.

In an attempt to overcome some of these problems my colleague Dr. George Rowland has attached e.g. PDM or Melphalan to a carrier molecule that is subsequently attached to the Ig. One of the carriers studied from this point of view has been polyglutamic acid (PGA), and this complex also favourably influences tumours in the mouse model (ROWLAND et al., 1975, 1976). While studies of this kind are in progress, we are troubled by controls to demonstrate the true interpretation of the benefit accruing to treated mice because the effect may be implemented by drugged antibody behaving as antibody and drugged antibody (or drugged non-antibody Ig) behaving as drug, and giving the synergism (ADS) of the kind referred to below (ROWLAND, 1977).

One patient with advanced secondary melanoma was treated (*) with a Melphalan-PDM-anti-Melanoma Ig and did very well over a year of intermittent treatment after surgery, but no conclusions can be drawn from this instance (EVERALL *et al.*, 1977).

ADS

I believe in the use of "easy models" to seek clues for what may be effective in cancer, such that the conditions can be made more exacting as required when a clue is being followed up. A difficult ("more realistic") model such as a solid spontaneous mouse tumour e.g., might easily fail to reveal a clue. Thus it was that the phenomenona of ADS was revealed and this has been studied because I believe in providing directly what patients appear unable to provide for themselves. Thus if the progress of cancer growth is, even in part, due to the failure of the patient's immune response against his own tumour specificity, then for passive immunotherapy specific antibody must be provided. Attempts to provide specifically immune cells have run into serious trouble.

In the mouse model, rabbit serum against C57/BL lymphoma EL4 was absorbed, as described above, until the cytotoxicity for normal C57BL cells was totally removed. This absorbed serum was still cytotoxic (as measured by ^{51}Cr release) for EL4 tumour cell targets and such a reaction provides a test system to monitor antigen isolation. This aspect was followed to the point of identifying a component by column chromatography with characteristics differing from known normal tissue alloantigens of the mouse (DAVIES *et al.*, 1974). There appeared to be significant progress until EL4 specific antibody was isolated from the Ig on an EL4 CNBr-Sepharose column, after which the protective power of the serum was increased, its immunofluorescence increased, but its cytotoxicity decreased. Thus the antigen visualised on columns was not a relevant one for mediation of ADS. When mice are challenged with EL4 cells and treated with sub-toxic doses of cyclophosphamide, or a few mgs of anti-EL4 Ig, each given daily for 4 days and beginning a few days

---

(*) Treated at the Royal Marsden Hospital, London by Dr. J. EVERALL.

after challenge, then in either case the lifespan of mice is only slightly increased. When both cyclophosphamide and specific Ig are provided in the same amounts, then a considerable increase of lifespan is achieved. A subsequent experiment using chlorambucil revealed that actual permanent survival could be obtained for a proportion of the challenged mice and subsequently using melphalan it was shown that all mice could be saved even when the treatment began as much as 4 days after challenge. The phenomenon was not restricted to nitrogen mustards. A dose response relationship was established for the Ig administered in the presence of drug and the phenomenon was specific, i.e. e.g. anti-EL4 Ig was not effective against other lymphomas, nor vice versa. Antibody against alpha-fetoprotein was not a mediator of ADS. A large number of experiments now form the background to this subject (DAVIES and O'NEILL, 1973; DAVIES, 1974; DAVIES, BUCKHAM and MANSTONE, 1974).

As was briefly referred to already, the history of use of anti body in cancer has been a lack of effectiveness, which may be overcome by the phenomena of ADS, and problems of tumour enhancement, which now require serious consideration. This is especially the case because lymphomas are particularly difficult to enhance in mice and lymphomas might not be the tumour of choice to make a clinical trial. It is my view that enhancement of normal tissues is not due to antibody directed against the foreignness of the transplant (example, H-2 in the mouse and HLA in man). On the contrary, it is due to antibody against the trigger for the recognition process (Ia antibody in the mouse, non-SD antibody in man) (DAVIES and ALKINS, 1974; DAVIES and STAINES, 1976). This being the case any enhancing antibody elicited in animals by immunisation with tumour cells (cell suspensions of which are inevitably mixed in with normal cells which would carry non-SD antigen) would be removed by the absorptions which have been consistently carried out with great thoroughness in these studies to leave only antibody which would be directed against the foreignness of the tumour and hence not tumour-enhancing.

On this basis, some clinical studies were carried out; initially in advanced secondary melanoma using goat anti-melanoma Ig raised specifically for each patient. The patients accepted this treatment very well and there were minimal problems in providing it. The benefit was difficult to assess and quite limited, as would be expected in such a situation (EVERALL et al., 1977).

With this background, a new situation was sought where the tumour load would be very small but the prognosis sufficiently bad to justify a more extended pilot study. Post lung-resection bronchial carcinoma seemed to provide just that situation and the resected lung was made available as the immunogen for goats and Ig raised on a personal basis as described above. The patients all received polychemotherapy 4 weeks after surgery, and again 8 weeks after surgery. In the 8th week, half of the patients, randomly allotted, received, in addition, the Ig in 4 doses over a week. The distribution of possible prognostic factors and the results as at November 1976, and at May 1977 have been described (NEWMAN et al., 1977).

At all times over nearly three years that this study was running, the ADS patients have been at an advantage over those having polychemotherapy alone, until the present time when the figures are not visibly different. This is not surprising, because a 50% benefit would be needed to show 95% confidence even in 200 patients and the amount of specific antibody treatment is admittedly trivial.

There are various ways in which more antibody could be provided; the amount could clearly be increased if it were possible to use cross-reactive antibody. Thus, e.g. serological studies of the goat antisera against lung carcinoma patients' tumours show a considerable degree of cross-reactivity (NEWMAN et al., 1977). This is not due to CEA and suggests that possibly a pool of sera should be tried. It is clear from the work of Milstein's group (KÖHLER and MILSTEIN, 1975; GALFRE et al., 1977) that antibody will become available in gram amounts within the foreseeable future which might put an entirely new light on this approach and the use of antibodies clinically in general.

The drugs used for clinical chemotherapy are more or less nonspecific poisons and it may be that they work with a measurable degree of success because of collaboration with antibody which the patients have provided for themselves. Furthermore, it may be

[21] Davies, O'Neill - p. 6

that when antibody is no longer available for such a role, but is complexed with antigen or there is a condition of antigen excess, that chemotherapy then fails and tumour growth progresses.

In the context of Burkett's lymphoma, described by George Klein, ADS may account for the regression which sometimes follows "inadequate" chemotherapy and also for the coincidence in time of relapse with a fall in the antibody against membrane antigen (one of the 4 antibodies he referred to) and which was accounted for by complexing with antigen.

REFERENCES

Davies D. A. L., « Cancer Res. », *34*, 3040 (1974).

Davies D. A. L. and Alkins B. J., « Nature (Lond.) », *247*, 294 (1974).

Davies D. A. L., Baugh V. S. G., Buckham Sue and Manstone A. J., « Europ. J. Cancer », *10*, 781 (1974).

Davies D. A. L., Manstone A. J. and Buckham Sue, « Br. J. Cancer », *30*, 297.

Davies D. A. L. and O'Neill G. J., in: *Proc. of the XI Int. Cancer Congress*, Florence, Vol. 1, 218 (1974).

Davies D. A. L. and O'Neill G. J., « Br. J. Cancer », *28*, Supp. 1, 285 (1973).

Davies D. A. L. and Staines N. A., « Transplant. Rev. », *30*, 18 (1976).

Ehrlich P., in: *Studies in Immunity* (translated by C. Bolderan). Publ. J. Willey and Sons, New York, p. 441 (1906).

Everall J. D., Dowd P., Davies D. A. L., O'Neill G. J. and Rowland G. F., « Lancet », May 21, p. 1105 (1977).

Galfre G., Howe S. C., Milstein C., Butcher G. W. and Howard J. C., « Nature, (Lond.) », *266*, 550 (1977).

Ghose T., Norell S. T., Guclu A., Cameron D., Bodurtha A. and MacDonald A. S., « Brit. med. J. », *3*, 495 (1972).

Köhler G. and Milstein C., « Nature, (Lond.) », *256*, 49 (1975).

Mathé G., Loc T. B. and Bernard J., « C. R. Acad. Sci. (D), Paris », *246*, 1626 (1958).

Newman C. E., Ford C. H. J., Davies D. A. L. and O'Neill G. J., « Lancet », July 23, p. 163 (1977).

Newman C. E., Ford C. H. J., Stokes H. J., O'Neill G. J. and Thompson R. A., « Br. J. Cancer », *36*, 407 (1977).

O'Neill G. J., Pearson B. A. and Davies D. A. L., « Immunol. », *28*, 323 (1975).

Rowland G. F., « Europ. J. Cancer », *13*, 593 (1977).

Rowland G. F., O'Neill G J. and Davies D. A. L., « Nature », *255*, 487 (1975).

DISCUSSION

OETTGEN

I am not quite clear about dosages used. I think you said that this is the best possible chemotherapy, improved upon by antibody.

DAVIES

Yes, drugs alone will not prevent tumor growth to save the animals.

OETTGEN

Under the best possible conditions?

DAVIES

That is right; most of these tests used just submaximal dosages of drugs. Also we have a reasonable amount of evidence to suggest that the best drug for any particular kind of tumor in any particular mouse strain is the best drug to give synergism with antibody.

ROSENBERG

Could you comment on the specificity of this antibody? Does it react with only EL4? Does it not react with other lymphomas in the B6 mouse?

DAVIES

The EL4 Ig will not mediate this effect for ERLD for instance, which is one of Teddy Boyse's lymphomas also specific for C57 black mice.

OETTGEN

But an antibody against this other tumor will work?

DAVIES

Yes. For instance if we use a lymphoma in BALB/c (one we have of rather recent origin), then that is also equally specific for that tumor, yes.

TERRY

You told us about subcutaneous administration. If you put the tumor intraperitoneally, can you treat intravenously and get cure?

DAVIES

Yes.

TERRY

If you put the tumor intravenously, can you treat intraperitoneally and get cure?

DAVIES

I am not sure that that exactly has been done; but most of the combinations were tested subcutaneous i.p. and i.v.

TERRY

And one last question: you made a quick comment about an anti-alphaphetoprotein not mediating the effect. Was this true for a tumor that expressed alphaphetoprotein? — I mean that was an alphaphetoprotein positive tumor?

DAVIES

That is an interesting question. It was using EL4. Now I am not sure that EL4 is alphaphetoprotein positive.

[21] *Davies, O'Neill* · p. 10

TERRY

That does not express alphaphetoprotein.

DAVIES

Well, are you sure of that? — because I can recall immunizing rabbits with a variety of mouse tumors many years ago and I do not recall that EL4 was an exception, i.e. was negative.

NORTH

Have you tried to absorb this activity out with EL4 cells *in vitro*?

DAVIES

Oh, yes.

NORTH

You can absorb it out?

DAVIES

Yes.

MATHÉ

Is EL4 a T-lymphoma?

DAVIES

Yes, it is.

MATHÉ

So if it is, there may be a common antigen with brain?

[21] *Davies, O'Neill* - p. 11

DAVIES

Not necessarily.

TERRY

There are many lines of EL4 in different laboratories that have different cell surface characteristics. You cannot answer the question in general; you have to know what the characteristics are of the line that you are working with. I do not think anybody can give a categorical answer to that question.

MATHÉ

So if it is a T-lymphoma and if there is a common antigen with brain and T cells, what about brain specificity?

DAVIES

Well, I do not know about that. The thing is that mice are very happy to have this stuff, and their brains do not seem to be adversely influenced. And then of course, in this context, there is the blood-brain barrier that might save them CNS side effects; but on the other hand, that is also an embarrassment because we would like sometimes for things to go past the blood-brain barrier to impinge on metastases in the brain, for example.

ROSENBERG

What can you say about the specificity of the xenogeneic antibodies?

DAVIES

All I can say is what I said: that they are almost all reactive with their own patients' tumor samples, and that there is 70% cross-reactivity between them — we know also that if you absorb the serum with purified CEA, that does not take away fluorescence.

[21] *Davies, O'Neill* · p. 12

OETTGEN

In the melanoma system we find that some antibodies which do not react in direct tests with normal fibroblasts but do react with melanoma cells, and cannot be absorbed out with normal lymphoid cells of the same patient, can still be absorbed out with normal fibroblasts. I wonder if you have absorbed your goat antibody with normal fibroblasts and yet retained reactivity with lung cancer tissue. The autologous melanoma antibody cannot be absorbed out with normal lymphoid cells of the same patient, does not react in direct tests with his own fibroblasts, but in some instances can still be absorbed out by the same normal fibroblasts with which it does not react in direct tests. You say that the goat antibody reacts with 60% of the lung cancer cells. Does it still react after being absorbed with normal human fibroblast rather than lymphoid cells?

DAVIES

That I do not know, we have not absorbed with fibroblasts because it could not be done on the necessary scale for clinical use.

MARINI-BETTÒLO

Have you any evidence about the type of conjugation between the drug and the antibody?

DAVIES

Do you mean the chance that they may complex *in vivo* after injection?

MARINI-BETTÒLO

No, I mean if you have any kind of binding before injection.

DAVIES

No, nothing — there is none — no binding. The drug and antiserum are injected in parallel.

[21] *Davies, O'Neill* · p. 13

MARINI-BETTÒLO

But perhaps there may be some kind of binding of the drug and the tumor specific Ig adsorbed into the syringe.

DAVIES

I doubt it. They are normally injected at different times of the day: e.g. drug in the morning, antibodies in the afternoon.

MARINI-BETTÒLO

Are you really sure that there is no binding of the drug with the Ig in the patient?

DAVIES

We cannot be sure, but if there is a rather nonspecific kind of binding, there is an enormous amount of normal Ig in the patient anyway, so I do not see why the drug should bind to the fraction which matters, i.e. the injected tumour-specific Ig.

[21] *Davies, O'Neill* - p. 14

BCG IN THE TREATMENT AND PREVENTION
OF HUMAN CANCER

WILLIAM D. TERRY, M.D.

Associate Director for Immunology, Division of Cancer Biology & Diagnosis
National Cancer Institute, National Institutes of Health
Bethesda, Maryland 20014 U.S.A.

Bacteria and bacterial products having immunologic adjuvant activities have been tested for therapeutic effects in human cancer for almost 100 years. This paper will review some recent clinical investigations and will attempt to place in perspective the current role of BCG in the current treatment of human cancer, as well as its usefulness in the prevention of human cancer.

From a conceptual point of view, adjuvants can be used in two different, although not mutually exclusive, approaches to cancer treatment. They can be used to help stimulate specific tumor immunity in a manner analogous to the classical use of adjuvants to increase the magnitude of specific immune responses.

Adjuvants can also be used to induce a delayed hypersensitivity reaction against themselves or to increase the general level of reactivity of certain components of the immune system. If the consequence of adjuvant administration is the suppression of tumor growth in circumstances where there are not known to be tumor specific immune reactions, the process is referred to as non-specific immunotherapy. Thus, adjuvants can be used in specific as well as non-specific immunotherapy.

At the present time, it is not known whether any human tumor contains tumor-associated antigens that are of importance in terms of potential immunotherapy. Such antigens would have to be located on the tumor cell surface, would have to have the ability or potential to stimulate a cellular and/or a humoral immune response of cytolytic type, and would have to act as a suitable target site through which immune damage could be mediated. Finally, these hypothetical antigens would have to be expressed only on tumor cells or, if expressed on normal cells also, would have to differ qualitatively or quantitatively in expression on normal and tumor cells so that immune mechanisms would lead to tumor cell destruction without extensive damage of normal tissue. The existence of this type of tumor antigen is the fundamental requirement for any form of specific immunotherapy. Unequivocal proof that such antigens occur on human tumors remains to be provided. Until such proof is available, all attempts at specific immunotherapy must be considered acts of faith.

Non-specific immunotherapy by definition does not require that there be tumor specific antigens. This type of immunotherapy depends rather on the concept that activation of some part of the immune system of a tumor-bearing animal will lead to destruction of tumor cells with little or no destruction of normal cells. The remainder of this paper will be concerned only with the application of BCG as a non-specific immunotherapeutic agent.

Adjuvants have been tested for therapeutic efficacy following administration intratumorally, regionally, or systemically.

1. *Intratumoral Immunotherapy*

The injection of living BCG organisms into metastatic melanoma tumor deposits in the skin has caused regression of injected nodules in a high percentage of cases (MORTON et al., 1970, 1974; PINSKY et al., 1973; reviewed in ROSENBERG and RAPP, 1976). Patients must be capable of developing delayed hypersensitivity skin reactions in order for treatment to be effective. In general, therapeutic response has been limited to the injected nodule, although occasionally regression has been seen in uninjected nodules within the lymphatic drainage area of the injected nodule. There have been rare reports of regressions of uninjected visceral metastases (MASTRANGELO, 1975). BCG has also been injected into other types of cancer. Bronchogenic carcinoma lesions have been injected through a bronchoscope and lesions are reported to regress (HAYATA).

No study has yet been performed to determine whether intratumoral immunotherapy causes improved survival effect. Patients with melanoma entering remission following intratumoral injection and destruction of multiple melanoma skin nodules have survived for prolonged periods of time (MORTON, 1974). It is not known whether their survival was any longer than it would have been had all lesions been removed by surgery or other forms of local therapy. Until such studies are performed, it can only be concluded that intratumoral injection of BCG is a form of local treatment, one that may on occasion be preferable to surgery (e.g. large multiplicity of lesions that are more easily injected than resected, cosmetic reasons, etc.), but one that has not yet been tested for effect on survival relative to other forms of local treatment.

The mechanisms whereby intratumoral BCG leads to tumor cell destruction are not known. If melanoma tumor cells have specific antigens and if the patient has made an ineffective immune response against these antigens, BCG may have the effect of stimulating the specific immune response to a level of clinical effectiveness.

Other mechanisms have been discussed. It can be speculated that the intense delayed hypersensitivity reaction generated against BCG organisms leads to the accumulation of inflammatory cells, the release of lymphokines and the subsequent accumulation and activation of macrophages, the release of cytotoxic substances, and finally the destruction of cells, including tumor cells, in the area of the delayed hypersensitivity reaction. Tumor cells would then be destroyed as "innocent bystanders" in the vicinity of the delayed hypersensitivity response to BCG. Destruction of uninjected nodules within the lymphatic drainage region of the tumor could be caused by the migration of BCG organisms through the lymphatics and their accumulation at these nearby tumor deposits. Additional delayed hypersensitivity reactions would then be generated at these additional tumor sites.

Another possible mechanism is one in which BCG organisms preferentially adhere to tumor cells, thus possibly sensitizing them for immune destruction by the cell-mediated response to BCG. Here the tumor cell is the not so completely "innocent bystander" serving rather as the physical carrier for large numbers of BCG organisms. A more sophisticated variant of this hypothesis is that BCG organisms adhere to the tumor cell surface causing modification of HLA antigens and inducing a state of altered self. Immune reactivity would then be directed not at BCG alone nor at tumor cells alone, but at a complex of cell surface antigens modified by BCG (for a review of immune reactions against altered self caused by exogenous antigens see SHEARER and SCHMITT-VERHULST).

Finally, several studies have suggested that the surface of BCG organisms contains antigens cross reactive with cell surface antigens of certain tumor cells (BORSOS and RAPP, 1973; BUCANA and HANNA, 1974; MINDEN et al., 1974). This raises the possibility that sensitization against BCG produces an immune response that can be directly cross reactive with at least some tumor cells. The presence of the cross reactive antigens seems to have been established — the biological role of these antigens is not yet clear.

All of the mechanisms discussed are speculative. Little has been done to clearly delineate the way in which intratumoral BCG leads to tumor cell destruction. It is unfortunate that this is so, since our ability to make this effect a clinically important one depends upon our understanding of the cellular and molecular mechanisms involved.

2. Regional Immunotherapy

Clinical effects have also been demonstrated when BCG is introduced into the area around a tumor. McKNEALLY et al have studied the effect of intrapleural administration of BCG on the remission duration and survival of patients with resectable Stage I lung cancer. Patients were randomly assigned to treatment with 10^7 colony forming units of BCG as a single intrapleural injection 2 or 3 days postoperatively, followed by isoniazide begun 14 days post-BCG and continued for 12 weeks, or were assigned to control. Control patients also received the same dose of isoniazide.

Of the 34 patients receiving BCG, 3 have had recurrence; while of the 35 patients not receiving BCG, 15 have recurred.

These values were obtained at a time when median duration of follow up was 2 years. Thus, the postoperative intrapleural administration of BCG appears to cause prolonged remission and survival in the relatively small number of Stage I patients studied. In order to ensure that this clinical effect is a reproducible one, this trial is being repeated with larger numbers of patients.

Assuming that the treatment effect is real, the mechanisms responsible are not known. All of the mechanisms discussed with regard to intratumoral BCG are equally applicable in this intrapleural setting. It is possible that tumors confined to body cavities lined by serosal membranes will be particularly vulnerable to treatment with regional immunotherapy since large numbers of immunologically active mononuclear cells accumulate in these cavities in response to injection of BCG or other adjuvants.

3. Systemic Immunotherapy

Most of the clinical uses of BCG have been in the form of systemic treatment; that is, application at some site distant from the tumor. Patients treated have included those rendered free of disease by other forms of treatment, as well as those with more advanced disease. Results in general have not been encouraging. Although there are many enthusiastic reports in the literature concerning apparent effects of BCG in the treatment of acute lymphocytic leukemia, melanoma, breast cancer, colon cancer, and acute myelogenous leukemia (AML), it is only in AML that a series of prospectively randomized studies with reasonable numbers of patients have been carried out and have shown a consistent treatment effect (Table 1). In these trials, chemotherapy was used to induce and maintain remission. BCG was given during maintenance and was applied intradermally either by scarification or some form of multi-puncture device. The one exception is the study by WHITTAKER and SLATER where BCG was administered intravenously. It should also be noted that in the studies of POWLES and PETO, irradiated allogeneic cells were given along with BCG. The results of all of these trials demonstrate a consistent trend toward improved remission duration (the trend does not achieve statistical significance), and a consistent trend toward prolongation in survival which is reported to be statistically significant in three of the trials (Table 1).

These results indicate that the addition of BCG to maintenance chemotherapy leads to survival that may be almost double that obtained with chemotherapy alone. It appears that most of this treatment effect occurs after first relapse, since the prolongation of first remission duration is not very great. The mechanism causing prolongation of survival is not known, and there is no a priori reason for considering this to be due to immunotherapy. BCG is known to have effects on a multiplicity of cell types including hematopoietic stem cells, and it is also known to alter liver function and thereby affect drug metabolism. Here again, the absence of information concerning the molecular and cellular mechanisms

TABLE 1

Reference		No. of Patients	Median Remission Duration (weeks)	Median Survival (weeks)
Powles	- Control	22	27	39
	Immunotherapy	28	44	73*
Peto	- Control	24	28	48
	Immunotherapy	47	36	68
Vogler	- Control	33	34	66
	Immunotherapy	25	41	83
Gutterman	- Control	24	52	96
	Immunotherapy	14	85	>145*
Whittaker	- Control	19	23	47
	Immunotherapy	18	30	65*

*p = or < 0.05

responsible for the treatment effect leaves us in a quandary as to how to achieve more significant clinical applications or even whether to include this as an example of immunotherapy.

BCG in the Prevention of Cancer

Several studies have been published in which it is alleged that children vaccinated early in life with BCG have a decreased incidence of acute lymphocytic leukemia and other childhood tumors (DAVI-GNON et al.; ROSENTHAL, et al.). The data from one of these studies (ROSENTHAL) were made available for analyses by other investigators. The original study indicated that vaccination reduced the death rate from acute lymphocytic leukemia from 2.02/100,000/year to 0.31/100,000/year. Reevaluation of these data did not support the original conclusions (HOOVER) and at the present time there is no convincing evidence that neonatal vaccination with BCG causes any decrease in incidence or mortality of any cancer.

SUMMARY

BCG has been administered to cancer patients intratumorally, regionally, and systemically. Regressions caused by intratumoral injections have been seen often enough to assure validity but the mechanism of the effect is not known. Regional administration has led to apparent clinical effects. These have been noted only recently and will have to be reproduced in a larger number of patients to assure validity. Systemic administration has had a therapeutic effect reproducibly demonstrated only in patients with AML. At the present time, it is not known whether the effect is mediated by the immune system.

BCG has also been alleged to reduce cancer mortality in vaccinated children but convincing evidence for this effect has not been produced.

Future progress in the use of BCG or other adjuvants as a form of immunotherapy of cancer will depend in large part on achieving a better understanding of the mechanisms responsible for observed clinical effects.

REFERENCES

BORSOS T. and RAPP H.J., *Antigenic relationship between* Mycobacterium bovis *(BCG) and guinea pig hepatoma.* « J. Natl. Cancer Inst. », *51*, 1085-1086 (1973).

BUCANA C. and HANNA M.G., *Immunoelectromicroscopic analysis of surface antigens common to* Mycobacterium bovis *(BCG) and tumor cells.* « J. Natl. Cancer Inst. », *53*, 1313-1318 (1974).

DAVIGNON L., LEMONDE P., ROBILLARD P. and FRAPPIER A., *B.C.G. Vaccination and leukaemia mortality.* « Lancet », *2*, 638 (1970).

GUTTERMAN J.U., RODRIGUEZ V., McCREDIE K.B., HESTER J.P., BODEY G.P., FREIREICH E.J. and HERSH E.M., *Chemoimmunotheraphy of acute myeloblastic leukemia: Four-year follow up with BCG.* In: Terry W.D. and Windhorst D.B. (Eds.): « Immunotherapy of Cancer: Present Status of Trials in Man. ». Raven Press, New York (1978).

HAYATA Y., OHO K., OGAWA I. and TAIRA O., *Immunotherapy for lung cancer cases using BCG and BCG cell wall skeleton.* « Gann » (submitted for publication).

HOOVER R.N., *BCG vaccination and cancer prevention: A critical evaluation of the human experience.* « Cancer Res. », *36*, 652-654 (1976).

MASTRANGELO M.J., BELLET R.E., BERKELHAMMER J. and CLARK W.H. Jr., *Regression of pulmonary metastatic disease associated with intralesional BCG therapy of dermal melanoma metastases.* « Cancer », *36*, 1305-1308 (1975).

McKNEALLY M.F., MAVER C.M. and KAUSEL H.W., *Regional immunotherapy of lung cancer using postoperative intrapleural BCG.* In: Terry W.D. and Windhorst D.B. (Eds.): « Immunotherapy of Cancer: Present Status of Trials in Man. ». Raven Press, New York (1978).

MINDEN P., McCLATCHY J.K., WAINBERG M. and WEISS D.W., *Shared antigens between* Mycobacterium bovis *(BCG) and neoplastic cells.* « J. Natl. Cancer Inst. », *53*, 1325-1331 (1974).

MORTON D.L., EILBER F.R., HOLMES E.C., *et al., BCG immunotherapy of malignant melanoma: Summary of a seven-year experience.* « Ann. Surg. », *180*, 635-643 (1974).

MORTON D.L., EILBER F.R., MALMGREN R.A., *et al., Immunological factors which influence response to immunotherapy in malignant melanoma.* « Surgery », *68*, 158-164 (1970).

PETO R., *Immunotherapy of acute myeloid leukaemia.* In: Terry W.D. and Windhorst D.B. (Eds.): « Immunotherapy of Cancer: Present Status of Trials in Man. ». Raven Press, New York (1978).

PINSKY C., HIRSHAUT Y. and OETTGEN H., *Treatment of malignant melanoma by intratumoral injection of BCG*. « Natl. Cancer Inst. Monogr. », *39*, 225-228 (1973).

POWLES R.L., RUSSELL J., LISTER T.A., OLIVER T., WHITEHOUSE J.M.A., MALPAS J., CHAPUIS B., CROWTHER D. and ALEXANDER P., *Immunotherapy for acute myelogenous leukaemia: Analysis of a controlled clinical study 2-1/2 years after entry of the last patient*. In: Terry W.D. and Windhorst D.B. (Eds.): « Immunotherapy of Cancer: Present Status of Trials in Man. ». Raven Press, New York (1978).

ROSENBERG S.A. and RAPP H.J., *Intralesional immunotherapy of melanoma with BCG*. « Med. Clin. North Am. », *60*, 419-430 (1976).

ROSENTHAL S.R., CRISPEN R.G., THORNE M.G., PIEKARSKI N., RAISYS N. and RETTIG P.G., *B.C.G. vaccination and leukemia mortality*. « J. Am. Med. Assoc. », *222*, 1543-1544 (1972).

SHEARER G.M. and SCHMITT-VERHULST A.M., *Major histocompatibility complex restricted cell mediated immunity*. « Adv. Immunol. », (In Press).

VOGLER W.R., BARTOLUCCI A.A., OMURA G.A., MILLER D., SMALLEY R.V., KNOSPE W.H. and GOLDSMITH A.S., *A randomized clinical trial of BCG in myeloblastic leukemia conducted by the Southeastern Cancer Study Group*. In: Terry W.D. and Windhorst D.B. (Eds.): « Immunotherapy of Cancer: Present Status of Trials in Man. ». Raven Press, New York (1978).

WHITTAKER J.A. and SLATER A.J., *The immunotherapy of acute myelogenous leukaemia using intravenous BCG*. In: Terry W.D. and Windhorst D.B. (Eds.): « Immunotherapy of Cancer: Present Status of Trials in Man. ». Raven Press, New York (1978).

DISCUSSION

TERRY

I think that in order to proceed with some order, what I would like to do would be to throw open for discussion the comments that I have made about clinical immunotherapy and the clinical trials and let us discuss that for a little bit. I would then like to proceed to the question of what we know about the mechanisms that might be operative in the animal experimental situations where we have shown that injection of adjuvant material into a tumor or around a tumor can lead to tumor destruction. The mechanism has been referred to marginally during the course of the week, but I think we ought to focus on that for a little bit to see what the accumulated wisdom is here in this room in terms of hard experimental fact, not speculation — what do we really know in experimental terms about the mechanisms that are involved; and then we can proceed to some other questions.

WEISS

I should like to emphasize once more several points that are emerging from the CALGB cooperative trials of MER in AML patients, in light of Dr. Terry's comments. The heightened proportion of patients that can be brought into remission by the addition of MER to induction chemotherapy is more apparent in certain age groups than in others. Second, there is a notable difference between patients who are responsive to one or more recall antigens in the routine skin hypersensitivity testing to which all patients are subjected, and those who are unresponsive to all four of the assay antigens. It is only the latter in whom MER acts appreciably to increase remission incidence. This is an interesting observation, in line with our information from many animal test systems that MER can prevent or reverse states of immunological deficiency of varied etiology, and that it is most effective as an immunopotentiator where host reactivity is low to begin with, or the antigenic stimulus a limited one. The finding that it is the anergic patient who stands most to benefit from MER immunological intervention thus falls attractively into place within our general perspective of the opportunities of nonspecific immunological intervention: It might not be possible to add much to a fully intact immunological functionality, but it may be possible to bring defective functionality to normal levels. I have never been able to accept the arguments of clinical investigators that immunologically deficient patients — deficient as judged by one or another arbitrary criterion — should not be considered for immunotherapy. We must take into account, of course, that the various tests employed to measure immunological function in patients are no more than stabs in the dark, and may correlate very poorly or not at all with those immunological functions that are required to inhibit a particular neoplastic process.

If the impression holds up that MER treatment is effective only in patients scoring low on certain immunological monitoring tests, it may be possible in the future to select at the outset those individuals likely to benefit from this, and from other, immunological manipulation.

With reference to Dr. Chedid's question, I want to restate the observation that the incidence of severe infections during second-cycle induction chemotherapy was markedly reduced in the AML patients who received a single pre-remission treatment with MER.

TERRY

If I can add to that, I think in terms of the non-MER trials that are on the board, the analysis, although limited, did not really suggest very much in the way of difference in infectious episodes in most of these trials, did not indicate any protection against the negative consequences of the chemotherapy; that is where it has been looked at, the amount of chemotherapy administered during maintenance appeared to be roughly comparable. There do not seem to be any very strong clues out of this from the analyses that have been done, with the one exception, which again is analyzed, and perhaps Jordan will have something more to say about that, that everybody seems to have the feeling, although I have not seen it documented, that induction of second remission is much easier in those patients who have been previously treated with BCG.

[22] *Terry* - p. 12

ROSENBERG

From McKneally's study, the BCG was administered regionally, but for it to have a positive effect would clearly imply a systemic effect of the BCG since patients with stage 1 lung cancer when they recur, recur at different sites; and so although the BCG was given in a regional manner, one would still have to assume, if that trial turns out to be repeatable, that the effects of BCG are at sites other than the local area.

TERRY

I think we could possibly take the reverse track and say that before the tumor got to some other place maybe it was localized within the chest, and maybe at the time the BCG was administered it was not yet disseminated and maybe therefore you are cutting it off before it has had a chance to disseminate. Now I think there is no evidence for that.

RAPP

Dr. Rosenberg does not understand your point. The BCG was given soon after surgery, at a time when the disease might have been localized. For stage 1 carcinoma there is a chance that disease is confined to the primary site. Treatment at that stage need not affect systemic disease in order to be effective.

TERRY

Possibly, but there is no more evidence on that side than there was on the other side.

RAPP

No, but it cannot be concluded from McKneally's results that his treatment has affected systemic disease.

TERRY

I think we have got to put this in the context for what it is worth. Again, I do not think we know what it means in terms of the biology

[22] *Terry* - p. 13

35

of cancer, — but everybody would agree that if you had looked hard enough at the time that hard surgery was done, there were circulating tumor cells. Maybe before the surgery was done — I do not mean to imply as a consequence of the surgery — that this already is a systemic disease and that therefore the argument in terms of whether this is a local effect or a systemic effect becomes rather difficult. I think we just do not have enough information.

RAPP

But that would apply to any cancer.

TERRY

I agree.

MATHÉ

The definition of stage 1 is the stage in which the surgeon does not find lymph nodes; and we know that the metastases may be far from the nodes. So if there is an effect in McKneally's work, it may be a systemic effect. He has systemic manifestations, hence dissemination of BCG, hence he uses systemic immunotherapy simultaneously with regional immunotherapy.

TERRY

Why do you say that, George?

MATHÉ

McKneally wrote in the *Lancet* that patients had fever and malaise.

TERRY

In a small percentage of the patients, yes.

[22] *Terry* - p. 14

MATHÉ

I do not think so. McKneally does not give the proportion of the patients who had fever and malaise, but he wrote that he gave aspirin and diphenhydramine for 48 h "to reduce the discomfort of the fever and malaise".

Moreover, in one bronchus carcinoma trial of immunotherapy, we only applied systemic BCG: the difference in favor of BCG is presently significant at $p \leqslant 0.07$.

There are other trials that you should have mentioned: those of Edwards and Whitwell, of EORTC bronchus group, of Stefani and Kerman with BCG, those of Pines with BCG and BGC and levamisole, that of Amery with levamisole.

TERRY

I think that in order to really make this discussion of some value, if you have data on those trials which you can put up for us, tell us how many patients, whether it was randomized, what the treatment was etc., etc.

MATHÉ

At time of publication, Edwards and Whitwell had 60 patients with BCG versus 60 controls: the survival rate was increased from 38% in the controls, from 52% in the BCG group. In Stefani's and Kerman's randomized trial concerning inoperable irradiated bronchus carcinoma, the median survival time of the BCG group is 52 weeks versus 33.5 weeks in the control group ($p < 0.01$). In randomized Amery's trial, there were 69 patients receiving levamisole versus 79 controls. In a recent publication, there were 51.2% patients free of disease in the placebo group versus 80% in the levamisole group. This difference was highly significant. In Decroix's trial which compares 54 patients submitted to *M. smegmatis* to historical controls, there were, at time of publication 80% of the patients in survival versus 35 to 45% of the different groups of historical controls.

TERRY

I would again say that the issue remains open, that it is not a question of whether or not the tumor cells are in the next lymph node but whether the tumor cells are in the pleural space and whether those tumor cells then are the ones which have been adapted to cut loose and to systematize, and where the treatment may therefore be local in the sense of sterilizing the pleural space and getting rid of those cells that have the capacity to spread. But I think that we should not pursue this much further because none of us have information and we are talking without data.

MATHÉ

You were in charge of the review and you should have the data. In order to answer the question concerning the kind of effect, only regional or regional and systemic which McNeally has obtained, you should have mentioned the sites of the relapses of the controls; you should know the data of their autopsies.

RAPP

In the guinea pig, when there are local microscopic lymph node metastases, regional or local treatment will get rid of them. Is that analogous to part of what you are talking about?

TERRY

Not necessarily.

RAPP

I did not think so.

NORTH

Doesn't that really put a lot of emphasis on the use of INH in these results? Didn't he have experimental work in the mouse which indicated that it was rather necessary? I do not know whether it was published yet.

[22] *Terry* - p. 16

TERRY

Dr. McKneally had some preliminary animal experiments in mice, suggesting that there might be a synergistic effect of INH on BCG, but the data were, as I recall, rather marginal; I do not think there was anything published, and I do not know that there is any other information in the literature that bears on that point.

OETTGEN

There is yet another problem with the interpretation of McKneally's trial: What is called stage 1 lung cancer depends on the extent of the lymph node dissection. It seems one has to consider the possibility, therefore, that there may be an uneven distribution of cases in the two arms which would have been classified as stage 2 after more extensive lymph node dissection.

TERRY

Dr. Oettgen raises a point which has really several different aspects, and in essence forms the rationale for needing to go ahead despite this rather impressive clinical observation, to attempt to reproduce the finding, with larger numbers of patients, because what you are suggesting is that by chance alone there might have been maldistribution of patients, such that patients who really were stage 2 or stage 3 occurred in his control group in a much higher proportion than they occurred in his test group. And with 35 or 40 patients that is certainly an easily possible happening. On the other hand, with 200 patients: 100 and 100 — it should not happen, and I think that it just will fall out that it proves I think again the important need for achieving confirmation with reasonable numbers of patients before accepting any single trial.

NOSSAL

A question on just that. It seems to me that nearly all the data that has been presented in summary form at this meeting has shown curves that look good at the beginning but look a lot less impressive at the end. Have any of the trials which you have put on the board progressed for long enough to allow us to say that one patient or two patients are at beyond, let us say, three standard deviations from the historical median of survival?

TERRY

Now of course that gets back to the point Dr. Oettgen was making: for stage 1 I believe it runs around 45% in terms of 2-year survival.

NOSSAL

Let us talk about the acute myeloid leukaemia. This is still a very lethal disease and I found De Duve's 80% DNA-daunorubicin very impressive. Now is there in any of those trials one patient with AML who is alive for five years, or six years?

TERRY

All of those patients are now dead, so that is a totally completed study. And I must say I cannot tell you what the longest survival was within that group in either the control or in the treated group.

NOSSAL

But the fact that you cannot tell us suggests that there has not been anything very dramatic — there are not a lot of cured people with AML walking around as a result of immunotherapy.

TERRY

This is adult AML, but there are not many cured adults walking around.

WEISS

There have actually been 3 clinical trials with MER in AML so far. The first was initiated by Dr. G. Izak of Hadassah Hospital in Jerusalem, about 7 years ago. There are now ca. 60 patients in this study, alternated into treatment schedules of standard chemotherapy, with or without monthly intradermal applications of 1.0 mg MER. The second study was a pilot trial of MER conducted in AML patients by Drs. James Holland and Janet Cuttner at Mt. Sinai Hospital in New York, involving ca. 25 patients. In both of these small studies, MER displayed an appreciable effect in prolonging remission and survival time. The third investigation is the large trial mounted by CALGB, with concurrent randomized controls. There are now over 800 patients in this study, and more are being introduced. There is a new investigation now under way under CALGB auspices, in which AML patients will be given MER only during remission induction, rather than both during induction and maintenance or in maintenance only, as has been the case in the earlier trials. Taken together, one strong impression is emerging from these clinical experiments: The number of patients treated with MER who have very long remissions — more than two years — is greater than has been the experience with the best schedules of chemotherapy alone. As I have mentioned previously, other areas of benefit are being noted as well, i.e. an increase in the numbers of patients who can be brought into remission, a reduction in the incidence of infections, and, seemingly, a facilitation of induction of second remissions in relapsed patients. At least in some patients, then, MER immunotherapy is of value.

NOSSAL

Thank you very much — that was just the sort of response that I was after, and now I would like somebody who is experienced in chemotherapy to tell me whether in AML they know of any substantial group of patients still alive six years into a trial, purely from chemotherapy.

TERRY

I would like specific answers to Dr. Nossal's question.

OETTGEN

In the randomized Pseudomonas trial 6 out of 13 vaccinated patients have remained in complete remission for 5 to 6½ years, and only 1 of 17 non-vaccinated patients has remained in remission, for almost 5 years.

GUTTERMAN

I agree with what David Weiss said; that it sounds like a MER effect. However, it should be put in perspective that there are patients in our AML series, I think between 10 and 13, maybe as high as 15%, which were treated with cytostatic drugs without immunotherapy which are in remission at 5 years. Now in our trial on 14 patients in our initial study receiving chemotherapy plus BCG, 6 of the 14 (around 40%) are still in remission for 3 to 5 years after the start. I do not think the real number is going to be quite that high, but I have to emphasize that you do see remission durations and survival well beyond 5 years with chemotherapy alone, but it appears from the Pseudomonas, MER and BCG from our own series, that we will probably be able to push that up.

MATHÉ

One must consider with reserve the results of large cooperative group trials because of the well known compromise phenomenon and the dilution phenomenon. What is the meaning of a significant increase of remission induction compared to 45% in the controls when the specialized centers have 75%? What do the results mean which Terry presented on the survival medians, comparing the results obtained with polycentric trials. I am not surprised that some are significant and some (mainly those presenting the dilution phenomenon) are not. You should have mentioned the Swedish trial on BCG and cells and that of Holland in which neuraminidase which persists after cell washing probably works as an immunity adjuvant: his curve of remission presents a plateau which concerns between 45% and 50% of the patients.

TERRY

Dr. Mathé, there is no question about that, but I think it is totally off the topic of our conversation this afternoon. I think we are not concerned about the group trial dilution effect because what we are looking at here are randomized trials where we are looking at what they do one arm against the other, and the dilution applies to both arms. It may not be optimal but it lets us see the difference. I am also sure that you did not mean to imply that Dr. Gutterman was not one of the best centers around for treating adult AML.

MATHÉ

But he has a significant result.

GUTTERMAN

Just for the record, before bringing up a question, I just wanted to add to George Mathé's list. I think, as you know, that you are a little bit more pessimistic than I am and several of us are. I think there is a randomized trial in lymphoma from Bordeaux that is now statistically significant and also in melanoma, although that is highly controversial, and possibly in breast cancer.

TERRY

Before you go on with your comment, I think this might be the time to introduce an element that I know Dr. Oettgen is very familiar with and that I think we all see and we need to make very clear as we are talking about trials that have now achieved significance. Everyone of these trials on the board, with the exception of the Whittaker trial (there I simply do not know), originally during their early publication reported significant prolongation of median remission duration. As the trials progressed, the differences were no longer significant. The trends are there but no longer significant. The actuarial curve of Dr. Paulz's trial went right on across the slide, when it was published in 1973, and everybody said: "Dr. Paulz has cured AML". I think that there is great danger, given the present level of either a lack of sophistication of statisticians or the lack of our sophistication in understanding what the statistics are telling us, in interpreting either too early or too vigorously trials before they have reached a real stage of maturity. And I think that Dr. Oettgen at his institution has a trial which has gone several years as being statistically significant which now is no longer statistically significant but which, at its next evaluation, may again be statistically significant. We are dealing with small numbers usually, where the fluctuation of one or two or three patients can make all the difference in the world between "Oh, this is marvelous" and "Oh, it is not working".

GUTTERMAN

I do not entirely agree with you, since I do not think that the actual biological results are changing that much with time. The P value changes — it is .04 one month and .07 with the death of the patient in one arm or the other — but I do not think that the real significance is really changing.

Well, this is always in the context — a trial has been going for X number of years, and that is all you can say about it. You are correct, we are always looking for plateaus but 95% of the time we do not achieve them.

DE DUVE

I would like to make a very brief comment as a complete outsider. I think it is a little dangerous to speak of "not significant" and "significant" statistically. I think you are right in saying that the only thing is the P value, which is an assessment of the probability that the observed difference may be fortuitous. The difference between a P value of 0.10 and one of 0.05 is not the all-or-none difference indicated by nonsignificant and significant. It is the difference between a 90% and a 95% chance of the observed difference being real.

TERRY

That is absolutely correct — terribly important but must be remembered in the context of what you said: that 10% of the time this could be due to chance alone and when there are 40 trials or 400 trials in AML, then the statistics start becoming very important in terms of with what random incidence or with what random frequency we are going to find a trial that shows that difference.

OETTGEN

Randomization in clinical trials aims at distributing patients into comparable groups. Factors other than stage of disease, which we know to be of prognostic significance, have to be taken into account. Even if we do this very carefully as I believe we have done in the breast cancer trial that was quoted here, there are obviously factors affecting the outcome about which we do not know enough, factors which make survival esti-mates unreliable at an early stage of a trial with small numbers of patients.

TERRY

I suppose it is worth pointing out again in the context of Dr. de Duve's comment that the implications are not academic. What one is confronted with is the fact that when the paper is published and it says that this trial has now achieved significance, the implication of this for the medical community is: this is a treatment now that all patients with that category disease should receive and that obviously creates a very difficult situation, where you do not want to commit the patients for the indefinite future to a treatment form that may really be of no value; and it creates great difficulties I think for the clinicians in trying to decide when they have reached the point where they know: yes, this now should be incorporated as a standard part of the treatment.

ROSENBERG

While we have talked about the possible benefits of BCG, we have not really spent a lot of time talking about its dangers. And in the absence of positive effect, BCG can not only be dangerous but can be lethal. Unless a definite positive effect exists, then, as any other dan-gerous drug, it should not be used, and the dangers, especially in intra-lesional treatment that come from using viable BCG in terms of disse-minated BCG infection can be very serious. The dangers from using any BCG preparation — be it viable or not — that result from hyper-sensitivity have already resulted in deaths in humans and are a problem.

NORTH

What evidence do you have that you get generalized BCG infection?

ROSENBERG

Unfortunately, we have several patients that have been given viable BCG that have had the symptoms of disseminated BCG infection: high fever, liver function abnormalities, general malaise and so on, but, perhaps more objectively, we have grown BCG out of bone marrow biopsies, out of liver biopsies following BCG injection into a primary melanoma lesion.

MATHÉ

I completely agree on the fact that BCG, whatever the route of administration, disseminates and induces a bacteremia. But we have not lost one patient using BCG for systemic or local immunotherapy in more than 400 patients. The two or three deaths mentioned in the literature concern intratumoral injections of BCG in patients not controlled for their allergic state to BCG which is an error. This bacteremia seems necessary for systemic immunotherapy action, as we showed in mice the correlation of its presence with the antileukaemia efficiency.

TERRY

Dr. Mathé, at the beginning of your comment you said that when you inject BCG you get fever and that in fact you want fever. Would you enlarge on that? Why do you want fever?

MATHÉ

Yes, in man, we only consider as correct an application of BCG which induces $\geq$ 38°C fever after a few hours. If it does not, we repeat the application. Such a proof of an effective penetration and of the bacilli is generally not mentioned in so called "negative" trials.

TERRY

That is an interesting correlation, but is there anything further than that? — that is, is there any real experimental proof that it is necessary to induce a BCG septicemia in order to have a therapeutic effect in either animals or man?

MATHÉ

Let me comment the experiment I was quoting. We compared the pathological findings of two groups of leukaemia mice: those which received BCG i.v. and were cured, those who received it s.c. and were not cured.   There were many manifestations of BCG septicemia in the first, no or few manifestations of such a septicemia in the second.

RAPP

Well, clearly, since nonviable BCG can be made to work, successful therapy does not require an infection — at least in one animal model.

TERRY

Do you agree, Dr. Mathé?

MATHÉ

Dr. Rapp is speaking about intratumoral immunotherapy described by Morton in man and confirmed by him in guinea pigs.   As Rosenfeld mentioned, we observed that tumoral injection in man is usually followed by systemic dissemination.   I do not know if Zbar and coworkers studied carefully the pathology of their guinea pigs.

GUTTERMAN

I would like to get a clarification from Dr. Rapp, because I did not understand his point.   What Dr. Mathé is saying is that if you are using live BCG in acute leukemia both for man and experimentally, one needs to induce perhaps septicemia.   Now I gather that you have extrapolated from your guinea pig hepatoma model that since you do not use live bacteria, one does not need an infection as in Dr. Mathé's example or just — what exactly do you mean?

RAPP

I was speaking in general.   I thought that was the question: can you get an antitumor effect in general with killed BCG, and the answer is yes.   And to answer your question, Dr. Mathé would now have to try one of these nonviable preparations to see if it produces a cure.

GUTTERMAN

I think that has been tried by Mathé with MER, for example, and I believe it works. If you give MER i.v. compared to MER s.c., in your model, is there a difference or have you not done it?

RAPP

No, but MER would have to be tried in oil droplets the way the BCG works in the guinea pig.

WEISS

MER can be administered intravenously (i.v.). Mice tolerate such administration surprisingly well — this is work conducted in our laboratories — and Dr. Steve Vogel at Albert Einstein Medical Center in New York, and Drs. I. J. Fidler and M. Hanna of the Frederick Cancer Center have reported surprisingly little toxicity in dogs so treated. When we have tested macrophage and lymphoid cell functions of mice given MER i.v., potentiated activities were found in several test models.

i.v. injection has been administered to a series of patients by Dr. E. Robinson of Rambam Hospital in Haifa; this work is about to be published, and I believe that Dr. Robinson has concluded that this route of administration is a safe one in man. Phase I trials with MER injected i.v. are now being conducted by Drs. E. Hersh and J. Gutterman at M.D. Anderson Hospital and Tumor Institute in Houston, and by Dr. J. Holland at Mt. Sinai Hospital in New York.

Regarding the septicemia with BCG organism following administration of living BCG, this might be a necessary, albeit potentially hazardous, aspect of treatment with this preparation. As I have indicated above, the amount of material introduced with the usual inocula of living BCG is probably much below the threshold required for activation of immunological and immune functions, and progressive replication and spread of the living microorganisms in host tissues is required for a sufficient accumulation of the active principle(s).

CHEDID

At this level it seems to me that it is possible to get a clear answer since there exist enough animal models, murine or others, in which non-viable materials are active. So the question I put to Dr. Mathé is the following: In what models did you find that only viable BCG was effective?

MATHÉ

For example L1210 leukemia and Lewis tumor among the several tests of our screening.

CHEDID

Did you also try on the same models MER or cell walls or cord factor, that is, active non-viable material?

MATHÉ

Yes, and WSA and the hydrosoluble factor "Hiu II" did not work; only MER gave some positive results as we published in the Israelian Journal of Medical Sciences.

CHEDID

I must say that I find these differences in general difficult to understand. I am always extremely astonished by the simple fact that although we have such good evdience of strong immunostimulatory activity on animal models, it is so difficult to have similar results in clinical situations. In other terms this means to me: do we really have a good animal tumor model?

TERRY

I think this is a good point at which to sort of shift the discussion; let us spend a few minutes talking about animal models and about the relevance of the kinds of animal tumors and the kinds of animal experiments that are done — of the real relevance of those for the clinical situation.

RAPP

I am also outside of clinical cancer immunotherapy but I think the answer to Chedid's question — the first part of his question — is simple. In the human trials of cancer immunotherapy you have been treating patients who are at an advanced stage of disease. Everything I have ever done in animal models says you will not succeed — immunologic methods are not yet available to treat advanced cancer in humans. And I believe until you start learning how to treat patients at stages analogous to those that work in animals you are not going to be successful.

MATHÉ

We have been working on Gross virus induced E(Akr) leukemia and on spontaneous AkR leukemia on which we used cells and/or BCG; J. and F. Lacour worked on C₃H spontaneous mammary tumor with poly A-poly U, and in all these experiments systemic active immunotherapy obtained significant favorable results.

TERRY

What sort of immunotherapy was that?

MATHÉ

Either i.v. BCG and/or s.c. irradiated cells in my two experiments, or poly A- poly U i.v. in Lacour's experiments. These are the types of systemic immunotherapy which are reproduced in man.

DAVIES

There is no question about what Herbert Rapp said — he is right. We have tried to test antibody-drug synergism in spontaneous mammary carcinomas in mice, using individually raised antisera against each tumor, and treated the mice post-operatively but it was just too hard and we had to drop it. I think one has to make do with something less than the ideal model.

[22] *Terry* - p. 28

WEISS

In response to Dr. Chedid, it should be remembered that even in the most "successful" animal studies, for every effective treatment group, for every effective combination of treatment conditions, there are many which fail — and these may not be reported at all!   Syngeneic animals may be expensive, but they are expendable, and the only real limitation in animal investigations of this sort is the skill of the investigator as fund-raiser.   In clinical trials, to the contrary, we work under stringent restrictions, ethical and otherwise, and the variations of treatment which can be tested are always greatly limited.

From the lofty perspective of hindsight, it seems to me that in many instances the parameters of immunological intervention in patients have been precisely those which should have been employed had the aim been to encourage immunological tolerance rather than responsiveness, suppression rather than activation.   There has been treatment with overly great quantities of immunomodulators, too frequently, and at intervals in relation to chemotherapy when the effects of the drugs could be expected to cancel out any immunological activation or to lay the grounds for the induction of unresponsiveness.   The seemingly far greater success attained for nonspecific immunotherapy in animal models, and for specific immunization as well, may be largely due to the opportunity for wide variations of test conditions, and for a convenient relegation of the failures, which may indeed be far more frequent than the successes, to one or two sentences in the Discussion sections of our papers.   We can heighten our chances for success, even limited success, in clinical studies only by giving very careful attention to the design of the study, on the basis of *immunological* considerations; moreover, we must take the view that human neoplasia is a broad category of diseases, with certain features in common; we shall have to rely on a multitude of models of cancer in man as well as on numerous test systems in animals, and hope that we can learn something of relevance from each and thereby ultimately synthesize a set of principles of immunotherapy that will suggest *a range* of conditions under which we can expect certain accomplishments.   Searches for *the* ideal model or for *the* ideal set of treatment parameters are likely to be similar to the seeking for the Holy Grail — interesting journeys leading nowhere.

[22] *Terry* - p. 29

TERRY

I take chairman's prerogative and just say that experimental models
in which tumors are induced acutely injecting 10^3 and 10^5 tumor cells
into an animal and develop in few weeks cannot be compared to the
neoplasia in man which undoubtedly develops over decades for most tumors
and which does not start with an acute challenge. I think that there are
just such large biological differences, that we always know that we are
dealing with a highly artificial situation. There are other alternatives.

ROSENBERG

One of the most impressive models we have for positive regional
immunotherapy of local disease would be the guinea pig hepatoma model,
and I would like to pose a question to Dr. Rapp as to how he would put
together the experiments he has done over the years in terms of a
mechanism for how the local disease is eliminated and with a special
reference to how the disease in the training lymph node is eliminated.
What do we know about the mechanism of that immunotherapeutic
effect?

RAPP

Before answering that, I would like to take the prerogative of giving
a prelude which would speak, I think, to Dr. Weiss's comment and would
be relevant to what you are asking for. Again I am not a clinician but I
am aware of the fact that in the United States 96% of all cancer deaths
are due to only eight carcinomas. They all start as localized lesions,
they all are capable of metastasizing to draining lymph nodes, and many
of them metastasize hematogenously. In the guinea pig line 10 model,
unfortunately, there are no hematogenous metastases. Theoretically, we
could eliminate 96% of all cancer deaths in the USA if we could diagnose
them all at stage 1, even with occult metastasis in the draining lymph
node, if the guinea pig model is applicable.

TERRY

I am shaking my head because this is not fair — it is like a floating

[22] *Terry* · p. 30

crap game that we have been running for years — this is an inside discussion that goes on and on. It is the point that has been made repeatedly: the guinea pig model has the limit of the fact that it goes to the lymph node and stops. Human cancer goes to the lymph node — maybe does not go to the lymph node — but it disseminates, and it is a very different biologic system. So whatever conclusions we draw I think have to keep that limit in mind.

RAPP

But as I say, in some cancers hematogenous spread may be the problem and I do not know any way of dealing with that right now, except perhaps for some clues Mike Hanna has obtained in studies of "artificial" hematogenous spread in the guinea pig model. Hematogenously spread tumor cells might be effected by intratumorally administered BCG because after such treatment animals become systemically immune. What we do not know is whether that systemic immunity has anything to do with why the animal lives. One would hope that it did. So, when you put the BCG right into the tumor, you are creating a specific immunological response to the BCG antigens initially. We assume that specific response involves at least sensitized lymphocytes, which when they react with the BCG antigens, will release lymphokines, among which is migration inhibition factor, for example; and when the migration inhibition factor is released, its highest concentration will he right in the tumor because that is where we put the initiating agent. And as the macrophages come wandering by, they will be stopped by the migration inhibition factor and somehow become activated. The macrophages are doing the work, then, of destroying the local tumor, in the primary skin transplant. One possibility is that the macrophages somehow — perhaps by mechanisms that Dr. De Duve presented today — are promoting a lymphocyte mediated response by the host directed against tumor-specific antigens. When and if you have this second set of lymphocytes, which are sensitized against tumor-specific antigens, they provide a systemic mechanism to get rid of the remaining tumor.

TERRY

Suppose there are no tumor-specific antigens?

RAPP

Then my argument is down the drain.

TERRY

Dr. North, since the comment was about mechanisms that might be operative in the local immunotherapy do you have anything to add to that?

NORTH

I would like to make another comment — a general one — and that is that there is not much discrepancy really between animal and human tumors. There has been a lot said about the unsuitability of transplantable tumors. If you look at the literature in the mouse system and other systems, the situation is very artificial, in that the tumor is put in one day (transplant) and immunotherapy is started the next day, and the investigator knows very well that if they had left that tumor three days more, they would not get a result. So there is not much discrepancy. I think what one can say about most of the immunotherapy that has been performed is that there has been no real good attempt to correlate immunotherapeutic effect with immunogenicity of the tumor as defined by transplantation immunity. Until that is done we will not be able to say very much about whether you need tumor-specific antigens.

TERRY

I believe Dr. Baldwin has alluded to this the other day and I am pretty sure that he has data suggesting that those of his tumors that are poorly immunogenetic are also poorly responsive to his vaccine situation and are also poorly responsive to direct intralesional injections. Does everybody agree to that? I have heard him say that on a number of different occasions.

RAPP

We have also found that in several mouse tumors there is a rough correlation between responsiveness to immunotherapy and so-called immunogenicity — but unfortunately, with the guinea pig model we got the opposite results.

OETTGEN

One of the problems in clinical trials of BCG and other immuno-potentiators is that we have very little to indicate that immunopotentiation is in fact achieved. The tests which show immunopotentiation in the mouse are often quite different from the tests that we can use in man. We are certainly not increasing our patients' liver weight by a factor of 2 or 3, as we do in the mouse when we achieve optimal systemic thera-peutic activity. So I think that there is a great need for us to show that we in fact induce immunopotentiation, and test the principle rather than just giving BCG at a possibly insufficient dose.

TERRY

I wonder if I could sort of terminate this portion of the discussion by simply making the following comment. It seems to me that Dr. Chedid is right in one sense — there are a number of models around that have been used, that is animal models either for intratumoral or for systemic forms of immunotherapy, and I think one of the greatest failures of the field has been the fact that despite the rather long time that these models have been around, we know almost nothing about the mechanism involved. It has been the failure to proceed along the line of trying to carefully define why things work when they apparently do work; in the absence of having that kind of information, I think we really do not know how to generalize to the human system, and I think that this is one of the areas that we certainly have to pay more attention to in the future. Having said future, I would like, for the final part of this discussion, to turn this in the direction of the kind of question that Dr. Klein was asking and that Dr. Rapp has brought up several times: what of the future, where is the use of immuno-adjuvants as a cancer treatment going? Where should it go?

ED. KLEIN

I would like to be very blunt about it: by and large, immunological approaches to treating malignant diseases have received a rather black eye in the eyes of our colleagues in other types of medicine, or for that matter in other types of oncology, and I think it is quite undeserved. Being a little older than most of the others in this room, I am going back to the days when I was with Sidney Farber and when the chemotherapy area was under precisely the same attack, or more so, as immunotherapy is today, and I cannot help thinking, with some chagrin, that the very people who at that time were in the frying pan are the ones who are now putting the immunotherapy fraternity into the fire. Now I think one of the lessons is that we have not attempted to look at the simple and successful areas that offer the most promise and I do not mean to be parochial but naturally I am referring to what you have passed over very quickly as an anecdotal phenomenon, namely, local therapy. Albeit by vigorous standards it may be an anecdotal series of experiences although that is not so, it nevertheless has the vast advantage of (a) simplicity, (b) accessibility, (c) an adequate animal model, (d) the promise of actually showing both to our colleagues and to the public, who ultimately foots the bill for this, that there is something we can do in terms of real clinical accomplishment as well as paliation and possibly devote some of the energy that we are throwing away in fruitless chasing of rainbows into the study of mechanisms that are staring us in the face. It is possible that we are looking for the key under the lamp when we dropped it in the parking lot and that we will not learn from the local lesion what goes on inside the lung or inside the uterus. But the chances are that by looking at something that works you may find out more than by looking at something that does not work or we do not know whether it works.

Terry

How do you want to proceed to look at it? What needs to be done?

Ed. Klein

Well, there are a great many things that need to be done, like looking at the isolated systems, and at the cell composition, trying to find out *in vivo* what goes on, and looking at turnover rates of components of the immune system which are now available.

[22] *Terry* - p. 34

TERRY

So you are suggesting that, in terms of proceeding with mechanisms and trying to understand mechanisms, the local form of therapy is one which provides a good opportunity for doing that.

SELA

I hope I am not misquoting you, but I think that the suggestion made is that maybe the kind of skin cancer discussed here is not the major cancer, but it is one in which limited application of immunotherapy seems to be successful. Is this what you meant?

ED. KLEIN

Yes, and I would like to go a step further, because almost the entire spectrum of malignant diseases that we have looked at in the human skin has responded exactly the same way as the cancer derived from the epidermis, whether it is carcinoma of the breast, carcinoma of the stomach, carcinoma of the lung.

TERRY

O.K. Again, mechanistically, let us agree for now that it might be fruitful to look at local types of approaches that involve accessible tumors in the skin. I think the question on the floor is slightly different, and that is: besides that type of mechanistic approach, from the point of view of what the clinical immunotherapist should be doing now, where is this field, where is its application supposed to be going?

ED. KLEIN

I would like to address myself to that. When you have a large carcinoma of the breast and the patient is sinking away and you can shut it off within two weeks, it is worth doing it for its own sake even if you do not cure the bone or hepatic metastasis, and immunotherapy can do it and we have proved this, and nobody has picked it up.

[22] Terry - p. 35

MATHÉ

I would like to give my opinion on the future. First, there are more favorable clinical data concerning the results of systemic immunotherapy than those quoted incompletely by Terry: let me quote a) EORTC's Haemopathy Working Group's, Ekert's and Izawa's data on A.L.L.; b) Hoerni's data on lymphosarcoma; c) Gutterman's, Ikonopisov's, Morton's, Beretta's, Deutschman's, El Domeris, Serrou's data on melanoma; d) Hudson's data as well as Albert's data on ovary cancers which were neither in the program nor quoted by Terry.

Secondly, let me remind you that adjuvant chemotherapy results are getting deteriorated: a) in breast cancer, adjuvant chemotherapy does not work in post-menopausal women after a few years' follow-up; b) in osteo-sarcoma, the 80% relapse free rate has got down to 40% at the fourth year. Hence chemotherapists have to remember that chemotherapy, because it obeys first order kinetics and because of cell resistance, does not kill "the last cell". On the contrary, our experimental work showed that, if systemic immunotherapy does not affect large tumors, it may eradicate small population of tumor cells. Hence, we have to work on the combination of chemotherapy and systemic immunotherapy in the adjuvant treatment of post-surgical residual disease. Moreover, we have to try to reproduce the effects of fresh Pasteur BCG applied in the condition which we defined, by adjuvants which could be administered in Uganda or G.B. as in Paris, in any state of U.S. or as in Houston. There are some which are pure molecules, such as levamisole and interferon, which seems efficient, and we have to combine the many new ones in order to obtain, with pharmacologically well defined substances, at least the effect of BCG. We have new agents which work mainly on T-cells, others which work mainly on B-cells, other on macrophages: let us try to combine them. Finally, the researchocrats, if we eliminate from their quotations, the trials of which they do not like the statistical methodology, should also eliminate the trials of which experienced immunotherapists do not consider the immunotherapy technology suitable. The great merit of McKneally is to have really applied BCG to his patients.

RAPP

I agree that mechanism is an important thing to study and we do it, and I hope we all do it, but I think at the moment the most fruitful results will come from empiricism. Not entirely empiricism, however, thanks to Dr. Klein's pioneering work. The skin is an epithelial site; carcinomas are all epithelial tumors. I think I am justified in the assumption that epithelial tumors no matter where they are, will react the same way they react in the skin. Now, in order to best that hypothesis, I think the best way to proceed is to look for naturally occurring cancers in animals that are analogous to human disease — and there are many. I mentioned some Monday — for example, breast cancer in dogs; I have spoken to veterinarians who run hospitals for dogs and I have found one hospital that sees 200 breast cancers per year in dogs and 80% of those are at stage 1 — a perfect test ground for what I am suggesting. We have melanoma in horses that is naturally occurring and we can get it at any stage we like, the smallest to the largest lesion. We have bovine lymphosarcoma, perhaps an ideal disease in which to test treatments proposed for analogous human malignancies. We have to fractionate and purify the adjuvants, study their mechanism of action in animal models and test them in animal analogs of human disease.

TERRY

Now, does anybody want to speak to those parts — that is, to Dr. Rapp's suggestion that spontaneously arising tumors in animals are the place to proceed? Nobody wants to argue with him on that point?

ED. KLEIN

I would like to subscribe to it and I would like to add that we have some preliminary data on the combination of multiple sensitizing agents or immunopotentiators both locally and with systemic potentiation, and we do indeed find a more than additive effect — now Dr. Rapp will not accept my data, but he has not seen them all and I am sure he will subscribe to them if he does. I would further like to add to Dr. Mathé's suggestion that expands on Dr. Rapp's suggestion that there are a large number of tumors — and some of the large killer tumors like carcinoma in the cervix which have already been shown by several groups to respond to immunologic manipulation at the primary stage: at Hopkins, at Edinburgh, at the Sidney Farber, and at Roswell — and they are ready to be explored and I cannot for the world understand why this is not being pushed.

GUTTERMAN

Well, I agree with what has been said by Drs. Klein, Rapp and Mathé and I think we really have to make a very, very serious effort and persist on that, to begin to work with stage 1 carcinoma. Rapp pushed for that, Klein has also made a plea for it. I think the use of naturally occurring tumors is going to be very useful — stage 1 breast cancer in dogs, etc., but I think we primarily have to convince our surgical colleagues that we have achieved enough in very late disease — more than perhaps we anticipated. We have agents now of which we have a great deal more understanding than we did 5 or 10 years ago — certainly they are safe in terms of nonviable fractions. I think we have to make a very considered effort with our surgical colleagues to begin to look at prostate cancer, ovarian cancer, colon cancer, breast cancer, the tumors that Herb Rapp was referring to. Also, as George Mathé said, begin to look at the tumors that the chemotherapy colleagues now are using in adjuvant trials. I think those trials although very positive are not going to be cured in the long run, and we clearly have to begin to use immunotherapy, post-chemotherapy in those situations. Why we have not been able to succeed in getting these tumors, I think, is because of a little bit of what Ed. Klein said: there has been a wave of pessimism regarding immunotherapy. I think it did occur with chemotherapy 30 years ago — we have got to make every possible effort to be able to reverse this situation. And so I think if we work together we will be able to get these tumors, and I think if we can begin to get these tumors at the stage 1 level, we are going to see in the next decade with what I have heard this week, even if we do not understand the basic mechanisms yet, and we may never understand them in the next 20 or 30 years, I think in the next 20 or 30 years we should be able to see major progress in the use of nonspecific immunotherapy.

TERRY

Let me push you a little further on this because I think this is coming down to the crux of the issue. Can you outline a stage 1 trial on a particular tumor that you think is something that should be done, so that we can concretely deal with the question of what tumor it is that you are talking about, what the present survival is in the treatment of stage 1 of that disease by conventional treatment, how you would go about evaluating whether or not anything that you would choose to do would improve that significantly, and what the dimensions of the trial would be.

GUTTERMAN

Well, I am just looking at my notes on some of the tumors that we are talking about. I am going to leave out breast cancer for the moment. I think that is going to be a little difficult with stage 1 breast cancer because that is fairly cured although it is still a bad tumor. I think certain questions on the bladder, cervical cancer, Edmund Klein has already referred to.

TERRY

What is the treatment for stage 1 carcinoma of the cervix and what are the results?

ED. KLEIN

98%. Some of my friends in gynecology are prepared to put BCG into their carcinomas *in situ* and follow these patients for ten or twenty years, and they include some very notable gynecologists, and they are not afraid of it; that is why I asked Dr. Baldwin the question whether or not he has ever seen a metastasis. I have never seen a metastasis; Dr. Rapp has never seen a metastasis. You see the opposite, you see the prevention of metastasis. You cannot possibly, according to all the data that we have, hurt the patient by inundating the carcinoma *in situ* at the cervix with immunopotentiating agents locally, then go ahead, do the conization and then follow the patient.

TERRY

Is your suggestion that if you did that, your 98% might be better than 98%.

[22] *Terry* - p. 39

Ed. Klein

100% — the 2% of patients would greatly appreciate it — I assure you.

Terry

I am sure that that 2% of patients would appreciate it, but I also suggest that if you sit down and picture the clinical trial that would be involved, it is not one that is readily approachable.

Ed. Klein

I have faced that very situation with a 98% curable tumor, namely skin cancer, and we raised it to a higher percentage, and nobody, including all those who have been very opposed to it, would say a word against it now. I think that sound barrier has been broken. And I think it can be broken again. I think it is worthwhile.

Terry

I think we have got to take the final series of comments in order to stay within the scheduled time.

Gutterman

Well, let me just make a general comment on that. I cannot give you specific details but, for example, there are tumors like colon cancer, there may be tumors of stage 1 that are 95% curable by surgery, but there are intermediate stage tumors that are not metastatic to regional nodes. I think this is the type of tumor that one could clearly consider for local and/or systemic immunotherapy. I think prostate cancer is another one. Again, I do not know about stage 1 disease, but here is one of the major killers around the world and by the time patients get cancer of the prostate they are not going to be able to tolerate chemotherapy. I think it is a tumor that, if you got the right stage, could be quite amenable to immunotherapy, and there has already been suggested evidence of local immunotherapy working in this tumor.

TERRY

I think since the question that has been brought up relates mostly to surgical tumors, and since we have a surgeon in the room, we will give him a chance to make a comment.

ROSENBERG

What I would like to do is disagree with much of what has been said in the last 20 minutes or so. First, it is my belief that the problem with current immunotherapy is not that we do not have good models — it is that we do not know what to do. Switching to the dogs that have mammary cancer or the AKR mouse that has spontaneous leukemia really does not answer any question. The things that we have tried, even in poorer models, have basically not worked. We have tried things in the best model of human cancer — the human — and virtually nothing has worked. Dr. Rapp mentioned the need to emphasize models such as epithelial tumors which are more analogous to the majority of human tumors. The idea that he has worked with, taking a transplantable epithelial tumor and putting it into the skin, is far from reality in the human. Now, Dr. Klein has emphasized repeatedly his own work on the treatment of skin tumors. I think Dr. Klein has made a very significant contribution to the treatment of the tumors with which he has dealt; but I think it is unfair of Dr. Klein, to emphasize it as much as he has because of the extreme rarity of application of this approach.

Now, I do not in any sense wish to say that what has been done is not important. I consider it an immensely impressive and important achievement. But you know, and I know, that the overwhelming majority of all tumors in humans are not amenable directly to the approach that you have mentioned. The tumor in the breast of the woman that is ulcerating and causing cosmetic problems is not a problem. In the 99.9% of all women that die of breast cancer, they die with disseminated disease. I am not saying that local control is never a problem. You emphasize local control to the exclusion of our need to develop techniques for treating disseminated disease.

One final point: We talked about the treatment of local stage 1 disease, and discussed models in the experimental animal that treat local stage 1 disease as representing successes that might be applied to the human. No human dies of local stage 1 disease. For any major tumors that one might mention — be it breast, colon, lung, — local stage 1 disease is curable by local surgery. What kills patients with stage 1 disease is the undetected distant metastases that ultimately grow out and kill that patient. In other words, the patients that fail therapy with stage 1 disease in fact were never stage 1 — they had distant disease at the time of their local treatment. And so to talk about successes in animal models that truly are stage 1, such as the guinea pig model that never metastasizes hematogenously, I think can lead us down fruitless alleys.

WEISS

Perhaps we should view the very limited success achieved so far in clinical studies of immunotherapy as a source of encouragement rather than as one of diappointment. We have come to recognize the immunological apparatus as a labyrinthine maze of positive and negative signals, of forward and reverse reactions, of helper and suppressor factors, cellular and humoral. Within this interlocking network of reactivities which must be in fine equilibria with each other to permit the coexistence and integrity of the many tissue systems that make up higher animal organisms, the difficulties of altering the extent and direction of selected processes by nonspecific means loom very large. That we have made any headway at all with the crude tools now at our disposal is rather amazing. Instead of rushing into many more clinical trials empirically, I believe that our efforts should now be directed at gaining greater understanding of the phenomena we seek to control. Several main lines of approach have been accentuated at this conference. One is the purification and definition of action of the components of complex immunomodulators of microbial origin. A second lies with the characterization of the anti-tumor potentials of isolated components of the immune response, both cellular and humoral, alone and in combination; this approach may be facilitated considerably by the work I have described on *in vitro* sensitization of effector cells and on *in vitro* production of antibodies — by creating better defined immunological microcosms, we may be able not only to create various effector agents for passive/adoptive immunotherapy, but also to gain far greater insight into the intricacies of anti-tumor immunological responses. A third lies with the active recognition of neoplasia as a dynamic and labile host-parasite relationship, in which the pathogenetic entity and the host stand in continuous reaction and counteraction to each other, and in which each step and event represents the composite result of the interactions in a continuously changing tissue microenvironment. As an illustration of the immediate clinical implications of this perspective of neoplasia, there might be cited the recent observations of Lucien Israel that repeated plasma exchange may be beneficial in itself for cancer patients, presumably because of a diminution of various factors blocking immunological reactions. Such procedure might be a precondition for effective immunological intervention from without; the blocking factors, of host or of tumor origin, represent a dimension that cannot be ignored by the therapist; they make up one aspect of the total matrix of the situation of progressive neoplasia — and the view that must be taken can only be an inclusive one.

Marini-Bettòlo

We are just at the last hours of our very interesting meeting of this Study Week, and I think that the principal scope of this Study Week is to make somehow an assessment of what is the present state in this field and what are the possible future lines of research. I believe that we have learned a lot from each other in this interesting and very important rapport that we have had. But now, speaking as a man of the street, I think we should point out three or four questions to which we must give a definite answer, and this would be useful also for future research. I therefore put these questions. *First*, what are the present practical possibilities of successful use in man of the immunotherapy of cancer? *Second*, can other substances besides BCG, vaccines and toxins be used as cancer aspecific immunity elicitors? The examples we have heard concerning glycopolipeptide are very interesting, but I am asking whether other products could be considered, such as enzymes, protease, glycosidase, and other types of products. *Third*, how is it possible to envisage the preparation of specific antibodies for tumors? I think this is a key point in this immunity program. *Fourth*, do you not think that the study of the mode of action at the molecular level — not only through a great number of experiments but also through a theoretical approach — could be very important in order to understand better the mechanism and then to envisage new strategies for the future? I think we must consider at the molecular level the tumor inhibition or the lysis, and this could be extremely important.

CHAGAS

I think that at the last meeting we are going to trust Sir Gustav Nossal to give us his concluding remarks.

CHAGAS

We are nearing very much the closing hour. You must be quite tired after the many hours of intellectual excitation, hard work, early hours. I would like to close this meeting by expressing to you all my profound thanks for coming over from your countries, leaving your laboratories, to discuss, to observe, to debate, sometimes to quarrel and so to really help mankind in one of its very severe problems. And in the name of the Academy, express to you how thankful we are, for all the trouble, for all the fatigue you have undertaken to come and to light up this quite old room with your experiments, with your talents, and with your generosity. I want especially to say how grateful I am to Michael Sela, who has really engineered the meeting and has been the man who was responsible for our success. Most of all I believe that something has come out of this meeting which is also the establishment of ties between different groups, and even if there are here people who have known one another for many, many years and have worked together, I think that a new relationship and friendship has been established. And here I have probably a small complaint to make, that I am calling everyone by his first name and I am called back "Dr. Chagas". My next words will be said in the most cordial expression and that is: Thank you very much.

WESTPHAL

Dear Carlos... I hesitate to address you like that, but you allowed us all to call you in that way from now on. Somebody should finally express our gratitude to you. It was Gus Nossal, just because I am sitting next to him, who pushed me to do that. I feel very honored and, indeed, we have to thank you, first of all, for creating this very colleagual atmosphere. We thank you and Michael Sela for the organization of this meeting of which Gus already said: everybody goes home with ideas for further work in the laboratory or in the hospital. Individual action in this very field is certainly necessary, but much weaker than concerted action. Again and again people ask for meetings of this kind with the aim to create such concerted actions against cancer. It is perhaps the most important outcome of our meeting that 20 to 25 colleagues met — some of whom knew each other already, others did not — who got together in a way that everybody approaches everybody by forename. We, thus, have created a kind of scientists' family for this concerted approach. You, Carlos, have made this possible, and this is for what we should like to thank you most heartily. Furthermore, we would like to thank you for the few hours — I should say, because you kept us very busy — the few hours of relaxed, but stimulated being together in this beautiful cultural atmosphere of Art and History which the Vatican offers. Thank you very much, Carlos!

CHAGAS

Thank you very much. Before we close the meeting I want to make a special reference to Father di Rovasenda, Madame Michelle Porcelli, and to all those who have helped us because they have done their best to make the Study week a success.

[22] *Terry* - p. 45

37

CONCLUSIONS

SUMMARY AND PROSPECTS
FOR FUTURE RESEARCH

G.J.V. NOSSAL

The Walter and Eliza Hall Institute of Medical Research
Melbourne, Victoria 3050, Australia

While the kaleidoscopic images of this remarkable week tumble freshly around in our minds, I must now try to gather them into an orderly linear array. We have indeed ranged widely, yet I believe one can detect six threads, that have wound their way through our work; six themes that have recurred.

The first of these, the dominant motif on the first day and re-echoed repeatedly throughout the meeting, we might term the empirical action-oriented thread. Given that non-specific inflammatory stimuli can under some circumstances make cancer deposits shrink away, let us leap in and see how well immunotherapy can perform in various forms of human cancer. I remind you that such enlightened empiricism is nothing new. It stands in the mainstream of the tradition of medicine since Hippocrates, and of immunology since Jenner. It must and will continue while cancer kills one in six in many countries. No one needs to apologize for it. Our round table discussion revealed only too clearly that the early, heady enthusiasms about immunotherapy in general, and BCG in particular, have not produced a miraculous cure for advanced cancer. We parted company on how to regard the marginal benefits claimed in some trials or the undoubted palliation achieved in individual patients. We did achieve consensus that a ray of hope exists. To the acute myeloid leukaemia story so thoroughly discussed, we should add Strander's remarkable osteogenic sarcoma interferon trial, action-oriented empiricism of a heroic order. This has whetted my appetite both for early independent confirmation *and* for a trial of double-stranded RNA in this disease.

Overall, however, the extensive experience with immunotherapy in *advanced* malignancy may have a deeper significance. The toxicity, particularly of non-living materials, and the rarity of obvious enhancement, are gradually positioning us for an onslaught on earlier cancers. As Rapp emphasized so strongly, animal models give little support to immunotherapy as a cure for late, disseminated cancer. They tell us we have to step in earlier. Hopefully, as we learn more about the importance of bacterial strains, viability, dose, about the various non-living crude, semi-pure and pure preparations, about the apparent importance of producing fever, about synergy with drugs, we may design intelligent trials in various Stage 1 and Stage 2 cancers of relatively better prognosis. Dr. Gutterman put my position on this very well with his example of colon cancer groups that are 65% curable. Perhaps we could have tried harder to answer questions which will shortly confront us. Do we all agree with Rapp and Edmund Klein that intralesional immunotherapy is safe, that it will not spread disease? Do non-living preparations avoid the dangers of intralesional live BCG? If immunotherapy is to be given after putatively curative surgery, what sort, by what route, how often and for how long after apparent cure? Surely this debate, which we initiated all too late in our deliberations, must be resumed at a very early date.

The next two threads of our story represent the basic scientist's intuitive responses to an empirical discovery. If non-specific cellular immunity can lead to killing of cancer cells, how does this work (thread 2); and how can we create useful and realistic animal models to extend the discovery (thread 3)?

Our search for how tumor immunotherapy might work took us in two directions, one constructive and one more disappointing. The first was the definition of purer substances that retained some or all of the bioactivities of living immunostimulant microorganisms. I think we all accepted muramyl dipeptide and the lysolecithin analogs as offering enormous potential, both theoretical and practical. The adjuvant properties and resistance-promoting capacities of both approaches were sufficiently remarkable to suggest a role in both specific and non-specific tumor immunotherapy. MDP's high solubility and rapid renal clearance, limiting factors today, should surely soon be overcome through appropriate conjugations and modifications.

Not quite so encouraging was our progress as regards mechanisms of tumor regression. Otto Westphal reminded us that the field was two centuries old yet we can do little better than murmur: "perhaps the macrophages have become a bit angry". We have learnt much about how macrophages can become activated following specific T lymphocyte-antigen interactions and lymphokine release, but once activated, how do they kill tumor cells? By what molecular mechanisms can an activated macrophage discriminate a tumor cell from a normal cell — or can it? Perhaps tumor necrosis factor will take us a giant leap forward. We were told that TNF can kill some tumors directly, while normal cells escape unharmed. Much as I appreciated Oettgen's elegant dissection of the many immunological effects of TNF, which left me with the distinct feeling that it may be a mixture of molecules, I would have been even more grateful for some clues as to how it killed the villains of our drama. The non-specificity of the susceptible targets for TNF, even to the extent of a crossing of species barriers, argues against macromolecular recognition and for the exploitation by TNF of some metabolic quirk of tumor cells, but I urge Oettgen and Old pursue this question with diligence. If it turns out, as well it might, that there are two aspects, namely direct effects of TNF on tumor cells and effects enhancing the specific immune response, so much the better.

The problem of the mode of action of BCG and its analogs is clearly most vexing, and no one could quarrel with Rapp's frustration that a patient search through virtually all known in vitro tests correlated so poorly with observed in vivo tumor regression effects. Westphal's suggestion that some portion of the action of lysolecithin analogs may be on the tumor cell itself, the final killing depending on synergistic effects of macrophage activation and deleterious LLA accumulation on tumor cell membranes, offers a new possibility. It certainly lends evidence to Rapp's pleas for an intralesional approach to immunotherapy. But on the whole, I was left

[23] *Nossal* - p. 3

with the impression that we need far more basic research on tumor regression mechanisms.

Our third thread was that of credible model systems in animals, which mimic the clinical situations we face. It is perhaps a pity that neither Hewitt nor Prehn were here, to deliver their usual salutory reminders about the relatively low immunogenicity of spontaneous tumors when compared with those beloved by tumor immunologists and filling all the best cancer journals. However, Baldwin saved the day, but only up to a point. He told us first that about 7 of 17 spontaneous tumors in rats were immunogenic when thoroughly investigated. Having raised our hopes, he dashed them by saying that standard specific immunotherapy protocols, perfectly capable of causing rejection of the more immunogenic, carcinogen induced tumors, mostly failed with these less immunogenic spontaneous tumors. Having thus depressed us, however, he raised our spirits again by reminding us of the concept of contact suppression. BCG or C. parvum mixed with the tumor cell inoculum, even a non-immunogenic line, suppresses tumor growth by a T-cell-independent, presumably macrophage-dependent mechanism which works even when the recovered host is left subsequently non-immune. I believe his examples were as clear an indication as we could hope for that non-specific elements acting alone can kill tumor cells. Most other speakers defended their favorite models but none, I believe, approached with sufficient fortitude the Hewitt-Prehn dilemma. Mathé's L1210 leukaemia, Rapp's line 10 hepatoma, North's SA 1 sarcoma, all of these have their virtues. But all represent artificially "hot" situations, the battle between host and tumor starkly dramatized with one side or the other winning quickly and clearly; a far cry from the fascinating slow and balanced interplay of forces in spontaneous human cancer, which grows, after all, so slowly and can be held in check for so long. I offer no solution to this problem, but feel it should be posed and faced more often and more squarely.

The keynote of our fourth theme was sounded by David Weiss, who reminded us that the areas of specific and non-specific immunity are closely related and spill over into each other. The same agent, for example MER, can simultaneously stimulate each.

Of course, it was George Mackaness and his colleagues at the Trudeau Institute who first showed us how the specific interaction of an antigen with its specifically sensitized T cell led to the production of lymphokines which activated macrophages to a non-specifically heightened bacteriocidal and, we presume, tumoricidal state. This week, we looked at cytotoxic T cell killing and antibody-dependent lymphocyte-mediated cytotoxicity by K cells as examples of specific resistance. Circulating complexes of tumor antigen and antibody probably also fall into this group as immunodepressive agents. Activated macrophages and tumor necrosis factor represent non-specific examples. The so-called natural killer cells, with their wide but not unrestricted target cell range, and their capacity to be considerably heightened in activity through co-cultivation with a susceptible cell line, fit somewhere in between, an intriguing observation not yet comfortably settled into our framework.

To explore the specific response in any detail, we need to have a tumor antigen. I don't think any of us could avoid a tinge of envy as George Klein described for us, with his usual brilliance, the veritable galaxy of sequentially expressed EBV-induced antigens, EBNA, EA, VCA and MA coming out strongly and to order in virus-transformed B lymphocytes. Think of all we could do in human tumor immunology if most cancers possessed such antigens! But they do not, and for the immediate future it looks as though we may have to content ourselves with a hard, patient search for weak antigens, frequently displaying individual specificity. After many disappointments, it was very heartening to hear the paper of Rosenberg on human sarcoma antigens and the brief intervention of Oettgen on malignant melanoma antigens. In the sarcoma story, we heard that once the problem of virtually ubiquitous natural antibodies to widely-expressed foetal antigens was disposed of by absorption, the sarcoma patient displays, though in small amounts, an antibody reactive with cells from his own sarcoma but not with any other sarcoma. In melanoma, the analysis is a little more advanced, and individual-specific as well as shared tumor specific antigens have been identified. I cannot stress too strongly how important continued painstaking survey work of this sort will be, to allow a serology of human malignancy gradually to emerge.

[23] *Nossal* - p. 5

I am much reminded of the status of HLA antigens when Dausset first published his pioneering studies 20 years ago. He and his many colleagues then attacked the enormous task of sorting out the incredible complexities of the highly polymorphic human HLA system. In the tumor field, we may face still greater problems but there will be no short cuts. We received hints from Baldwin and from George Klein that isolation and dissection of immune complexes in cancer patients might speed us on our way, and the practical potential of pure antibodies, as revealed by Sela and by Davies present a further lure. Surely the Rosenberg approach must soon be taken up by 50 laboratories on a dozen different kinds of human tumors. We may well need better assays such as radio-immunoassays. Certainly serum banks with repeated bleeds from the one patient will be required. Before leaving this fourth thread, we should pause for a moment at the interface of tumor resistance and resistance to infection. The way we have brought this interface to the fore has been another highlight of our week. Particularly encouraging has been the trend, initiated by Wolff and maintained throughout, for better molecular definition of the resistance enhancing factors. The interface was greatly enriched by our consideration of interferon and interferon inducers. Interferon itself can retard growth of tumor lines. Interferon inducers can have powerful effects on tumors, both via their action on the host immune system, and, intriguingly, perhaps via an antagonism of tumor angiogenesis factor. Again, as for lysolecithin analogs, multiple synergistic mechanisms may be at work.

Though it is early days in respect of cellular and molecular mechanisms, one "fringe benefit" of the infection — cancer resistance interface did not elude us. It is that any help which cancer patients get in throwing off their infections may in itself be life-prolonging. I found it a little disappointing that Dr. Terry could not substantiate this logical pre-supposition.

Our fifth thread also harks back to an honoured tradition, namely the concept of a magic bullet, a targeted missile to track down and destroy the tumor. The three specific approaches of this morning are fresh in our minds and need no further annotation. The antibody molecule as a magic bullet for isotopes and drugs looks interesting in animal models, but if human tumor antigens are largely individual-specific, this will impose great constraints of a logistic and financial nature on the wide application of the principle. The lysosomotropic drug approach employs a wider principle and certainly directs our attention in a new and sharper way to the pinocytotic rate and specificity in different tumors and tumor lines.

Our sixth and final thread, on which we touched all too lightly, is of absolutely crucial importance. It is that of escape mechanisms; ways by which the tumor can foil specific and non-specific immune defences. If there is one dominant pictorial image which I shall take away from this conference, it is the recurring refrain of human patient survival curves where control and treated groups set off at pleasingly separated rates, only to approach each other within an all too brief period of two or three years. What is at the root of this escape? We discussed the postulated immuno-depressive effects of immune complexes; we heard of local antagonists to effective macrophage function existing within established tumors; we discussed briefly the possibility that metastases may represent antigenic variants. But by far the most important reminder that we had concerning this disastrous phenomenon of escape came from George Klein when he told us that Burkitt lymphoma induction was a multi-stage process, not a *single* catastrophe but a series of separate sequential steps. First, the EBV transformed B lymphocytes into immortalized cell lines, the number of which was normally kept in check by host immune defences and other homeostatic forces. Secondly, promoting factor, perhaps chronic holoendemic malaria, enters the picture to diminish the efficacy of host surveillance. Thirdly, the cells now partially released from control accumulate somatic mutations till one lethal variant, with its telltale cytogenetic change in chromosome 14, emerges, now refractory to in vivo stop signals. This multi-stage progression is probably the rule in all cancers, and moreover the process of progressive refractoriness to homeostasis does not stop once the malignant state is reached. In fact, mutation and selection continues at an accelerated rate, in established malignancies, as anyone who has followed the cytogenetics of leukemic cells from patients undergoing chemotherapy knows only too well. In the face of vigorous tumor immunotherapy, the selection must inevitably be towards immunoresistance, towards the emergence and selective survival of mutants that have lost antigens or lost the capacity to be killed by specific or non-specific immunocytes or factors from them. Were we to think of tumor antigens as immutable entities within the cancer of a given patient, we would be ignoring the whole history of genetics and Darwinian evolution. I believe this inevitable drift towards escape gives the greatest possible boost to Dr. Spreafico's plea for rational combinations of treatment modalities. The immunotherapist must learn from the chemotherapist and be prepared to switch his weapons as many times as it is reasonable to believe that separate tumoricidal mechanisms are at work. Thus, perhaps the immunotherapist of the future will construct his acronyms for sequential treatments as confidently as today's leukemologist. We could have CLIM, for C. parvum. levamisole, interferon and muramyl dipeptide; or we could draw a BEAD on the tumor by BCG, endotoxin, adriamycin - DNA coacervates and double-stranded RNA. On a more serious note, though, the phenomenon of escape emphasizes the imperative need both to institute immunotherapy as early as possible, and to learn more about tumoricidal mechanisms so that our arsenal can attack at all the different possible weak points.

The end of this exciting study week is at hand. What final pleas might one make for the direction of future work? I have five to put forward.

1) To the basic scientists: let us strive much harder to find out what really happens when tumor immunotherapy shrinks those lumps. In particular, we must determine the discriminatory power of tumoricidal macrophages, if any, in clean and elegant in vitro systems.

2) To the creators of animal models of tumor immunotherapy: have the patience and the courage to do more with spontaneous tumors and transplants of low or absent immunogenicity.

3) To the students of human tumors: keep up the tedious search for antigens, help us gradually to create the Kaufmann-White scheme of tumor antigens not only for melanoma and sarcoma but for all the more important human malignancies.

4) To those who treat human malignancy: get together more and try to group around a somewhat smaller series of immunostimulants, preferably chiefly those of defined chemical structure. Then work out a courageous strategy for trials on earlier cancers.

5) To all of us: let us regard the escape from immunotherapy, which so often occurs, not as a cause for despair but as one of the ultimate challenges. After all, the central fact remains that manipulations of a purely immunological nature can lead to tumor necrosis and resolution in both animals and man. This extraordinary finding is here, it cannot be taken away from us. Here in the Vatican, it seems hardly necessary to point out the historic dimension of scientific research. A scientific discovery, accurately made and objectively reported, cannot be undiscovered. Interpretations may change, the framework of the discipline in which the discovery is embedded may undergo a total reshaping, but the discovery itself remains, one indestructible fragment of the history of our race. Herein lies the final justification of our work. This Study Week has pulled together many embellishments around the central theme. We return to our laboratories enriched and strengthened, ready to resume the search.